PLACEBOS FOR PETS?

THE TRUTH ABOUT ALTERNATIVE MEDICINE IN ANIMALS

BRENNEN MCKENZIE, VMD, MSc

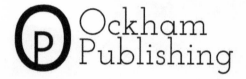

Published in 2019 by Ockham Publishing in the United Kingdom

ISBN 978-1-912701-36-0

Cover design by Claire Wood

www.ockham-publishing.com

ABOUT THE AUTHOR

Dr. McKenzie has been in small animal general practice for eighteen years. After completing a bachelor's degree with majors in English Literature and Biology at the University of California at Santa Cruz, he followed his dream of becoming a primatologist. He obtained a master's degree in Animal Behavior and worked for several years in environmental enrichment and primate behavior.

Switching gears, Dr. McKenzie attended the School of Veterinary Medicine at the University of Pennsylvania and began working as a vet in private practice. He has served as President of the Evidence-Based Veterinary Medicine Association and taught veterinary students as a clinical instructor for the College of Veterinary Medicine at Western University of Health Sciences. In 2015 he completed his MSc in Epidemiology at the London School of Hygiene and Tropical Medicine.

Dr. McKenzie has shared his expertise through lectures at numerous veterinary conferences and in a monthly column in *Veterinary Practice News* magazine. He runs the SkeptVet Blog and contributes to the Science-Based Medicine Blog.

In his sparse free time, he enjoys playing his mandolin, traveling with his family, and sitting on the couch with his dogs watching the hummingbirds and woodpeckers outside his living-room window.

CONTENTS

INTRODUCTION

As a veterinarian, I get to spend much of my day interacting with animals. This is one of the great pleasures of my work. However, some people are surprised to learn that vets spend as much, or more, time interacting with people as with animals. Talking with the owners and caretakers of my patients is critical to helping the animals I treat. Listening to my clients' concerns and observations, asking questions about their animals, and educating them about how to best care for their pets is a critical part of my job. While most vets enter the field eager to help animals, it turns out we get to help people too, and that is also quite rewarding!

A very important part of talking with my clients involves answering their questions and helping them make informed and effective decisions about the care of their animal companions. In order to do this I have to be informed myself, about many different kinds of medical problems and the bewildering variety of options for preventing or treating them. Many of the treatments I use are things I learned about in veterinary school. But in the eighteen years I have been in practice, much has changed in veterinary medicine. New therapies have been developed, and research has shown us that some treatments we used to rely on are not as safe or effective as we once thought. An important part of my responsibility is to keep up with the progress and research in medicine so I can give current and accurate information to my clients.

There are also many products and procedures available to animal patients that are not part of the mainstream medicine typically taught to veterinary students. These are sometimes collectively referred to as "complementary and alternative medicine" or CAM (though we will see a bit later that it is not at all clear or simple to determine exactly what that means). Even though these methods may not be part of the veterinary curriculum, it is important for me to know as much as possible about these options so I can counsel my clients and help my patients.

I have put a great deal of time and energy over my career into learning about such alternative therapies. I have asked questions of those offering these treatments; read the literature produced by CAM practitioners and the scientific research regarding these practices; considered the work of skeptics and critics of CAM; I have even been certified in one CAM method (acupuncture). In doing this, I discovered that figuring out what works and what doesn't in medicine is itself a fascinating and complicated business. This realization led me to completing a master's degree in epidemiology, the science of how we study health and disease and the medical treatments we use. Throughout my career I have tried to approach all the questions my clients ask, and all the treatments they ask about, with both an open mind and a commitment to providing the highest quality of scientific, evidence-based medicine to my patients.

I have been happy to discover that in the veterinary profession the learning never stops! I will never reach a place where I know all there is to know, about CAM or anything else. However, I have learned a lot over the years, both from my clients and patients, and from the time and effort I have put into studying and investigating all of the treatment options available. I share that knowledge individually with my clients every day. My hope is to share it with you in this book and to help you answer some of your questions about how to care for your own animal companions or, if you are also a veterinarian or veterinary nurse, how to give the best care to your patients.

Perhaps the best way to learn is to begin by asking questions. For each of the practices I discuss in this book, I will ask three basic questions:

1. What is it?
2. Does it work?
3. Is it safe?

These are the questions I always ask of any therapy I might use or recommend to my clients. One goal in this book is to answer these questions for some of the most common CAM practices my clients ask me about. Hopefully, you will find useful information about many of the products or techniques you might be interested in using to help your own pets or your patients.

However, another, and perhaps even more important, goal is to empower you to ask and answer these questions for yourself. As well as sharing what I have learned about specific alternative practices, I want to share what I have learned about how to evaluate new and unfamiliar treatment options. It turns out that the way we go about answering these questions has a huge impact on the reliability of the answers we come up with.

It is an exciting time in veterinary medicine, with new discoveries and improvements in our diagnostic and treatment abilities appearing all the time. No one can be an expert in every aspect of medicine, and both vets and pet owners can sometimes feel overwhelmed by the sheer number of choices and options available. A reliance on the best evidence available and a thoughtful, careful approach to evaluating claims about pet care products and medical treatments can help us make good choices. I hope you will find both the information and the strategies I present here useful and that they will help you to critically evaluate all the options you encounter in caring for your pets and patients.

Brennen McKenzie, MA, MSc, VMD, cVMA

1|
What is Complementary and Alternative Medicine?

There cannot be two kinds of medicine—conventional and alternative. There is only medicine that has been adequately tested and medicine that has not, medicine that works and medicine that may or may not work. Once a treatment has been tested rigorously, it no longer matters whether it was considered alternative at the outset. If it is found to be reasonably safe and effective, it will be accepted.

- Marcia Angell and Jerome Kassirer

A book about complementary and alternative medicine has to begin by at least trying to explain what that means. It turns out that isn't as simple as it might sound. This label is applied to a huge variety of very different practices. Proponents of CAM therapies often disagree with each other about what to call their approaches, about the theories behind them, about the details of how they should be used, and about the extent to which they are compatible or incompatible with mainstream scientific medicine. No one definition or description will satisfy everyone. However, to talk about CAM

5

we have to have at least some sense of what we mean, so I will try to give some pragmatic definitions of commonly used terms.

In each chapter of this book, I have provided references for scientific journal articles, books, websites, and other resources that provide more detailed information about specific topics. I have also created a bibliography at the end of the book suggesting other resources which discuss CAM, evidence-based medicine, psychology, and other related subjects. My hope is that these sources will be useful to you in exploring all of these topics.

WORDS, WORDS, WORDS

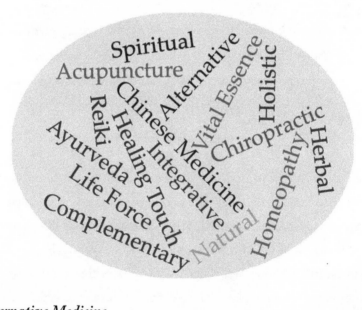

Alternative Medicine

This is an older term less commonly used alone today, though it is still often included as part of the phrase "complementary and alternative medicine."

Placebos for Pets?

This label originally identified practices fundamentally incompatible with scientific medicine and intended to replace it.

For example, some practitioners of homeopathy don't believe infectious organisms, such as viruses or bacteria, directly cause infectious diseases. They propose the alternative explanation that an imbalance in the nonphysical or spiritual energy they call the Vital Force underlies all disease, and that infectious organisms merely contribute to such an imbalance or are symptoms rather than causes of disease. This alternative theory leads to rejection of many medical practices based on conventional germ theory, such as the use of vaccines or antibiotics.[1]

Many other alternative therapies, such as Traditional Chinese Medicine, Indian Ayurvedic medicine, and Reiki or other types of "energy medicine," also reject the conventional explanations of disease as primarily physical, with roots in the sciences of chemistry, anatomy, physiology, and so on. Instead, these approaches have entirely separate explanations for how disease develops, often centered on spiritual forces that cannot be examined or manipulated through traditional scientific methods. This view is called "vitalism," and it is part of many alternative medical approaches.[2,3]

These alternative practices were often intended to replace mainstream medical care. However, because of the many apparent successes of scientific medicine in the twentieth century, few people have been willing to entirely abandon conventional scientific explanations for disease and scientific medical therapies, so truly alternative approaches are less commonly recommended these days. This has led to the development of the category of "complementary medicine."

Complementary Medicine

Many of the therapies initially promoted under the label "alternative medicine" are now more often identified as "complementary," or "complementary and alternative medicine," abbreviated for convenience as CAM (or CAVM for complementary and alternative veterinary medicine). This label suggests that the therapies under this umbrella can be used along with conventional scientific medicine and that they provide some additional benefits that complement mainstream treatment. The therapies themselves, and the theories behind them, however, are typically the same as those identified by the earlier label.

Integrative Medicine

Even the term "complementary" is disliked by some CAM practitioners however, because it implies that conventional medicine is the main treatment and alternative therapies simply "complement" or add something to it. This gives CAM the appearance of a subordinate or second-class status. To better convey their belief that alternative therapies should be viewed as equal to, or in some cases better than, conventional medicine, many of these practitioners now prefer the term "integrative medicine." The underlying idea here is that both conventional and alternative therapies are simply different but equally useful tools available to veterinarians, and they should each be chosen and employed when appropriate without any distinctions based on their underlying rationales of history. The alternative therapies themselves, however, are the same regardless of whether they are used under the banner of alterative, complementary, or integrative medicine.

Placebos for Pets?

Integrative medicine is, perhaps, the trickiest label for CAM because it obscures important differences between alternative and science-based therapies. The term suggests we can seamlessly blend alternative and conventional therapies, that they are equally useful and reliable tools we can select from for the medical job at hand. However, the reality is that there are practical and philosophical differences between how alternative and conventional therapies are developed, tested, and employed, and sometimes these differences matter.

There are several ways in which CAM approaches commonly differ from conventional medicine: they often rely on a theoretical foundation that is incompatible with established scientific knowledge; they usually lack substantial supporting scientific evidence; and they are frequently promoted by a committed group of supporters who believe a particular therapy is safe and effective based on anecdotal experience or historical and cultural tradition despite the absence of supporting scientific evidence.

There is no reason to integrate a plausible and scientifically proven therapy into mainstream medicine and still preserve for it a separate identity as "alternative." If we treat all proposed therapies equally, evaluating their mechanisms and clinical effects at every level through rigorous research, then we can simply accept those that prove their value and abandon the rest. As the editors of the *Journal of the American Medical Association* have put it: "There is no alternative medicine, only scientifically proven, evidence-based medicine supported by solid data or unproven medicine, for which scientific evidence is lacking."[4] The only use for a special category of integrative medicine is to present some therapies as equal in legitimacy to others before they have been properly tested and proven their worth. This is a subject I will discuss in more detail shortly.

Holistic Medicine

Holistic is an interesting term since its typical meaning in the area of CAM differs quite a bit from its strict definition. Formally defined, "holistic" simply means viewing things as complete, integrated wholes rather than collections of individual parts. It is often contrasted with "reductionism," which in its most extreme forms views complex systems such as living beings as only the sum of their separate parts. In medicine, a holistic approach means treating a patient as a complete individual, with attention to all relevant aspects of the patient's body, mind, and context or environment.

This is, of course, an approach every doctor should take. Imagine one of my patients comes in with a nosebleed. If I look only at the patient's nose and ignore the rest of the body and how the patient is feeling generally, or if I don't consider systemic diseases, genetic factors, or environmental causes that might be behind the problem, then I am practicing an extreme and ridiculous kind of reductionist medicine. Despite the suggestion that scientific medicine works this way, conventional doctors are taught to look at all relevant aspects of their patients' condition and context and to practice holistically in the strictest sense.

The tricky part of the concept of holism, though, is the question of what is relevant. It is impossible, and pointless, to consider everything in the universe when trying to understand and treat an individual's health problem. Some things are more relevant than others, and we often have good reason to know the difference. If I suddenly start vomiting profusely, the fact that I recently ate a piece of spoiled fish is likely quite relevant! The fact that I was wearing a blue shirt that day, on the other hand, is almost certainly not. The problem with the term holistic is that in most cases it is not used to suggest that understanding health and disease require a comprehensive evaluation of all relevant factors but to imply some specific factors are relevant which scientific medicine doesn't generally consider to be so.

Holistic medicine is often defined, for example, as including the influence of spiritual factors or other nonphysical energy forces among the most important variables in determining health or illness. As one CAM veterinarian and author has said: "Holistic practitioners believe that vital life energy is the most important factor in the health of the patient…Because medical science has defined itself on a strictly physical basis, it is true that vitalism is unscientific. By definition, vitalism embraces a concept about a nonphysical force that can never be understood within the current scientific, medical paradigm."[5]

Other CAM vets have somewhat different definitions of what must be considered to practice "holistically." Some may view all disease as caused by dietary factors; others may feel that many chronic diseases can be traced to the use of vaccines or antibiotics in a patient many years before; and still others may believe that electromagnetic radiation from modern electronic devices is a crucial factor in illness. These are all real claims I have heard from CAVM practitioners. Each individual would then say that a holistic approach must consider the particular factor he or she believes is relevant, and that any approach which does not is "reductionistic" and deficient.

In practice, "holistic" is most often a code for the use of alternative theories of disease and alternative therapies, intended to signal a distinction from conventional scientific medicine. The specific difference in what is considered relevant to health varies with the particular alternative theory or approach employed. I believe that all good vets should practice holistically in the sense of considering all likely relevant factors and treating every patient as a whole individual in a unique context. However, I think the specific factors that are relevant within this holistic approach have to be demonstrated through research and a sound scientific understanding of health and disease. The concept is legitimate, but the term should not be misused as a mere code for an alternative medical ideology.

Natural

This is one of the terms most commonly used to market and promote CAM approaches, yet it is surprisingly difficult to define consistently. A natural remedy, one would think, would be something found in nature in its original and final form, requiring no processing or alteration by humans to be useful. The opposite, then, would be a remedy that is artificially created and could not exist without human efforts. Yet it turns out that the boundary between the natural and artificial is more of a blurry region with no clear or sharp dividing line. And even when such a distinction can be made, it is often not meaningful.

Certainly, it is fair to consider many modern medical therapies as artificial in the sense that they could not exist without extensive human effort. Anesthesia and surgery, pharmaceuticals, artificial joints, and many other medical technologies are clearly not natural in any obvious sense. On the other hand, what therapies might be considered natural?

Placebos for Pets?

Perhaps feeding an animal raw plant leaves believed to have medicinal properties is using a natural therapy? What if those leaves are dried and combined with leaves from several other plants? How about if the leaves are powdered and placed into capsules or mixed into a liquid for injection? If a specific chemical compound is identified in a plant, isolated in a laboratory and then packaged into pills, is it still natural? What about manufacturing the exact same chemical, down to the last atom, in a laboratory rather than extracting it from a plant? Would it somehow not be safe or effective if made this way when it was before?

Can a herbal remedy be natural if it is identified and prescribed according to a complex set of theoretical principles and rules developed by humans over centuries? Can piercing the body with needles, as in acupuncture, be considered a natural therapy? How about extracting chemicals from natural substances, diluting them repeatedly until no actual molecules of the original substance remain, as is done in homeopathy? Is this a natural therapy? Is feeding raw meat to our pets natural while feeding cooked meat isn't? What if vitamins and minerals are added to the meat and it is frozen or canned?

As you can see, there is virtually nothing in medicine that doesn't involve some effort or alteration of natural materials by humans. It is not obvious what degree of human activity renders something no longer natural. Even more problematic, however, is the issue of why a natural treatment should be better than an artificial one.

Saying that something is natural is usually a way of implying it is inherently healthy and benign. Calling something artificial, by contrast, conveys a much more negative impression, implying it is unhealthy or even false and deceptive. However, it is easy to find examples that belie these connotations.

Nothing could be more natural than *E. coli* or *Salmonella*, bacterial organisms in raw foods that cause diarrhea and vomiting. Intestinal worms and malnutrition are ubiquitous among animals in nature. Even toxins such as radioactive uranium, asbestos, and cyanide are found, complete and functional, in nature. Yet all of these natural things are harmful to us and our pets.

In contrast, the vaccines which have eliminated smallpox and polio and greatly reduced the suffering once caused by many infectious diseases are clearly artificial, in the sense of being created by humans out of natural materials. Antibiotics, which have rendered many routinely fatal diseases curable, and vitamin supplementation of foods, which have eliminated dreadful and once common maladies like scurvy and rickets, do not exist in nature. Blood transfusions, organ transplants, prosthetic limbs, insulin for diabetics, and even such simple and unheralded public health technologies as indoor plumbing and toilet paper, have saved lives and reduced suffering for millions. Yet these could not be described as natural in the usual sense.

The term "natural" is ill-defined and largely meaningless when applied to medicine. It doesn't help us decide whether a therapy is safe or beneficial for our animals. It doesn't even reliably distinguish between conventional scientific and alternative approaches. Every day I remind my clients of the importance of providing plenty of exercise, healthy food and water, and appropriate social interaction for their pets. These are all beneficial, natural, and completely science-based healthcare recommendations.

The idea that something natural must automatically be good is so widespread and consistently mistaken that philosophers have given it its own name: The Appeal to Nature Fallacy. While things that are "natural," insofar as we can even define that, may be good, the fact that they are natural doesn't prove or predict their good qualities. This is an idea that will come up again and again in our discussions of alternative medicine, and it is pernicious because it is both intuitively appealing and completely unreliable.

MEDICINE AND PHILOSOPHY

When I first began to investigate CAM, I had the rather naïve view that all I needed to do to effectively help my clients was find the appropriate published research showing which therapies worked and which didn't. I initially saw CAM as just a set of medical treatments that, for some reason, got a special label but could otherwise be considered, tested, and then accepted or rejected in the same way as conventional treatments. It took some time for me to understand that much of the reason the category of complementary and alternative medicine exists at all is rooted in basic ideas about the world that are very different from those behind science-based medicine.

Some CAM therapies can be studied and used scientifically, of course, and I will talk about these when I get into specific CAM treatments. However, CAM in general is an ideological category, not merely a collection of individual treatments. It is a collection of different, sometimes even mutually incompatible, ideas and practices united by their status as outside the mainstream, and often by a few general philosophical concepts (though even these are not uniformly accepted by all practitioners of alternative therapies). Therefore, I think it will be useful to briefly introduce here some of the differences in the core philosophies of alternative and science-based medicine. This will help us a lot later when we come to evaluating the claims and evidence behind CAM practices and comparing them with conventional medicine.

Do Our Thoughts Make Our Reality?

One key idea taken as a given in the scientific view is that the world exists independent of what we humans think or believe about it. I may not understand how the world works all the time, but my beliefs about it don't change how it works. I would be surprised if many people seriously question this assumption, but there are some strains of CAM that don't accept that the natural world is independent of human beliefs.

Some CAM vets, for example, rely on the idea that we can influence the physical world directly with our thoughts, and that we can cause disease in our pets with our thoughts and feelings.

> ...the major influence that directs your pets' health and well being [sic] is your perceived state of being.... what my years of observation have taught me is that when our pet develops a chronic or fatal disease, the form of that disease often reflects our perspective on life.... the emotions we are experiencing, when we think about our pet's health condition, are likely the emotions that participated in the development of the problem in the first place. If I am frustrated with life and this perception persists long enough, the energy that is created will influence my reality.
>
> When I see a person who is chronically frustrated with their job, or relationships, it does not surprise me when their pet develops a chronic illness.[6]

Similarly, some CAM therapists believe that the key to curing disease is in how we direct our mental, emotional, and spiritual energies, and that the physical aspects of illness are secondary, if they matter at all.

Our energy field creates our reality, and if we can learn to take control of our energy, we change our lives. The concepts of resonance and entrainment form the basis for energy medicine modalities such as Healing Touch, Healing Touch for Animals, Therapeutic Touch, Reiki, Pranic and Reconnective Healing. The practitioner's energy field entrains the patient's energy field and changes its vibration, allowing the body's instinctive healing mechanisms to work more efficiently... So in order to be an effective practitioner of any type, we must create a healing state with our own energy field.[7]

It is nearly impossible to prove or disprove the existence of nonphysical energies or effects of our thoughts on the physical world. There is no good scientific evidence that such beliefs are true, but many people who believe in them claim this is because science simply doesn't have the ability to detect or understand such forces. The supernatural, by definition, transcends the natural world and so cannot be consistently controlled, manipulated or predicted. Whatever the truth may be about the existence of supernatural forces, science as a system for understanding the world only applies to aspects of the physical world—things that can be detected, measured, and that manifest regular, consistent behavior. Anything else must be accepted or rejected on faith alone.

Science assumes the physical world exists independent of the beliefs, or even the existence, of human beings. This means that for some CAM practices, especially those that rely on a belief in nonphysical energies or spiritual forces, it isn't very useful to study them scientifically. Individuals who believe in the importance of such metaphysical forces are unlikely to give up those beliefs regardless of the outcome of scientific research. These practices are fundamentally faith-based.

While I have no objection to personal faith or spiritual beliefs in general, I think they are an unreliable foundation for medicine. Historically, we based our medicine on personal experience and belief for thousands of years. This approach failed spectacularly, not producing in several millennia even a fraction of the improvements in our health and life expectancy science has given us in only a couple of centuries. Furthermore, if the foundation for how we treat our pets' illness is the personal belief of each individual doctor, then there is no shared understanding, no common ground to define veterinary medicine, just individual vets each making up their own system of healthcare. How, then, are pet owners to decide which of these varieties of faith-based medicine is most likely to help their pets? For reasons I will explore throughout this book, I think science is the best tool for deciding which treatments will really help our animal companions and which won't. Any method that excludes itself from scientific evaluation should be treated very skeptically indeed!

Can We Know Anything?

In addition to the view that the world has a real, physical nature that is independent of human beliefs, the scientific approach to understanding health and disease also relies on the assumption that we can develop practical, useful knowledge about how the natural world works and that we can use this knowledge to change things, including to influence health and disease. Just as the world is real, the knowledge we get through scientific investigation is real.

Placebos for Pets?

Sure, science makes mistakes all the time. It eventually corrects these given enough time and effort, but clearly our knowledge at any given moment is incomplete and imperfect. In the scientific view, however, there are such things as facts, and we can know some things with a pretty high degree of confidence. We may still have some tinkering to do with the theory of gravity, for example, but it is vanishingly unlikely that we will one day realize it was wrong all along and that we actually can fly using the power of our minds, just by thinking differently about our relationship to the ground.

While advocates of alternative approaches to health also often claim to have practical knowledge, to understand the causes of disease and how to prevent or treat them, some subscribe to a very different philosophy of knowledge than that of scientific medicine. CAM practitioners sometimes reject scientific facts that conflict with their beliefs by claiming that all human understanding of nature is just a collection of ideas in our heads, metaphors that don't have any objective reality. This means that any set of metaphors we choose to use is equally valid, and no approach to knowledge, scientific or otherwise, can claim superiority over other approaches.

This is an appealing notion in some ways. It is useful in other fields, such as art, politics, religion, and so on, in preventing ethnocentrism, the conviction that one's own cultural beliefs are inherently true and the beliefs of other cultures are false. Such ethnocentric views have caused no end of trouble in the world, and it is worthwhile trying to minimize them. Unfortunately, applied to medicine and other aspects of the natural world, this kind of relativism can quickly lead to absurdity. One defender of Traditional Chinese Medicine provides a good illustration of this:

If no paradigm [meaning a model of reality] does have absolute value, there is no absolute basis with which to judge another paradigm. Any paradigm will appear limited or incorrect from the perspective of a different paradigm, so Chinese medicine will seem incorrect from a biomedical point of view, and vice versa.

The invocation of a saint can cure intractable cancer; a voodoo curse can kill….A shaman applying a curse does not consider it to be a placebo, nor does his victim. To them, real magic is involved. To interpret it otherwise is to make a culturally, paradigmatically biased judgment. We can never prove the shaman wrong, only offer an alternative explanation.[8]

Clearly, relativism carried to this extreme rejects the possibility of any real knowledge and progress, in medicine or any other field.

THE POLITICS OF CAM

As we have seen, the question of what complementary and alternative medicine really is, and what distinguishes it from conventional medicine, is not a simple one. CAM is a diverse collection of beliefs and practices, some of which are compatible with scientific views of health and disease and some of which are not. Many of the specific CAM theories about what causes illness and how we should prevent or treat it conflict not only with a scientific understanding of the natural world but with each other. Accepting the core principles of homeopathy, for example, must mean Traditional Chinese Medicine is completely wrong, at least if we are to be intellectually consistent.

Placebos for Pets?

The category of complementary and alternative veterinary medicine, then, is not a set of beliefs about health and disease so much as an ideological construct. It links ideas and practices primarily through a shared status as outside the medical mainstream. And though there are some common philosophical themes that appear in many CAM approaches, these are by no means universal in the CAM community. Advocates of alternative therapies often disagree as vociferously with each other as with proponents of science-based medicine about the nature of health and the value of specific therapies. However, the CAM label provides a useful tool for joining together disparate approaches outside the scientific mainstream in advocacy, lobbying, and marketing efforts to obtain recognition and a larger role in veterinary medicine.

Part of the challenge of defining complementary and alternative medicine is that in some sense there really is no such thing. In terms of what matters most, whether a specific treatment is safe and works for patients, calling something CAM is meaningless. We don't distinguish treatments in scientific medicine on the basis of what country or historical period they originated in, because this tells us nothing useful about them. And we don't judge the safety and effectiveness of conventional treatments by different standards based on the theory of how they work, how old they are, how popular they are, and so on. These factors may matter in the marketing or promotion of a practice, but not in terms of judging whether that practice is useful to patients.

Ideally, all medical therapies we apply to our pets should have a plausible theory for how they might work that is consistent with well-established scientific principles. Our treatments should also be supported by a variety of forms of scientific evidence, from test tube and laboratory studies to trials with patients in the real world, showing they have benefits greater than their risks. If we can demonstrate a particular therapy is safe and effective using appropriate scientific testing, why does it require a separate category, such as "alternative" or "integrative," to be utilized as part of our overall treatment approach? If we test a therapy, show it works, and begin using it, how is it not simply another tool of conventional or science-based medicine?

DEFINING CAM BY EXAMPLE

Because of the complexity and inconsistency of CAM terminology, listing specific practices that are typically considered part of CAM is sometimes used as a substitute for defining the general category. This too is an imperfect strategy which often fails to achieve the truly important distinction vets and pet owners need, between safe and effective therapies and those which are ineffective or do more harm than good.

Confusion is also created when some conventional therapies are claimed as alternative by CAM practitioners because they are popular or well-supported scientifically and this makes the category as a whole seem more legitimate. In human medicine, for example, alternative practitioners often claim that recommending healthy nutrition, regular exercise, and attention to one's emotional and social needs as well as physical symptoms are features of CAM, even though these are established, routine practices in conventional medicine as well. And, as I've already argued, there really isn't much need for a list of alternative therapies if we simply apply the same standards of evidence to every practice and then accept the useful and reject the useless or harmful.

Placebos for Pets?

Nevertheless, some practices are consistently identified as alternative, for historical reasons or because of philosophical differences from science-based medicine such as I've discussed already. And since this book will be most useful to pet owners if I am able to select and discuss those alternative therapies that are most likely to be offered to them, it is worthwhile to make at least a rough list of the most common CAM practices. More detailed discussion of each approach and the theory and evidence concerning it can be found in the chapters addressing individual practices.

The approaches that almost everyone would agree are part of complementary and alternative medicine include homeopathy, herbal remedies, acupuncture, historical systems of folk medicine—such as Traditional Chinese Medicine or the Indian system of Ayurvedic Medicine—and any therapy that claims to work primarily by detecting and manipulating nonphysical "energy" of some kind or spiritual forces.

There is less agreement about the wide variety of practices often called "manual therapy" or "physical medicine." Certainly, direct extrapolation of human chiropractic to veterinary patients is an alternative practice. However, massage and many rehabilitative or physical therapy modalities, including hydrotherapy, cold laser therapy, therapies involving the use of electricity or ultrasound to treat musculoskeletal disease, and many others are in a grey area. Some are clearly incompatible in theory with scientific principles and have no real evidence to support claims that they work. Others, however, often offered by the same practitioners, have at least some plausible theoretical rationale or even some research evidence in humans or animals to suggest they may be effective for some problems.

In these unclear cases, the distinction between not yet tested or proven conventional therapy and alternative medicine is, once again, often more in the philosophical foundations than in the specific treatment itself. A science-based practitioner will make limited claims proportional to the available evidence and not rely primarily on anecdotes or speculate wildly about the effects of their therapies. If someone says a massage might make your pet feel better or that laser therapy is a possible, but not entirely proven, way to encourage wound healing, these claims are perfectly compatible with scientific veterinary medicine. It is not a form of alternative or integrative medicine to offer a plausible but unproven therapy, so long as the nature of the evidence is honestly disclosed.

However, if someone claims a massage will "release toxins" or slow the progression of cancer in your dog, or that laser therapy can reverse aging or adjust your pet's energy field, this person is promoting alternative medicine. Even if the specific treatments they use are nearly identical to those offered by a conventional veterinarian, this view of what these treatments do and how they do it is vastly different from, and incompatible with, the view of scientific medicine.

This may not seem an important distinction at first. Surely a massage is a massage regardless of whether one thinks it increases blood flow or removes "toxins?" And if cold laser therapy improves healing, who cares whether the vet offering it believes it works by stimulating cell regeneration or balancing Qi (a mystical spiritual energy important in Traditional Chinese Medicine)? However, these differences really do matter when deciding who to trust with the care of your pet.

Placebos for Pets?

Dramatic unsubstantiated claims and theories that conflict with established scientific knowledge, even when employed to justify a benign or even potentially useful therapy, are a warning sign. Practitioners who don't rely on science and evidence-based medicine are unlikely to distinguish between promising but unproven treatments and completely ineffective ones. If you believe one can balance Qi using laser light, you are likely to also believe unbalanced Qi is a cause of illness. When this is true, you may be less interested in identifying and treating real causes of illness, such as infectious agents or cancer. And if wild and unlikely claims for massage are acceptable without good evidence, why wouldn't such claims for homeopathy or "energy medicine" or any other ineffective method be just as acceptable?

BOTTOM LINE

Ultimately, calling a specific practice alternative or holistic, natural or integrative, tells us very little about whether that practice is safe or whether it will be beneficial for our pets. As usual, the devil is in the details, and most of this book will be about exploring the details. To determine which claims about CAM are likely true, which are false, and which we don't yet have enough information to judge, we need to look closely at specific practices and claims made for them.

But what's the best way to figure out if such claims are true or if a CAM treatment really works? Should we ask a conventional vet or one who practices alternative therapies? Should we ask other pet owners who have tried CAM treatments? Or do we have to try each one for ourselves to really know whether or not it works?

As you likely already suspect, my approach to evaluating CAM is to look to science. Though science can produce facts, bits of knowledge in which we can have a pretty high degree of confidence, science is not primarily a collection of facts. Science is a method for testing what we guess or think we know about the world. In the next chapter, I'll introduce you to some of the ways science can help us understand alternative therapies, and how it can help us make the best decisions possible in caring for our animal friends.

By definition...complementary and alternative medicine...has either not been proved to work or been proved not to work. Do you know what they call alternative medicine that's been proved to work? Medicine.

- Tim Minchin

[1] Morrell P. Triumph of the light--isopathy and the rise of transcendental homeopathy, 1830-1920. *Med Humanit.* 2003;29(1):22-32. doi:10.1136/mh.29.1.22

[2] McKenzie BA. Is complementary and alternative medicine compatible with evidence-based medicine? *J Am Vet Med Assoc.* 2012;241(4). doi:10.2460/javma.241.4.421

[3] TJ K. Historical context of the concept of vitalism in complementary and alternative medicine. In: MS M, ed. *Fundamentals of Complementary and Alternative Medicine.* New York N.Y.: Churchill Livingstone; 1996.

[4] Fontanarosa PB, Lundberg GD. Alternative medicine meets science. *JAMA.* 1998;280(18):1618-1619.

[5] Knueven D. An introduction to holistic medicine. In: *The Holistic Health Guide: Natural Care for the Whole Dog.* Neptune City, NJ: T.F.H. Publications; 2008:9-13.

[6] Thomas D. Discover the most powerful pet medicine Available at: https://www.healyourlife.com/discover-the-most-powerful-pet-medicine-available. Published 2015. Accessed September 11, 2018.

[7] Wagner S. Energy Medicine. In: *American Holisic Veterinary Medical Association Annual Meeting.* Birmingham, AL; 2012.

[8] Churchill W. Implications of evidence-based medicine for complementary and alternative medicine. *J Chinese Med.* 1999;59:32-35.

2|
How to Evaluate Medical Therapies for our Pets

Another source of fallacy is the vicious circle of illusions which consist on the one hand of believing what we see and on the other seeing what we believe.

\- Sir Clifford Allbutt

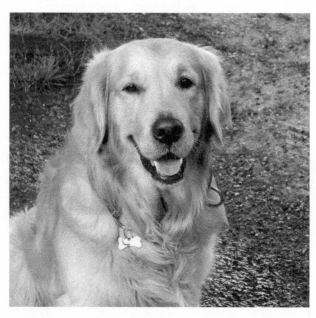

Placebos for Pets?

Missy's Story

Missy was a perfect golden retriever, with beautiful red-gold hair and a friendly, joyful demeanor. She seemed the picture of health when I walked into the exam room. Her owner, though, was worried and had brought her to see me because she was concerned that Missy might have leukemia.

Leukemia is a relatively rare blood cancer, but golden retrievers are more prone to a variety of cancers than some breeds, and at eight years old, Missy was old enough for cancer to be a potential concern. Usually, however, dogs with leukemia are sick: not eating, losing weight, with a listless, sad demeanor. Missy looked nothing like a dog with cancer.

When I asked her owner about her behavior at home, she told me Missy was eating well, playful, energetic, and showing no symptoms. Puzzled, I asked the owner why she thought Missy might have leukemia. The answer was that an energy healer had told her that Missy had this disease.

I briefly mentioned energy medicine in the last chapter, and I will evaluate the concept in more detail later. The vague term "energy" is used to refer to everything from the chemical reactions in cells that fuel normal metabolism, to nonphysical spiritual forces some CAM practitioners believe are responsible for health and disease. Such forces cannot be objectively detected or measured, so there is no scientific evidence for their existence or their role in health. This means that any claim about them has to be taken on faith since it cannot be tested in any objective way.

Though I was skeptical of the idea that Missy might have such a serious illness that had created no symptoms but could only be detected by subjective or intuitive methods, I certainly took her owner's concern seriously. Leukemia is a cancer of blood cells, and it is usually diagnosed by taking a blood sample and looking for abnormal cells. So I ran a number of blood tests on Missy to check for leukemia and other possible diseases. Fortunately, all the test results were normal.

I expected Missy's owner would be relieved to hear that there was no evidence her companion had cancer, but she still seemed uneasy, not satisfied by the good news. Believing Missy had a specific illness gave her owner a focus for her fears about her pet's well-being and an opportunity to take action to help her beloved companion. Being told there was nothing wrong, especially when she did not necessarily understand why the blood test should be more reliable than her energy healer's methods, left Missy's owner anxious and unsure about what she could do to take control and ensure her pet's welfare.

I checked in on Missy from time to time after her visit, and the owner always reported she was doing well. Then about a year later, Missy came back to the hospital again. This time, she had a cough, and her energy practitioner had determined she most likely had a lung tumor.

As before, Missy was joyful and energetic. She was eating well, breathing comfortably, and seemed overall in perfect condition. Her cough and other symptoms were typical for an upper respiratory infection, something which is rarely serious and is easily treated. Still, I did not wish to overlook the possibility of something more serious, so I took an X-ray of her chest to look for possible causes of Missy's cough.

Happily, her chest X-rays showed no tumor, and after a few days of antibiotics her cough went away. I couldn't help asking Missy's owner what her energy practitioner had said about the failure of any sign of leukemia to develop after her previous visit, thinking that perhaps two mistaken diagnoses of life-threatening illness might have shaken the client's confidence in the practitioner's methods. How naïve I was! Missy's owner informed me, without any hint of doubt, that not only had her energy healer detected the leukemia even before it was possible to see it in the blood, but that she had cured it using homeopathy!

Missy's story illustrates a number of the ways in which people can develop and maintain dubious beliefs about health and disease, and how alternative medicine for pets often appears to work even when it really has no effect. We are all naturally worried about the possibility our pets may become ill, and we want to be able to do something to prevent this. Though there is reason to believe that our pets, like us, are living longer and healthier lives than ever before, it is hard not to fear the inevitable loss of our companions, and we naturally want to do everything we can to keep them well and put off that loss.

Unfortunately, this desire for control over our pets' fate can lead us to believing in the power of alternative therapies even when there is little reason to believe they actually work. Humans readily see what we want or expect to see in the world around us, and this tendency can be dangerously misleading. Things are all too often not what they seem.

The purpose of this chapter is to address some of the ways we typically judge claims about medical therapies, and how we can improve the process to make better decisions for our pets. Some kinds of evidence are more trustworthy than others. And while all information should be viewed critically and skeptically, some sources are more reliable than others. By understanding how our own thoughts and perceptions can fool us, and which methods are most effective at guarding against these errors, we can make the best healthcare choices for our pets.

ANECDOTAL EVIDENCE: IS SEEING BELIEVING?

Can you tell which of these two people is a woman and which a man?

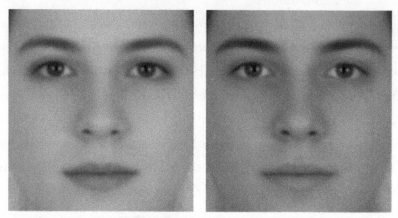

Image from Russell R. Perception. 2009;38(8):1211-1219.[1]) © R. Russell

Would you be surprised to be told these are both pictures of the same person? The apparent gender difference is just a trick created by changing the level of contrast in the photos.[1] You shouldn't feel bad if you guessed wrong because most people do. But more importantly, you shouldn't feel too confident if you guessed right, since you had a 50/50 chance! This image illustrates how easily our judgement can be mistaken, even about something as basic as identifying the sex of another human.

Most people are familiar with the large variety of optical illusions and how our vision can fool us. However, every aspect of our processes for perceiving and evaluating the world, from our senses to our reasoning and memory, has quirks and weaknesses like those that make us susceptible to optical illusions. This means that for all our talents as a species, and all our intelligence, education, and experience as individuals, we can still come to the wrong conclusion in an astounding number of ways!

Despite the abundant evidence from the fields of psychology and neuroscience that our direct experiences often can't be trusted, much of what we believe about the world still comes from such experiences.[2-6] Anyone who has ever been stung by a bee or burned their hand on a hot stove has a compelling set of beliefs about bees and stoves, and these beliefs don't seem to require any scientific data or the opinions of experts on entomology or thermodynamics to validate them. Beliefs founded in direct experience are deeply compelling and often seem incontrovertible. The problem is that our sense of certainty about such beliefs doesn't have anything to do with how likely they are to be correct.[7]

In the world of medicine, personal narratives used to support claims about medical practices are called anecdotes. By far the most common response I get when I question a claim about an alternative therapy is an anecdote supposedly proving that the therapy really does work. If you have ever had a sick pet and tried a number of different treatments without success, and then seen your pet get better following a particular treatment, you almost certainly believe that final therapy worked. What else could any reasonable person conclude?

You have probably heard the term "anecdotal evidence," and you may know that doctors and scientists don't put a lot of stock in it. So why don't scientists or your vet always agree with what seems the obvious conclusion from personal experience?

Well, the frustrating truth is that such experiences tell us very little about what works and what doesn't in medicine. After all, it is possible to find positive anecdotes, often quite a few, for every treatment anyone has ever tried. You can find stories of miraculous cures for everything from herbal remedies to homeopathy, from raw diets to prayer and even, of course, for the therapies of science-based medicine. Do they all work? Are they all the same? If a test always shows everything works, perhaps it's not a very reliable test? Anecdotes are a test no therapy has ever failed.

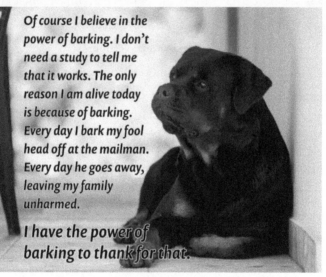

Of course I believe in the power of barking. I don't need a study to tell me that it works. The only reason I am alive today is because of barking. Every day I bark my fool head off at the mailman. Every day he goes away, leaving my family unharmed.

I have the power of barking to thank for that.

2018 By Paul Ingraham, used with permission

Unfortunately, because of their emotionally compelling nature, anecdotes sway us far more than dry, cold statistics, even if the numbers are more trustworthy. This is as true for doctors as it is for pet owners, which is why a story told by someone with lots of academic degrees or clinical experience isn't necessarily any more reliable than one told by anyone else.

Obviously, not every story is wrong. Quite often, anecdotes may illustrate the truth, even though they cannot prove it. And expertise and experience can reduce the chances of our falling into error, but not by as much as we like to think. I will certainly tell stories in this book because they are an efficient and enjoyable way to illustrate ideas. But I will repeatedly caution you not to imagine that stories alone, mine or anyone else's, can prove an idea true or false.

WHAT CAN WE LEARN FROM HISTORY?

In addition to anecdotes and testimonials, another common way in which proponents of alternative therapies support their claims is by referring to historical tradition. If some groups of people have practiced acupuncture, used herbal remedies, or relied some other alternative healing method for decades, maybe even centuries, those treatments must do something useful, right?! Unfortunately, once again this seemingly simple and obvious conclusion turns out not to be very reliable.

Bloodletting is a classic example of a medical practice that endured for thousands of years and was widely believed to be effective based on the experience of millions of people. However, it ultimately proved not only useless but actively dangerous. Many cultures around the world, from Ancient Egypt to China to Europe to pre-Colombian North America, practiced some form of bloodletting as a medical therapy. With a limited understanding of anatomy and little idea of the function of blood or internal organs, these cultures had a variety of theoretical ideas about the role of blood and other bodily fluids in health, and these ideas were often connected to the prevailing religious beliefs.[8]

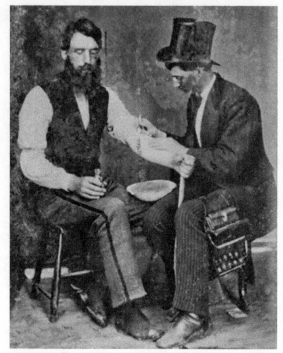

Illustration of nineteenth-century bloodletting. Image from the Burns Archive

The theories underlying the practice of bloodletting were intricate and varied with the specific time and place. In medieval Europe, for example, it was believed that our bodies contained four major fluids or "humors," and these had to be in balance for good health. These humors were names for fluids observed in the body at a time when people did not understand their real origin or function: yellow bile, black bile, blood, and phlegm. These were thought to be connected to the seasons, to the "elements" thought at the time to make up everything in the universe (earth, air, fire, and water), and to specific patterns of symptoms in people with illness. The four humors formed the core of a complex set of theories and metaphors that dominated

Western medical thought from the days of Ancient Greece until the 1800s.[9,10]

According to this theory bloodletting was useful as a medical therapy because it removed excess blood and kept the humors in balance. The same theory was also used to justify other now-abandoned therapies, such as inducing vomiting (emesis) or diarrhea (purging) in order to balance humors other than blood.

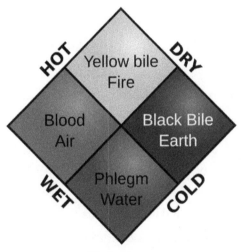

The four humors

In scientific medicine around the world, the humoral theory has been replaced by a more detailed and sophisticated understanding of physiology and disease supported by experimental scientific evidence. However, humorism is still a prominent concept in several modern schools of alternative medicine. There are the Five Elements in so-called Traditional Chinese Medicine, the three Doshas of Ayurvedic practices of India, and the four humors of some folk medicine practices in Tibet and parts of Latin America.[11-15]

These folk beliefs often have historical connections with those of Ancient Greece and with each other that contribute to the similarities in their theories. The same theories have also been applied to veterinary patients in these traditions, historically and even today.[16,17,18]

For thousands of years, millions of people had blood drained from their bodies to cure almost every condition imaginable, and for all this time both ordinary people and the most respected medical authorities believed this was an effective practice. And then, little more than a hundred years ago, bloodletting was abandoned by virtually everyone over the course of a few decades; almost overnight by the standards of history. Why? [8,19,20]

In the late eighteenth and early nineteenth centuries, the developing methods of science began to provide evidence which ultimately led to the rejection of bloodletting and other practices based on humorism in most of the world. First, our understanding of how the human body works grew more accurate, and it gradually became clear that the notion of physiology as simply the maintenance of balance between a small number of humors didn't fit the facts. Origins and functions were found for various bodily fluids that didn't match the guesses of Ancient Egyptian and Greek healers.

For example, the redness and swelling associated with inflammation in one part of the body was once seen as an excessive accumulation of blood in that body part. The sensible treatment for this, according to humoral theory, was to drain blood from that part of the body, through cutting nearby veins or lacerating the skin. Once it was shown, however, that blood circulates everywhere in the body and does not accumulate or stagnate at sites of inflammation, this practiced couldn't be justified by humoral theories anymore. And once, much later, the true causes and processes of inflammation were understood, humoral theory turned out to be completely wrong about the nature of this symptom.

However, the practice of bloodletting outlasted the replacement of humoral theory. As elements of the theory were disproven, proponents of bloodletting rearranged their arguments to defend the practice. Personal experience is very persuasive, and these doctors had thousands of years of anecdotes showing miraculous benefits from bloodletting. One late defender of the practice wrote in 1829 "Who is there with ten or twenty years experience in the profession, that has not seen the most marked advantages from bleeding..."[21] Another learned physician wrote even later, in 1875, that "He thought it really saying too much...that we should assume to be so much wiser than our fathers, who had lent their approval to a custom that had been sanctioned by ages of experience." With so many anecdotes accumulated over so many years, and in light of their own experience practicing bloodletting, it was simply impossible for these advocates of the therapy to accept the growing evidence that the practice made no sense and didn't work.

Of course, there were always anecdotes which suggested bloodletting wasn't beneficial, and even that it was harmful. One of the most famous victims of bloodletting was George Washington, first president of the United States.[22] After contracting what is now believed to be a case of the bacterial disease strep throat, Washington was fed various concoctions and drained of a significant quantity of blood. This certainly didn't help his infection, and it likely caused, or at least hastened, his death. Even at the time, there were doctors who doubted the wisdom of bloodletting based on such experiences.

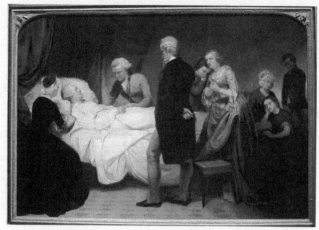

Washington on his Deathbed. Junius Brutus Stearns, 1851

However, our natural tendency is to look for ways to support and confirm what we believe, rather than undermine and reject it. This makes our lives feel a lot more stable and predictable. Over the years, we weave a tapestry of ideas that is complex and forms a consistent picture. Undoing individual threads threatens the coherence of the whole thing and makes the world seem harder to understand and predict, and so harder to control. We instinctively cling to anecdotes and evidence that fit our pictures and dismiss or ignore those that do not.

For these and other reasons, practitioners of bloodletting fought hard to continue the practice even when the core ideas it was based on were proven untrue. Ultimately, the practice was abandoned, however; not because science showed its basic theories to be false, but because science proved that it was not helping patients but actually harming them. Scientists began systematically comparing patients who were treated with bloodletting and patients with the same diseases who weren't. The results consistently showed that not only did bloodletting not help patients, in many cases it made them worse and even led to their death, as it had for George Washington.[8,19] This kind of evidence helped to convince many doctors that bloodletting did more harm than good, though there were some who continued to swear by the practice even in the face of such clear facts. Eventually, we ceased to teach this harmful practice to new doctors. Those who could not let it go despite the powerful evidence against it passed away, and the practice died out.

While it may seem a bizarre relic of history, bloodletting exemplifies the dangers of trusting our own observations and experiences when better evidence is available. It was used and trusted faithfully as a curative treatment, and millions of people could have provided stories of miraculous recoveries attributed to bloodletting. Yet even simple scientific studies, small and crude by the standards of research today, quickly showed it was worse than useless and sometimes deadly.

There is little difference between how people maintained their faith in bloodletting over millennia, and the way people maintain their belief in many modern healthcare practices. This is true for conventional medical practices as well as CAM. However, alternative medicine is especially vulnerable to this because of some of the philosophical differences I discussed in the last chapter. Many CAM practitioners reject the idea that controlled research is more reliable than personal experience, and cling to the belief that the historical use of a therapy is good reason to believe it works. These views make it even harder for practitioners of alternative therapies than for conventional vets to accept the verdict of science when it goes against their preferred beliefs.

IS THERE A PLACEBO EFFECT FOR ANIMALS?

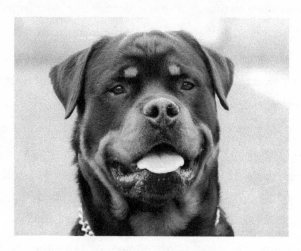

Titan was a solid, powerful 110-pound Rottweiler with a gentle, affectionate personality. When I met him, he was suffering from a painful and incurable bone tumor in his right front leg. Though he was a stoic dog, he was clearly in great pain. He would not put his paw on the ground to walk, and he whimpered at even the lightest touch on his tumor.

His owner was deeply distressed by the idea that she would very soon lose Titan. She had a strong personal faith in what she thought of as "natural" medical therapies, and a deep distrust of conventional medicine, especially drugs. Despite this, she had come to me to see if I could offer any hope for a cure for Titan, or at least a long-term delay in his death.

Unfortunately, I had to tell her honestly that even the most aggressive treatments for this type of cancer would only delay its spread by a few months, and these treatments consist of surgery and chemotherapy, treatments she was not willing to consider in any case. However, I did have a number of pain control therapies to offer Titan that would have greatly decreased his discomfort.

His owner seemed surprised, and a bit offended, when I mentioned the subject of pain control. She explained that she was already using a homeopathic remedy and acupuncture, and that she believed Titan's pain had almost completely gone away thanks to these therapies. When I gently pointed out that he could not walk on his affected leg and cried when it was touched, she became angry. My observations felt like an accusation to her that she wasn't taking good care of the pet she clearly loved very much. Her reaction illustrates one aspect of a phenomenon most people think doesn't exist in veterinary medicine: the placebo effect.

What is the Placebo Effect?

Though it has been known for a long time that our expectations and beliefs can affect the symptoms of disease, the first really scientific investigation of what we now call the placebo effect didn't occur until the eighteenth century. The best known early example of such investigations were conducted by a physician named Henry Beecher, who first became interested in the effect while working as an army doctor during World War II.[23,24]

While treating wounded soldiers in North Africa, Dr. Beecher was sometimes forced to cope with shortages of vital supplies, including painkillers like morphine. On more than one occasion when he had no morphine available to give his patients who were suffering, he instead gave them injections of saline, essentially salt water, and told them they were getting morphine. This seemed to produce a dramatic decrease in the soldiers' pain, even though the saline is just a component of our normal body fluids and doesn't have any effect when injected. Interestingly, Beecher discovered that for this trick to work, the patients had to believe they were getting a genuine pain-killer.

After the war, Beecher spent years conducting studies on the effects of fake drugs and treatments on pain and many other symptoms. Other doctors and scientists have also investigated placebos, often in ways we cannot imagine being permitted today. Not only have fake injections and fake pills been shown to make people feel better while not actually doing anything to their bodies, but fake surgeries have shown that even surgical procedures that are widely accepted as effective can sometimes turn out to be nothing more than placebos. The features of the human brain that fooled our ancestors into believing bloodletting was effective are still present in our brains today, and we can still be easily fooled in the same ways.

Additional research has shown that procedures and drugs which do nothing at all themselves can make people feel less pain, nausea, anxiety, and depression. And it turns out that many factors influence how effective a placebo treatment is. Big pills work better than small pills. Expensive fake treatments work better than cheap fake treatments. Placebos work better if offered by doctors rather than nurses, but they are less effective if the doctor wears a T-shirt instead of a white coat.[25,26] In general, however, placebos of any kind seem to work much better if people believe they are real, effective medical treatments. If you tell someone they are getting a useless sugar pill, then they aren't likely to feel much better after taking it.

This raises some interesting and important questions. Are the effects of placebos on symptoms of illness "real?" Sure the effect is "all in your head," because the treatments don't themselves do anything to your body. But if you feel better anyway, isn't that "real?"

Well, yes and no. If a treatment is truly inert, meaning it does nothing but change the person's perception of their symptoms, this can still have some value for a human patient. Unfortunately, there are also risks associated with the placebo effect. If you feel better, it's hard not to believe your disease is actually getting better, even when it's not. And that can affect your decisions about treatments that might actually make your disease better. And if your doctors, or researchers studying the effect of a new treatment, believe a placebo is actually making your illness go away because you feel better, this can lead to mistakes in understanding how your disease works and what treatments might really make it better.

Another problem with placebo effects is that they are usually small and temporary. They are consistently much less effective than treatments which actually work on your body, not only on your mind.[27-30] And placebos also raise serious ethical problems for doctors. To use a placebo effectively, your doctor has to lie to you, or they have to believe the placebo is a real treatment, which either means they have been lied to or they don't understand your disease very well. As a society, we're past the time when we thought it was okay for doctors to lie to their patients "for their own good." And presumably we want our doctors to be smart and well-informed about our illnesses. So it's hard to see how we can ethically make much use of placebo treatments.

In veterinary medicine, the question that naturally arises is, if placebo effects in humans seem to rely on a false belief that the person is getting a real medicine, how can animals experience placebo effects when they do not appear to have explicit beliefs about their own health? It turns out placebo effects *are* relevant to pets, and placebo-controlled studies are critical to an accurate understanding of whether medical therapies truly work for our animal companions.

The most significant aspect of placebo effects in animals is what is known as the "caregiver placebo effect."[31,32] Our pets cannot directly report their subjective symptoms, such as pain or nausea, so veterinarians and owners must observe animal patients and decide whether they are responding to treatment. Often, the humans will perceive improvement even when objective measures show none or when the animal is actually getting a placebo treatment. This is likely part of why Titan's owner felt his pain had responded to alternative therapies even when he still seemed obviously in pain to me. Humans are notorious for seeing what we want and expect to see, whether it is there or not.

In several studies of arthritis treatments in dogs, veterinarians reported improvement 40-45% of the time, and owners up to 57% of the time, even when the dogs were actually getting a placebo.[31] The same kind of effect has been found in studies of pain medications for cats.[32] Even when all objective measures of disease suggest a therapy isn't working, vets and owners who are hoping for the best will tend to see improvement in subjective symptoms of their animals.

This makes it especially important to have objective evidence that our therapies are helping our pets. If a treatment fools us into thinking our pets are feeling better when they really aren't, they can be left enduring unnecessary suffering. This certainly was the case for Titan. I might get some undeserved credit for an ineffective treatment that appears to work, and my clients might feel better about their pet's apparent improvement, but the patient is likely to still be suffering, and none of us wants that.

While the caregiver placebo is probably the most significant reason ineffective therapies can seem to work in pets, there are other ways we get fooled as well. One fascinating research study found that placebos could even appear to stop seizures in dogs with epilepsy![33] Almost 80% of the dogs showed a decrease in the number of seizures they had when put on a placebo treatment. Almost a third of the dogs in these studies had their seizure rate decrease by half, which is the usual cutoff for deciding a seizure drug is effective. Clearly, this isn't something owners can easily imagine, so how is this an example of the placebo effect?

There are other reasons, besides mistaken beliefs, that ineffective or placebo therapies might appear to work in animals. For example, when animals are in research studies, they tend to get overall better care and closer monitoring. As a result, many patients show improvement even if they are on a placebo treatment. The dogs in the epilepsy studies were likely getting their other medications more consistently and receiving more monitoring and better care when involved in the study than they had been, which explains some of the improvement in their condition. For this reason, if a study that shows benefits for a particular treatment *doesn't* include a placebo control group, those results are not a reliable measure of whether that therapy actually works. Such uncontrolled trials are, unfortunately, commonly part of the evidence cited to claim alternative therapies have been proven to work.

Many chronic diseases also vary over time, with symptoms being better at some times and worse at others. This variation can happen regardless of anything we might be doing to manage the disease. Of course, people don't take their pets to the doctor when the symptoms are mild. They tend to go in seeking more treatment when things have been getting worse for a while. So often the symptoms may get better after such a visit because they were going to get better anyway as part of the natural cycle of symptoms.[30] However, this can make any new treatment used look like it is working even if it isn't.

Other common reasons why the apparent cause of improvement or worsening in a medical problem might not be the real cause include: natural improvement with time (some conditions, even ones which are usually incurable, can resolve spontaneously even when we do nothing at all); misdiagnosis (if your pet is misdiagnosed with a disease and then gets better with an alternative therapy, the therapy will look like it cured a disease he or she never had); the effect of multiple therapies (it is common for alternative practitioners to use both conventional and alternative treatments and then give the credit for any improvement to the alternative therapy); and many other kinds of perception and reasoning errors built into our brains which I haven't discussed. All of these factors contribute to the appearance of benefits from therapies which do nothing at all or even harm patients, and all are part of what is commonly called the placebo effect.[34]

Placebo effects, of course, operate for all medical therapies, effective or ineffective, conventional or alternative. But when considering alternative therapies, it is especially important to be aware of such effects because these therapies most often lack convincing scientific evidence that they have benefits beyond that of a placebo. Because the false impression of a benefit from an ineffective therapy can truly harm our animal companions, who cannot speak for themselves or tell us directly when we have failed to relieve their symptoms, it is especially important to insist on reliable, controlled scientific evidence for the safety and efficacy of the therapies we use for our pets.

HOW SCIENCE HELPS US TO FIND THE BEST MEDICINE

So now that we know a bit about how our own observations can fool us, how do we decide whether a medical treatment is a good choice for our animals? I've talked a bit already about the role of science in helping us understand nature, and specifically in helping us figure out the causes of disease and the best ways to treat or prevent it. Now I want to talk briefly about why I think science deserves a special role in evaluating medical therapies.

Science is imperfect and deeply flawed, as are all human endeavors. Science is not a perfect oracle that can clearly and correctly answer all our questions. It is a slow, cumbersome, halting process of discovery, refinement and rejection which leaves us uncertain, ignorant, or even misinformed about many things at any given moment in time. However, Winston Churchill reportedly said, "Democracy is the worst form of government, except for all those other forms that have been tried." And this principle also applies to science. As a path to knowledge, it is long and winding, but it is far more likely to get us where we want to go than any other road we've tried.

People have been seeking ways to stay healthy and combat disease for thousands of years. And for most of this time, we relied on our own experience and the stories others told to help us choose the best preventative care and the best medical treatments. But early on we came up against a wall, and for most of human history we couldn't get over it. From the days of hunting and gathering to the early twentieth century, our average life expectancy stayed in the thirties. This was mostly because a huge proportion of our children died before reaching adulthood, and many women died young in childbirth.[35,36] We were also plagued with parasites and infectious diseases, malnutrition, and a host of other chronic ills that were mostly accepted as inevitable. While a few lucky in each generation managed to live to old age, the great majority could expect only the Hobbesian reality of a "poor, nasty, brutish, and short" life. And then, in a mere handful of centuries, we changed all that.

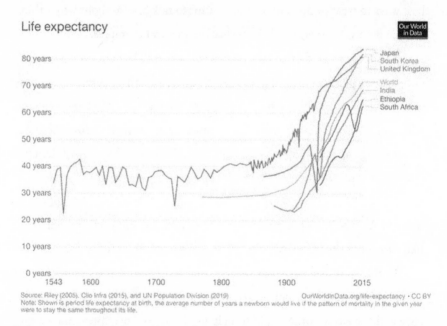

Life expectancy around the world. 2019. Image from OurWorldInData. Used with permission

This graph shows the life expectancy of humans around the world over the last 200 years. Average life expectancy in 1800 was less than 40 years in almost every country in the world, unchanged for thousands of years. Most of us couldn't expect a life much longer than what is now hardly even considered "middle aged."

A mere 200 years later, even those living in the poorest countries can expect to live longer than most humans could have dreamed for all of the tens of thousands of years that had gone before. And those of us in the richest nations, with the best access to the fruits of science and technology, now routinely live more than twice as long as most human beings who ever lived. This is not because we are fundamentally different from those who went before, but because we have developed ways to understand the world and use that understanding to reduce suffering and death more effectively than ever before.

The same pattern holds true for almost every measure of human health.

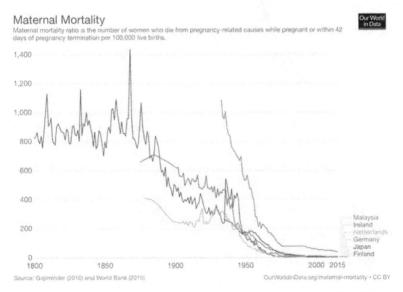

Maternal mortality in selected countries 1800-2015. 2019. Image from OurWorldInData.
Used with permission

For example, historically women have lived shorter lives than men on average, and a major reason has been the risk of dying in childbirth. Now, women outlive men in nearly every country in the world because we have dramatically reduced this risk.

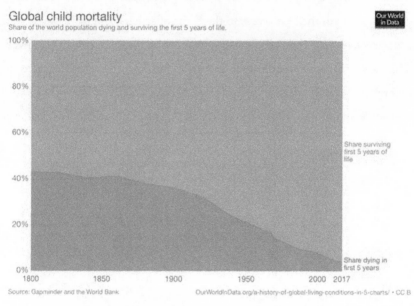

Global Child Mortality 1800-2017. 2019 Image from OurWorldInData. Used with permission.

And the greatest reason for the rise in overall life expectancy is the dramatic decline in early childhood mortality. Once again, in every part of the world where economic conditions allow the methods of sanitation, agriculture, and healthcare developed through science to be employed, it quickly becomes normal to expect our children to live to adulthood, something rarely to be hoped for at any other time in history.

Placebos for Pets?

Once again, the difference is due to the use of science as a way to understand what the risks are and what really works to combat them. In less than two centuries, we have accomplished what humankind had tried and failed to achieve for millennia, and the scientific method is why. The details of how that method is applied to testing medical practices are enormously complex, but the core idea is simple: controlled scientific research makes fewer mistakes than ordinary human observation and judgement.

In the long run, science gives us a more trustworthy and useful understanding of health and disease than any other approach. And it doesn't even take very long, by the standards of history, though a few decades to solve a particular medical problem can seem long to us as individuals, especially when the solution is unlikely to come soon enough to benefit us or our beloved companions.

There is much one can fairly criticize about science itself, as a method for understanding nature, and even more about the choices we have made in how to use the knowledge science has provided. However, my goal as a vet is to understand disease as accurately as possible so I can preserve and restore the health of my patients. Though science is an imperfect tool in this effort, it has earned its place as the foundation of modern veterinary medicine. Any alternative therapy that can truly benefit my patients should be able to show its worth through scientific testing, just as I expect of all the treatments I use.

Brennen McKenzie

HOW DOES SCIENCE WORK?

Wow, that's a big question! Since entire careers spanning decades have been spent trying to understand and explain how science works to help us understand the natural world, I'm not likely to be able to do much more than scratch the surface of the subject here. However, since hopefully I've made the case for you that our uncontrolled personal observations, and the anecdotes we tell about them, don't give us a very reliable picture of what works and what doesn't in medicine, I should at least introduce some of the tools science uses to do a better job.

Medical research proceeds through a general series of stages. A hypothesis or idea about how a disease works or about a possible treatment is developed based on what we know, or think we know about the problem right now. Since our knowledge is imperfect, and since in the early stages of understanding new medical problems and novel treatments this knowledge often comes from observation and intuition, most of our hypotheses turn out to be wrong. Maybe they are a little bit wrong and can be modified to be useful, or maybe they are totally off the mark and have to be discarded, but the important thing is that new ideas, even when based on the best available understanding, often fail to lead to useful explanations and effective therapies.

The best chance we have for developing hypotheses that have a chance of leading to effective treatments is to base them on soundly established scientific knowledge. If scientists have spent decades understanding each step in how a disease starts, progresses, spreads, and harms patients, then this understanding opens up many potential avenues for developing treatments that stop the disease at one or more of these steps.

Placebos for Pets?

If, on the other hand, we come up with a therapy by studying the practices of ancient folk healers who knew nothing about how the disease works, or by haphazardly trying ideas suggested by intuition or anecdotal experience, our odds of success are lower. Improbable guesses can be right, they are just right a lot less often than carefully developed hypotheses based on a sound basic understanding of the problem.

The type of hypothesis least likely to be useful is the one which is what we call implausible, meaning it can only be true if lots of other things we already know are wrong. Again, such implausible ideas do turn out to be right once in a while, and such exceptions are very exciting and make great stories. But most implausible ideas turn out to be wrong and are appropriately discarded and forgotten.

Unfortunately, many theories underlying popular alternative therapies turn out to be implausible and require us to believe that well-established principles of biology, chemistry, and other scientific fields are just plain wrong. While this is not impossible, these principles have led to a lot of successes, in medicine and in other fields, so betting that they are wrong and the implausible theories of ancient folk traditions or individual maverick geniuses are right is not a smart bet.

After developing a hypothesis, let's say about a new medical treatment, the medical research process moves forward to the preclinical stage. This means we try to see whether the treatment could work based on how it performs under artificially controlled conditions rather than jumping right to testing it in actual patients. We might test a medicine for cancer against cancer cells in a test tube. Or we could feed a diet intended for controlling diabetes in humans to diabetic mice and see what happens. Such preclinical testing is a great way of weeding out dangerous or useless treatments without the risk of giving them to actual patients. However, they are only an extremely simplified model of the real world, and most treatments which look promising at this stage still fail to work, or have unexpected dangers, when given to real patients.

For those ideas that do survive the preclinical stage, clinical trials in real-world patients is often the next step. There is a lot of complexity to how this is done, and as I will emphasize repeatedly throughout this book, the devil is in the details. Clinical trials can be utterly useless in understanding the value or risks of a therapy if they are done incorrectly or in ways that don't allow us to generalize to the patients we are actually interested in treating. A dietary supplement, for instance, may be effective in young humans with simple urinary tract infections, but this doesn't tell us if it is safe or effective in old cats with kidney infections who have chronic kidney disease and may have other conditions or be using other therapies at the same time. If we want to be as certain as possible that a medical therapy will work in a given patient, we need to have tested that therapy in a high-quality clinical trial using patients as similar to our patient as possible.

What do I mean by a high-quality clinical trial? Well, there are many features of a medical research study we can look at to evaluate how trustworthy the results may be. Small studies, for example, are often less reliable than large studies because a small group of patients may not fairly represent the overall population of patients we want to treat. And because of all the ways in which our beliefs and expectations mislead us into seeing what we hope or expect to see, a study in which researchers and patients know who is getting the test treatment, or one in which the measure of whether or not the treatment works is highly subjective, and tends to lead to predictably biased and unreliable results. We can reduce this risk by including a placebo treatment or other control and hiding from everyone involved in the study who is getting which treatment.

Such "blinding" and placebo controls, as well as many other factors in how clinical studies are designed, carried out, and analyzed, can give us some sense of how reliable the results are. But a great rule of thumb in scientific research is that no single study ever proves anything. Our confidence in any hypothesis should stay pretty low if only one study, or a small number of studies conducted by a single group of researchers, is available to support that hypothesis. Multiple large studies in different places, at different times, by different groups of researchers which all consistently find the same results is the gold standard for having real confidence in medical treatments. Lots of ideas that seemed promising, even in early clinical testing, have proven untrue once other people with different biases asked the same questions and got different answers.

In human medicine, we often have this level of evidence, so we can frequently turn to a subset of the scientific literature that reviews and analyzes many clinical studies to sort out the truth on a particular question. Systematic reviews and meta-analyses are technical terms for research that evaluates research and sifts through all the evidence to give us the most reliable answers. Unfortunately, we rarely have this level or quality of evidence in veterinary medicine, mostly because of the expense involved in developing it. As we discuss specific alternative therapies, I will talk about the review evidence in human medicine, and occasionally I will be able to point to reviews of veterinary studies, but in most cases the evidence is going to be limited and incomplete.

Without this evidence, we cannot have strong confidence in our conclusions. There is often room for uncertainty in veterinary medicine. But we want to make the best choices for our pets' health we can, so we need to place a bet at some point for or against the treatments we are considering. If we look at these therapies at every level, from the plausibility of the ideas behind them, to the preclinical and human clinical evidence, to the research done on them in the animals we actually want to treat, we can ensure that the bets we place are as safe and rational as possible.

NOW WHAT?

Hopefully, I've now laid the proper foundation for the rest of this book to be useful to you and your pets. Having now at least some idea of what is meant by complementary and alternative medicine, and a sense of how we should approach the claims made for it, we can begin the work of investigating specific methods and deciding what value they might have for our pets.

From here, I will look in detail at some of the most common CAVM approaches you might encounter. For each, I will try to faithfully explain the principles and methods as they are typically represented by practitioners of each. I will then look at whether the principles are plausible, that is consistent with what science has revealed about chemistry, physiology, and other relevant aspects of how nature works. And finally, I will summarize the evidence concerning the safety and effectiveness of these methods, from studies in humans and in veterinary species. The shorthand I will use for evaluating each category of CAM consists of the three questions I introduced earlier, that should always be asked of any medical therapy offered for our pets.

What Is It?

Does It Work?

Is It Safe?

Many of the themes and ideas I've already touched on will appear again and again in the coming chapters. My goal in this book is not only to share what science tells us about the CAVM methods I explore, but also to give you a framework for your own future investigations of other practices I may not touch on. There is a plethora of alternative therapies available, and the claims and evidence are always changing. As a caregiver and advocate for your pet, I want you to be able to ask these three useful questions and have the tools to find and critically evaluate the answers whenever you have to make a choice about what treatments to use for your animal companions.

The real purpose of the scientific method is to make sure Nature hasn't misled you into thinking you know something you actually don't know.

- Robert Pirsig

[1] Russell R. A sex difference in facial contrast and its exaggeration by cosmetics. *Perception*. 2009;38(8):1211-1219. doi:10.1068/p6331

[2] Kahneman D. *Thinking, Fast and Slow*. New York: Farrar, Straus and Giroux; 2011.

[3] Gilovich T. *How We Know What Isn't so : The Fallibility of Human Reason in Everyday Life*. New York N.Y.: Free Press; 1991.

[4] Kida T. *Don't Believe Everything You Think : The 6 Basic Mistakes We Make in Thinking*. Amherst N.Y.: Prometheus Books; 2006.

[5] Shermer M. *Why People Believe Weird Things : Pseudoscience, Superstition, and Other Confusions of Our Time*. New York: W.H. Freeman; 1997.

[6] Aschwanden C. Your Brain Is Primed To Reach False Conclusions | FiveThirtyEight. Available at: http://fivethirtyeight.com/features/your-brain-is-primed-to-reach-false-conclusions/. Published 2015. Accessed July 23, 2015.

[7] Burton R. *On Being Certain : Believing You Are Right Even When You're Not*. New York: St. Martin's Press; 2008.

[8] Greenstone G. The history of bloodletting. *B C Med J*. 2010;52(1):12-14.

[9] Jackson WA. A short guide to humoral medicine. *Trends Pharmacol Sci*. 2001;22(9):487-489. doi:10.1016/S0165-6147(00)01804-6

[10] Lagay F. The Legacy of Humoral Medicine. *AMA J Ethics*. 2002;4(7). doi:10.1001/virtualmentor.2002.4.7.mhst1-0207.

[11] Aranzeta AE De. From Hippocrates to Adams County : Tracing Humoral Medicine in Literature and Practice. *Int J Healthc Humanit*. 2008;2(2):25-29.

[12] Zhu B. *Basic theories of traditional Chinese medicine*. London; People's Military Medical Pressl; 2010.

[13] Patwardhan B, Warude D, Pushpangadan P, Bhatt N. Ayurveda and traditional Chinese medicine: a comparative overview. *Evid Based Complement Alternat Med*. 2005;2(4):465-473. doi:10.1093/ecam/neh140

[14] Chopra A, Doiphode V V. Ayurvedic medicine. Core concept, therapeutic principles, and current relevance. *Med Clin North Am*. 2002;86(1):75-89, vii.

[15] Finckh E. Tibetan medicine--constitutional types. *Am J Chin Med*. 1984;12(1-4):44-49. doi:10.1142/S0192415X84000040

[16] Buell PD, May T, Ramey D. Greek and Chinese horse medicine: déjà vu all over again. *Sudhoffs Arch*. 2010;94(1):31-56..

[17] Xie H. *Traditional Chinese Veterinary Medicine : Fundamental Principles*. Reddick Fla.: Chi Institute; 2007.

[18] Wynn S. *Veterinary Herbal Medicine*. St. Louis Mo.: Mosby Elsevier; 2007.

[19] Seigworth GR. Bloodletting over the centuries. *N Y State J Med*. 1980;80(13):2022-2028.

[20] Thomas D. The demise of bloodletting. *J R Coll Physicians Edinb*. 2014;44(1):72-77. doi:10.4997/JRCPE.2014.117

[21] Jameson HG. Review of Dewees' Practice of Physic. *Maryl Med Rec.* 1829;1(1):702-738.

[22] V. V. The Asphyxiating and Exsanguinating Death of President George Washington. *Perm J.* 2004;8(2):2002-2005.

[23] Beecher HK. The Powerful Placebo. *Am Med Assoc.* 1955;159(17):1602. doi:10.1001/jama.1955.02960340022006

[24] Best M, Neuhauser D. Henry K Beecher: Pain, belief and truth at the bedside. The powerful placebo, ethical research and anaesthesia safety. *Qual Saf Health Care.* 2010;19(5):466-468. doi:10.1136/qshc.2010.042200

[25] Singh S, Ernst E (Edzard). *Trick or Treatment? : Alternative Medicine on Trial.* London: Corgi; 2009.

[26] Köteles F, Fodor D, Cziboly Á, Bárdos G. Expectations of drug effects based on colours and sizes: The importance of learning. *Clin Exp Med J.* 2009; 3(1):99-107 doi:10.1556/CEMED.3.2009.1.9

[27] Howick J, Friedemann C, Tsakok M, et al. Are treatments more effective than placebos? A Systematic Review and Meta-Analysis. Manchikanti L, ed. *PLoS One.* 2013;8(5):e62599. doi:10.1371/journal.pone.0062599

[28] Hróbjartsson A, Gøtzsche PC. Placebo interventions for all clinical conditions. In: Hróbjartsson A, ed. *Cochrane Database of Systematic Reviews.* Chichester, UK: John Wiley & Sons, Ltd; 2004:CD003974. doi:10.1002/14651858.CD003974.pub2

[29] Jenkins DJA, Spence JD, Giovannucci EL, et al. Supplemental vitamins and minerals for cvd prevention and treatment. *J Am Coll Cardiol.* 2018;71(22):2570-2584. doi:10.1016/J.JACC.2018.04.020

[30] McDonald CJ, Mazzuca SA, McCabe GP. How much of the placebo "effect" is really statistical regression? *Stat Med.* 2(4):417-427.

[31] Conzemius MG, Evans RB. Caregiver placebo effect for dogs with lameness from osteoarthritis. *J Am Vet Med Assoc.* 2012;241(10):1314-1319. doi:10.2460/javma.241.10.1314

[32] Gruen ME, Dorman DC, Lascelles BDX. Caregiver placebo effect in analgesic clinical trials for cats with naturally occurring degenerative joint disease-associated pain. *Vet Rec.* 2017;180(19):473-473. doi:10.1136/vr.104168

[33] Muñana KR, Zhang D, Patterson EE. Placebo effect in canine epilepsy trials. *J Vet Intern Med.* 24(1):166-170. doi:10.1111/j.1939-1676.2009.0407.x

[34] McKenzie. What is a placebo? *Vet Pract News.* July 2018:32-33.

[35] Gurven M, Kaplan H. Longevity among hunter-gatherers: A cross-cultural examination. *Popul Dev Rev.* 33:321-365. doi:10.2307/25434609

[36] Roser M. Life Expectancy. OurWorldInData. https://ourworldindata.org/life-expectancy/. Published 2018. Accessed November 11, 2018.

3 |
HOMEOPATHY

As I understand it, the claim is that the less you use Homeopathy,
the better it works. Sounds plausible to me.

- David Deutsch

In many ways, homeopathy is a perfect place to begin our exploration of complementary and alternative veterinary medicine. It is not the most popular or widely used form of CAM. Surveys, for example, consistently show less than 5% of people in most countries report having tried it, and in the UK homeopathic prescriptions in the National Health Service have declined by over 90% in the last ten years.[1-4] However, from its theoretical foundations and history to how it is currently promoted, homeopathy illustrates nearly all of the issues I have touched on so far in the evaluation of CAM.

Homeopathy is a truly alternative medical approach in the sense that it operates on the basis of theories of health and disease that are incompatible with established scientific understandings of chemistry and biology. From its inception at the beginning of the nineteenth century, it was intended as a replacement for conventional medicine, and traditional doctrine states that homeopathic remedies should be used alone, not combined with other medical treatments (though this principle is often ignored by less orthodox homeopaths practicing integrative medicine). Homeopaths frequently claim that the practices of modern, scientific medicine are ineffective or even actively harmful, and they commonly discourage even the most demonstrably successful medical practices, such as vaccination and the use of antibiotics or other pharmaceutical medicines. On the level of basic theory and principles, then, homeopathy illustrates many of the core conflicts between alternative and mainstream medicine.

On a practical level, there are also significant differences between how homeopaths and conventional veterinarians diagnose and treat patients, and these differences also illustrate the relationship, and many of the conflicts, between mainstream medicine and CAM. And there has been a large volume of ostensibly scientific research on homeopathy. This literature is instructive in that it illustrates the challenges in conducting high-quality CAM research and in making effective use of the findings. So while homeopathy may not be the first or most common variety of CAM you will be offered for your animal companions, it serves as an excellent introduction to the issues and the methods involved in evaluating CAM approaches.

WHAT IS IT?

Let's try a little thought experiment. Imagine you have a glass of fresh water. Now put a pinch of salt into the glass and mix it well until the salt is completely dissolved. Does the water taste salty? Probably a little. Now, take a single drop from that glass and put it into another full glass of fresh water. Can you still taste the salt? Now do that one hundred more times, each time taking one drop from the glass and mixing it well in another full glass of fresh water. What do you end up with? Fresh water or salt water? Can you taste any salt in the hundredth glass? The thousandth or ten thousandth?

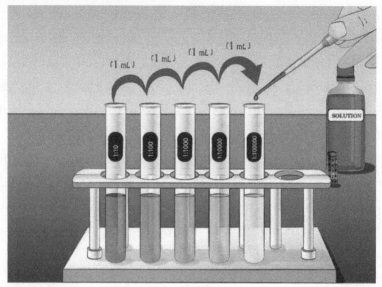

Logarithmic Dilution by Luigi Grasso under Creative Commons license by SA 4.0

This example illustrates one of the core principles of homeopathy, the idea of dilution. In contrast to the ordinary understanding of dilution as something which weakens the effects of whatever we are diluting (such as the effect of salt on the taste of water) homeopathy relies on the notion that extreme dilutions of substances with undesirable effects on health turn those substances, or more precisely the water or alcohol with which those materials are diluted, into powerful medicines. How this principle, and the concepts that underlie homeopathy and distinguish it from modern scientific medicine, were developed and sustained is a fascinating chapter in the history of medicine.

Homeopathy is a set of theories and practices largely invented by one man. Samuel Hahnemann was a doctor in the late eighteenth and early nineteenth centuries, and he practiced at a time when medicine was not yet based

64

on any truly scientific understanding of health and disease[5,6] The treatments in common use then, like bleeding patients and giving them laxatives, emetics, and poisonous potions of all kinds, were based on centuries of tradition and on the writings of revered individuals going back to Ancient Greek and Roman physicians. These treatments often did more harm than good. When President James Garfield was shot in 1881, and died of his wounds almost three months later, the assassin tried to use the well-known failings of medicine in his defense, claiming "The doctors killed Garfield, I just shot him."

Disturbed by the often brutal and ineffective methods of medicine at the time, Hahnemann looked for an entirely new way to approach treating disease. He was investigating a herbal remedy called Cinchona bark, which was used as a treatment for various kinds of fevers, and he experienced some unpleasant symptoms when he took the remedy himself:

My feet, finger ends, etc., at first became cold; I grew languid and drowsy, then my heart began to palpitate, and my pulse grew hard and small; intolerable anxiety, trembling, prostration, throughout all my limbs; then pulsation in the head, redness of my cheeks, thirst, and in short, all these symptoms which are ordinarily characteristic of intermittent fever, made their appearance, one after the other, yet without the peculiar chilly, shivering rigor, briefly, even those symptoms which are of regular occurrence and especially characteristic – as the dullness of mind, the kind of rigidity in all the limbs, but above all the numb, disagreeable sensation, which seems to have its seed in the periosteum, over every bone in the body – all these made their appearance. This paroxysm lasted two or three hours each time, and recurred if I repeated this dose.[7]

These symptoms reminded him of those experienced by sufferers of "intermittent fever," a condition sometimes due to the disease known today as malaria, though many other diseases create similar symptoms. It is theorized that Hahnemann may have had an allergy to the active chemical in the bark, quinine, since his symptoms were characteristic of such an allergic reaction experienced by patients who took quinine in the nineteenth and twentieth centuries, when this compound was isolated and used as a malaria treatment. In any case, Hahnemann decided that his experience represented a fundamental principle of medicine which would form the cornerstone of his system of homeopathy, *similia similibus curantur* or "like cures like."

Law of Similars

The first rule of homeopathy is that something which causes certain symptoms in a healthy person is the best treatment for those symptoms in someone who is sick. So if Cinchona bark made Hahnemann shake with fever and chills and caused pain in his bones, then a person suffering these symptoms, regardless of the cause, should take Cinchona bark as a medicine.

There is an obvious problem with this approach, of course, which Hahnemann soon encountered. If you give a sick patient a medicine which makes healthy people ill, the patient is likely to get even worse! Through trial-and-error experimentation, he discovered that the less of a substance he gave a patient, the fewer negative symptoms they would experience (not a very surprising finding). And since the "medicine" wasn't making them sicker when it was greatly diluted, patients were more likely to get better when given these heavily diluted remedies than when given ordinary Cinchona or other popular remedies used at the time, such as bloodletting. From this, Hahnemann derived the second basic law of homeopathy, the idea of potentization by dilution and succussion.

The Law of Infinitesimals: Potentization by Dilution and Succussion

Hahnemann decided that since patients seemed to do better the less medicine they got, something about diluting the original ingredients must actually be making the medicine more potent. And in the course of his travels, over unpaved roads on horseback or in a horse-drawn carriage, he decided that vigorous shaking of a diluted remedy (called succussion) made it even more effective. The process of making a medicine stronger by diluting it hundreds or even thousands of times, and shaking it each time, became known in homeopathy as "potentization."

Provings and the Materia Medica

Hahnemann tried out a wide variety of substances on himself, his family, and healthy volunteers and compiled a list of the symptoms caused by each substance. These experiments were called "provings," an English word coined as a translation of the German word Hahnemann used: "prufung," meaning "test." The way these tests worked is that the person would take the remedy and then for days or weeks afterwards they would keep a diary of any physical or mental experiences they had. Hahnemann would then look through these diaries and try to identify any patterns or similarities that would indicate to him what symptoms the substance could be expected to cure. He compiled a dictionary, the *Materia Medica Pura*, which listed the remedies and the symptoms they were to be used for, once properly prepared through dilution and succussion. [8] Hahnemann's successors expanded this list, which now includes over a thousand materials.

Homeopathic remedies are not made only from plants like Cinchona bark. They can also be made from animal tissues or body fluids, minerals, and even from so-called "imponderables," non-material ingredients such as sunlight, X-rays, magnetic fields, and even vacuum. "Nosodes" are homeopathic products intended to prevent or treat specific illness, and they are often made from materials obtained from sufferers of the malady they are supposed to prevent, such as the mucus from a patient with tuberculosis, cells from a cancerous tumor, diarrhea from a puppy with parvovirus, and so on.

Homeopathic Treatment

Hahnemann was very clear about the fundamental nature and rules of homeopathic treatment. He believed diseases were not ultimately physical problems but disorders of the spirit, what he called the "Vital Force" of the patient. Bacterial and viral infections, genetic mutations leading to cancer, clogging of the arteries with fat leading to heart attacks, are all examples of the physical causes medicine now tries to prevent or treat. However, according to the principles of homeopathy, these physical abnormalities are not actually causes of disease but only symptoms in the body of a disharmony originating in the spirit. The goal of homeopathic treatment is not to fix the particular problems in the body but to cure the patient and restore complete health by restoring balance to his or her vital force.

Placebos for Pets?

Hahnemann was also clear that homeopathy should not be combined with other therapeutic methods because these would have a disruptive influence on the vital force and so interfere with the effects of homeopathic treatment. He believed only one homeopathic remedy should be given at a time, and he established detailed criteria for judging the effects.

Since Hahnemann's time, there have been a number of different ideas and approaches developed by individual homeopaths, and while Hahnemann and his "classical" approach is still the most respected and dominant practice, there are variations. It is especially common for homeopaths to mix homeopathic treatment with other unrelated forms of alternative medicine, such as herbal remedies (which Hahnemann particularly objected to) as well as chiropractic, acupuncture, and so on.

Homeopaths generally begin treatment of an individual patient by collecting as much information as possible about them. They inquire at length into all the physical and emotional symptoms the patient has experienced as well as the details of all aspects of the patient's life, whether they seem immediately relevant or not. When a comprehensive list of symptoms is ready, the practitioner consults the *Materia Medica Pura* or other list of remedies to try and find the one that most closely matches the particular symptoms of the patient. A homeopath may also consult a dictionary of symptoms which lists the various remedies associated with each. There is a great deal of variation in this process and in the pattern of symptoms individual practitioners recognize in a patient, so the particular remedy chosen for a patient will likely be different for each homeopath consulted.

The conventional diagnosis is considered irrelevant from the perspective of classical homeopathy. Whether an animal has rabies or cancer or heatstroke is less important than the list of specific symptoms, the order of their appearance, the time of day or month in which they appeared, and many other such criteria unique to the homeopathic approach. In its classical form, homeopathy is truly an alternative to conventional medicine.

Some homeopaths and other integrative practitioners who utilize homeopathic remedies will use conventional diagnosis to guide the selection of homeopathic treatments, and they may combine these treatments with other alternative or even conventional remedies. However, this is a source of dissention in the homeopathic community. The official standards of practice for the Academy of Veterinary Homeopathy in the US, for example, state:

Only the remedy that is homeopathic to the patient is to be used. Drugs and methods of treatment which are not homeopathic to the case are to be avoided because of the possibility of interference with the progress of cure.

Use of acupuncture and moxa [the practice of burning dried mugwort at the tip of acupuncture needles inserted into patients] is not compatible with homeopathic treatment because of its effect on the vital force of the patient.

Symptoms on the skin or surface of the body that have expressed as a localized lesion are not to be treated in a vigorous way with the intent to cause their disappearance or by surgery to remove them. These are to be treated primarily by internal homeopathic treatment.[9]

Classical homeopathy is also an example of the principle of vitalism I discussed earlier. Hahnemann saw disease as fundamentally spiritual in origin, and he viewed treatment by homeopathy as less about repairing the body than about bringing balance and harmony back to the spirit.

During health a spiritual power (autocracy, vital force) animates the organism and keeps it in harmonious order. Without this animating, spirit-like power, the organism is dead.

In disease the vital force is primarily morbidly deranged and expresses its sufferings (the internal change) by abnormal sensations and functions of the organism.

The affection of the diseased vital force and the disease symptoms thereby produced constitute an inseparable whole—they are one and the same. It is only by the spiritual influences of morbific noxae [causes of illness that are part physical and part spiritual] that our spirit-like vital force can become ill; and in like manner, only by the spirit-like (dynamic) operation of medicines that it can be again restored to health.[6]

Many modern homeopaths practicing on humans and veterinary patients also hold this view of health and disease. For example, in a 2014 online introductory homeopathy course offered by the British Academy of Veterinary Homeopathy, the instructor distinguishes conventional medicine from homeopathy in terms of the spiritual orientation of the latter, using the same terminology as Hahnemann (the word "dynamic" being a synonym for spiritual or vital forces).

Conventional thinking is based in the material world, with most current treatments and research being centered around genes and the biochemical pathways that are altered in the expression of disease.

Homeopathic thinking is based in the dynamic world with treatments based on symptom expression of the whole individual with symptoms and material changes being a consequence of dynamic disturbance and not a cause of disease.

I am often asked why I talk about vitalism as a problem. Most people believe there is an essential spiritual dimension to our existence, and to that of our animal companions and other living beings. It seems reasonable, therefore, that spiritual forces might be important in health and disease, and it might be necessary to address these to fight disease and achieve wellness.

Contrary to what some people think, science and scientific thinking do not necessarily require abandoning belief in spiritual or nonphysical aspects of existence. Science does, however, employ the principle of methodological naturalism. This fancy philosophical term just means that when using science as a tool for investigating and explaining the natural world, we stick to considering physical objects and processes that can be measured and manipulated and that obey laws of nature that can potentially be deduced. Anything "supernatural," that is outside of nature and not subject to predictable laws and patterns, is also outside the bounds of scientific investigations and explanations of health and disease. Methodological naturalism does not require taking a position on the existence or importance of supernatural forces; it merely excludes consideration of these from scientific investigation.

So why should we do this even if we personally believe that a spiritual dimension to life is important? The value of this approach is that it ensures that the data used to defend or challenge explanations for natural phenomena can be evaluated critically by everyone. In contrast, the information used to challenge or defend claims based on supernatural phenomena come from inherently subjective sources, such as intuition, revelation, and faith. When belief itself becomes the basis for defending and challenging claims about the world, no objective standard of evidence can be persuasive. If a theory about a disease, or a claim about how to treat it, is based on evidence, you can disprove this theory by producing better evidence. You can never disprove an explanation or claim based on faith or personal insight because there is no way to contradict this kind of evidence except with your own faith or insight, which just leads to a circular debate about beliefs with no resolution.

Methodological naturalism has allowed great progress in our understanding of the natural world, and all the improvements in health and well-being brought about by scientific discovery, despite a rich variety of incompatible beliefs among scientists about the supernatural. This approach allows for a common ground of objective evidence when debating claims about the natural world, and it allows such debates to be settled by objective evidence.

Vitalism effectively places any claims or beliefs based on it beyond any objective proof or disproof and makes medicine, like religion, a matter of personal faith rather than objective fact. Historically, this has not been effective at improving health and healthcare, which is why it has been largely replaced by the scientific approach. Those who still invoke vitalistic explanations to support their claims about various approaches to medicine do so primarily to preempt any effort to prove those claims wrong with scientific evidence. Many alternative medical practitioners, such as homeopaths, cling to vitalism precisely because it makes their practices a matter of personal faith not to be disputed by others.

Unfortunately, this is not in the best interests of patients, who need the power of scientific methods to identify which treatments will truly help them and which are useless or even dangerous. Regardless of our personal spiritual beliefs, those of us privileged to treat animal patients have a responsibility to rely on scientific methods to test our treatments and to reject vitalism as a basis for the medical care we offer.

DOES IT WORK?

The underlying theories of homeopathy, the Law of Similars and the Law of Infinitesimals, are inconsistent with well-established principles of basic science. Put another way, for these homeopathic theories to be true, fundamental principles of chemistry and biology would have to be wrong, and all the evident successes in medicine and technology based on these principles must be merely lucky accidents. Homeopathy is the purest example of a system of medicine based on implausible ideas.

The Law of Similars

The concept of "like cures like" has an appealing logic and symmetry to it. It is essentially a variation of "sympathetic magic," the idea that things which resemble one another in some superficial way must be meaningfully related and that one can influence the other.[10] One can make an effigy or figure resembling an individual, a "voodoo doll" for example, and then use it to indirectly affect the health of that individual. Or one can use yellow plants as herbal remedies for jaundice, a yellowing of the skin caused by several different diseases. Walnuts may be eaten to treat problems in the brain because walnuts look a little like the human brain. Or preparations of mandrake root can be used to aid fertility because the root looks a little like a human penis. These are all examples of sympathetic magic which can be found in folk medicine traditions throughout the world.

Scientific investigation has not, however, found the idea of sympathetic magic to be a reliable principle for deciding which substances in the natural world will be useful as medicines. As it turns out, Cinchona bark was actually useful in the treatment of malaria, but not because it caused fever and chills in healthy people. It contains the chemical quinine, which kills the blood parasite that causes malaria.[11]

None of the other substances that Hahnemann decided had medicinal value based on the symptoms he felt they caused in healthy subjects, nor any of those his successors have added to the *Materia Medica Pura*, have turned out to actually be useful for treating the symptoms they supposedly cause. That Cinchona bark caused symptoms similar to malaria in Hahnemann, and that it was also a useful treatment for malaria, turns out to have been a lucky fluke. Or perhaps not so lucky, as it set Hahnemann firmly on the wrong path to understanding the causes and treatments of disease!

The Law of Infinitesimals: Potentization by Dilution and Succussion

The concept from homeopathy that most dramatically fails the test of basic plausibility is the notion that diluting and shaking a substance repeatedly makes it stronger as a medicine. As I pointed out earlier, the medical treatments other doctors were using in Hahnemann's day were often more likely to harm patients than to help them. So those patients who received no therapy at all, or who received ultra-diluted remedies with no active ingredients, likely had a better chance of recovering simply because they were not subjected to bloodletting, toxic compounds, and other treatments that weakened them. It is easy to see how Hahnemann could have mistakenly thought that because his patients did better with more diluted remedies that somehow the act of diluting them was making the remedies better, but now that we understand more about chemistry and the nature of molecules and solutions, it is clear why this cannot be true.[12]

Homeopathic remedies generally start with a "mother tincture." This is usually a solution of water or alcohol in which a piece of some material has been placed and allowed to sit for several weeks. For substances that don't dissolve in water or alcohol, they are often first ground up with milk powder or some other solid before being mixed with water. With "imponderables," the water may simply be exposed to the sunlight, X-rays, or other agent intended as the basis for a remedy.

These mother tinctures, already containing only a little of the original material, are then frequently diluted by a factor of 10 (that is, 1 part of the original substance in 9 parts of water or alcohol) many, many times over. The most concentrated remedies may be described as 1X, 2X, 4X, and so on. A 4X remedy means that the original liquid in which the starting substance was dissolved has subsequently been diluted four times by a factor of 10. The resulting solution is therefore 10,000 times more dilute than the starting solution. These "low potency" remedies, which according to Hahnemann's theories must be the weakest medicines, may actually contain miniscule amounts of the starting substance, depending on what was in the original mother tincture.

However, high potency remedies have been repeatedly diluted not by a factor of 10 but by a factor of 100 (1 part of the original solution to 100 parts of water or alcohol). A typical product would be labeled 30C, meaning it will have been diluted thirty times by a factor of 100. Such a solution is 1,000,000,000,000,000,000,000,000,000,000,000,000,000,000,000,00 0,000,000,000 times more dilute than the original solution. Another way of looking at such a huge number is that the chance of finding a single molecule of the original substance in a 30C dilution is not 1 in a million, not 1 in a trillion, but it is 1 in a billion billion billion billion. And if even that is not close enough to zero for you, many homeopathic solutions are not given directly as liquids but instead dripped onto sugar pills for the patient to swallow.

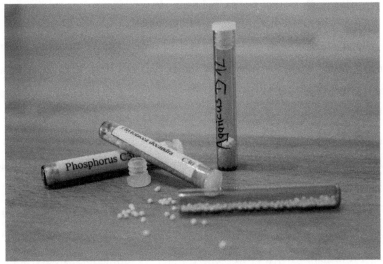

Homeopathic globuli (sugar pills infused with dilute homeopathic preparations)

Now many homeopaths will acknowledge that the majority of their remedies could not possibly contain any of the original substance. So how do they explain how these medicines supposedly work? Well, some have invented the concept of "water memory."[13,14] Remember, homeopaths don't believe that the physical causes of disease that scientific medicine identifies and treats are the true causes of illness. They believe illness is fundamentally a spiritual problem, an imbalance in the vital force. So the fact that their remedies contain only water or alcohol, or sometimes are only sugar pills which were once moistened with this water or alcohol, isn't an insurmountable problem for remedies that are intended to work on the spirit rather than the body anyway. Modern homeopaths often claim that water somehow remembers the "energy" of the original substance even after it is no longer present, and that it is this remembered energy that corrects the imbalance in the patient's vital force.

There are a lot of problems with the idea of water memory.[15,16] For one thing, if water remembers every substance that has been in it, how do homeopathic remedies only remember the substance from the mother tincture and forget everything else their water has been exposed to? And why isn't all water medicinal, since all water has had all kinds of substances dissolved in it at some time? For that matter, why has no one ever been poisoned or made ill by water that remembers some toxin or bacteria that used to be in it?

Other explanations have been proposed by homeopaths for how a remedy with all the active ingredient diluted out of it could be a powerful medicine. From nanoparticles[17] to quantum physics, homeopaths have pointed to all the strangest, least understood, and hardest to evaluate ideas in science as possible explanations for how homeopathy might work. However, none of these ideas have passed the test of rigorous and objective scientific investigation. The research into water structure and behavior has failed to demonstrate that homeopathic remedies remember the substances they were made from or get stronger when diluted and shaken. And research into nanoparticles and other theories has numerous methodological flaws that make it unconvincing. There is simply no way to consistently tell a homeopathic remedy from any other water or alcohol, and no reason to think these remedies have any special properties or effects. [18-22]

In contrast, the conventional scientific idea that higher concentrations of a chemical have greater biological effects than lower concentrations has not only been validated experimentally, it is the principle behind the use of all non-homeopathic medicines. If this principle is wrong, then none of these medicines should work. The concept of potentization by dilution simply cannot be true without the rejection of solidly established ideas in chemistry and biology, ideas which have proven themselves both in laboratory experiments and in serving as the foundation for all kinds of practical treatments that are known to work. [12,23,24]

Provings and Homeopathic Treatment

Apart from the issues of whether "like cures like" and how dilution could make a remedy more potent, there are problems with other aspects of homeopathic theory and practice. For one thing, the methods by which potentially medicinal compounds are identified in the first place are not reliable. In a proving, intended to identify which symptoms a substance causes so the homeopath can know which symptoms it might be useful to treat, the procedures followed are entirely subjective, and no attempt is made to control for any of the biases or blind spots I discussed in Chapter 1.

If you wake up one morning with a headache, do you start trying to figure out why? I certainly do. Maybe I didn't sleep long enough. Or maybe I had a little too much wine the night before. Could I have been clenching my teeth in my sleep because I'm worried about a deadline at work? No, it must have been the wine! Yes, that has to be it. If I try hard enough, I can always find a likely cause for my headache.

But, if you wake up without a headache, do you ever think about all the things you did that didn't give you a headache? Gee, I had two glasses of wine last night and only slept six hours, but I don't have a headache! Of course you don't do this. The fact is that the kind of casual guessing game we play trying to explain the minor, ordinary physical experiences of being alive isn't a very reliable guide to what actually causes these experiences. And yet a proving is exactly this kind of guessing game. The claim that a given substance causes certain symptoms in healthy people is based entirely on giving it to subjects and then looking at what they experience afterwards and guessing which experiences are due to the substance.

The unreliability of this method was recognized early on by critics of homeopathy. In his lectures *Homeopathy and Its Kindred Delusions*,[25] given in 1842, Oliver Wendell Holmes discussed some examples of homeopathic provings to make this point.

> The following list [of symptoms] was taken literally from the Materia Medica of Hahnemann...

'After stooping some time, sense of painful weight about the head upon resuming the erect posture.'

'An itching, tickling sensation at the outer edge of the palm of the left hand, which obliges the person to scratch.'

The medicine was acetate of lime, and as the action of the globule taken is said to last twenty-eight days, you may judge how many such symptoms as the last might be supposed to happen...

I have not cited these specimens with any view to exciting a sense of the ridiculous, which many others of those mentioned would not fail to do, but to show that the common accidents of sensation, the little bodily inconveniences to which all of us are subject, are seriously and systematically ascribed to whatever medicine may have been exhibited, even in the minute doses I have mentioned, whole days or weeks previously.

To these are added all the symptoms ever said by anybody, whether deserving confidence or not....

It's not at all clear how homeopathic provings are supposed to work in veterinary patients. They obviously can't report their feelings or experiences when taking a purported homeopathic remedy. Pet owners could keep a symptom diary on behalf of their pets for the purposes of such a proving, but it would obviously be quite different from Hahnemann's initial concept as applied to people. In reality, the use of homeopathic remedies for animals is typically based on provings conducted in humans, which adds one more layer of uncertainty to the process. Even in humans it is not clear that these proving experiments are consistent or reliable.

Attempts to repeat some of the proving Hahnemann reported, by giving homeopathic remedies to healthy people, have not shown that these remedies can elicit consistent, or even detectable, symptoms.[20, 26-30] In fact, a common gimmick used by critics of homeopathy, to illustrate both the lack of any active ingredient in ultra-dilute homeopathic products and to demonstrate the unreliability of provings, is to "overdose" on large quantities of a homeopathic sleeping remedy. The remedy usually consists of sugar pills on which an extremely diluted preparation of coffee has been dripped. If the Law of Similars and the Law of Infinitesimals were correct, taking such a remedy should make people who are unable to sleep feel sleepy, and it should make normally alert people hyperactive. So far, none of the participants in these demonstrations has reported any noticeable symptoms at all.

The methods of a homeopathic interview and the choice of a remedy are as subjective and inconsistent as the proving process.[27] While it is often comforting to a patient, or their owner in the case of a pet, to talk at length about their feelings and experiences and all the details of their daily lives, it is impossible to separate the relevant details from the irrelevant without a reliable theory about the causes of illness.

If you take a stroll in your garden after breakfast and are bitten by a rattlesnake, and then your leg becomes extremely painful and swollen, is it more likely your symptoms are due to the snake bite or to an allergy to something in your breakfast cereal? The answer seems obvious, but it is only obvious because you know something about the possible effects of snake bites and how they differ from the effects of eating something you are allergic to. This knowledge, the theory you have about how your symptoms came about, allows you to ignore the irrelevant matter of what you ate for breakfast and focus on the more likely cause of your problem.

However, since the principles of homeopathy do not accept that physical symptoms have primarily physical causes, or that the theories of conventional medicine correctly explain the causes of illness, there is no way to exclude some symptoms as irrelevant. Homeopaths make selections of particular remedies based on catalogues of symptoms that each remedy is to be used with and their personal intuition about which symptoms are most important and which remedies are appropriate. Homeopaths often advertise the fact that they individualize their treatment for each patient and each problem, but behind this claim is the fact that such treatment decisions are inherently subjective, basically guesswork. Every homeopath you see for the same problem will make a different assessment and a different prescription based on what they feel is relevant about your experiences. It is difficult to see how this differs from consulting an astrologer or palm reader. The process might be comforting, but this doesn't make it rational or objectively effective.[31]

What's the Evidence?

Despite how farfetched many of the basic ideas behind homeopathy are, it has been subjected to extensive scientific study. Homeopaths, of course, have done most of these studies in order to convince scientists, healthcare professionals, and the general public, that homeopathy works. Science is a powerful marketing tool because almost everyone acknowledges to at least some extent how effective it has been in improving healthcare, for people and their animals. Some research has also been done by skeptics of homeopathy and scientists curious about the claims made for the practice.

Evaluating a large body of research is challenging and requires an understanding of how scientific studies are done and where potential errors, biases, or other misleading factors can hide. As is the case for almost every proposed medical therapy that has been studied, it is possible to find reports of clinical trials that support the claim that homeopathy is an effective therapy. These studies are reported almost exclusively in journals devoted to homeopathy or other alternative therapies, and of course they are conducted by people who believe strongly in the safety and efficacy of homeopathy, so they are at significant risk of bias. But as I discussed at the outset, there are reliable ways to control for these biases, as well as nonspecific placebo effects on human patients, or the human owners of veterinary patients. This makes it especially important that such trials be conducted in a way that accounts for this potential bias. But even if individual studies may be unreliable, it is possible to look at the total of the evidence and draw some conclusions about whether or not homeopathy actually works.

The theoretical and laboratory studies done for homeopathy are unconvincing. Negative results, poor methodology, and an inability to reproduce results, especially when investigators who are not already believers in homeopathy are involved, makes the basic, preclinical research insufficient to even support the assertion that homeopathy *could* work.[12,23,28–30, 32–38] Of course, it takes clinical trial evidence to assess whether or not it actually does work.

The pattern to the evidence from clinical studies of homeopathy in humans is familiar and common to the research literature for many alternative therapies. Studies with few patients, studies conducted by homeopaths or funded by the makers of homeopathic products, studies published in homeopathic or alternative medicine journals, and studies with flawed methods and poor control for bias tend to show positive results. These results are still often slight, and not as dramatic as either the results seen with indisputably effective therapies or with the powerful testimonials offered by individual homeopaths or their patients, but they do sometimes appear to show measurable differences between homeopathic treatment and whatever it is compared with (placebo, standard therapy, or no therapy). This can create the false impression that homeopathy is an effective treatment.[39]

However, as is so often the case, when hundreds of these trials are examined together, the picture changes. The results are frequently inconsistent, so that one may show a positive effect for a certain disease while another does not. Or a single positive study may be repeated by other investigators who are then unable to get the same positive result. And when the studies are separated by size and the quality of their methods, the larger and better controlled a study is, the less likely it is to report a positive result. The multitude of systematic reviews of the many hundreds of clinical studies of homeopathy in humans consistently find a lack of convincing evidence for any real effect when reasonable efforts are made to control for bias and error.[39-54]

Of course, this is true of all clinical trials, not just those having to do with homeopathy. However, an analysis published in the prestigious journal *Lancet* compared high-quality trials of homeopathy with high-quality trials for conventional medical treatments and found that the very best studies for conventional therapies showed clear differences between the treatment and the placebo, but that the best homeopathy trials did not show homeopathic treatment to be any better than a placebo.[46] In other words, if something in scientific medicine works, it is possible to show clearly and consistently that it works in high-quality scientific studies. However, high-quality studies of homeopathy do not show any measurable superiority to a placebo.

There are, as always, far fewer clinical studies specifically investigating homeopathy for animals, and none that can match the size or quality of the best studies done in humans. Some studies have reported positive results and others have found no benefit to homeopathic treatment. But well-designed, high-quality studies comparing homeopathic treatment to placebo and/or standard therapy simply don't exist. Reviews of the existing literature do not find good evidence of real benefits. Even reviews conducted by homeopaths dedicated to promoting homeopathy have had to acknowledge that, after more than 150 years of use and study, almost no evidence exists to support the practice. Unfortunately, they still try valiantly to explain this in any way that does not involve the most obvious and likely reason—the practice simply doesn't work.[55–59]

IS IT SAFE?

Since I've already argued that most homeopathic remedies are nothing but water, or sugar pills dipped in water or alcohol, it might seem obvious that they are safe. And it is almost certainly true that high potency homeopathic remedies, which contains no trace of the original substance they are made from, are harmless. The "overdose" with homeopathic sleeping pills I described earlier is a pretty good illustration of this.

Near absolute safety seems like it would be a good quality in a medical therapy, and it is certainly one of the aspects of homeopathy that homeopaths often cite in trying to persuade people to use their remedies. Unfortunately, nothing that actually does anything at all is going to be completely safe. The body of a living organism is an amazingly intricate system, with every part of the system interacting with other parts in a beautiful, bewildering complexity. The idea that we could tinker with one part of such a system and have only the effect we desire without setting off any unintended consequences in other parts is naïve and unrealistic. In fact, the concept that any truly effective therapy must have some side effects is so important, I've given it a name: McKenzie's Law.

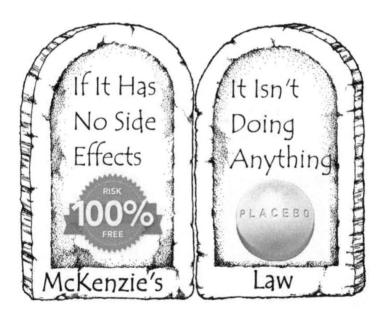

Okay, not a very humble name for the issue, I admit. I'm hoping it will catch on and become part of the vocabulary of scientific medicine, but that doesn't seem very likely. Regardless, it is surprising but true that the absence of established direct side effects from the use of properly constituted homeopathic remedies is actually a point against the value of these remedies.

Unfortunately, there are still some dangers associated with homeopathy that may not be immediately apparent. For one thing, not all remedies marketed as homeopathic are ultra-diluted. Some are herbal products or low potency remedies that might actually contain biologically active ingredients. Several homeopathic products have been recalled from the market after complaints about adverse effects. In June 2009 the Food and Drug Administration (FDA) warned consumers not to use Zicam, a cold remedy consisting of nasal swabs or an intranasal gel containing zinc, after a number of people permanently lost their sense of smell while using it.[60] This condition can be caused by zinc destroying the cells in the nose responsible for our sense of smell, so it is possible the remedy contained enough zinc to have an actual, and obviously undesirable, effect on users.

Similarly, in October 2010 the FDA ordered a recall of Hyland's Teething Tablets, a homeopathic remedy based on the plant toxin belladonna and intended for use in teething children. FDA testing had found measurable but inconsistent amounts of the toxin in the tablets and had received reports of symptoms in children taking them.[61] Belladonna can be a deadly poison, and it has been responsible for other cases of harm from homeopathic remedies.[62,63,64] Reviews of the scientific literature have found additional examples of people being harmed by homeopathic remedies that were either not truly ultra-dilute or that were contaminated with harmful substances.[65]

Certainly, recalls and serious adverse reactions can happen with conventional medicines as well. However, the risks of scientific medicines must be considered in light of the proven benefits. Given the implausibility of the theories behind homeopathy, and the absence of any convincing research evidence that it is effective, it is hard to justify any risk at all when using these products.

The more common, and more serious, risk posed by the use of homeopathy is that of not seeking and using truly effective treatments for serious illness.[66,67] Do you remember Titan, the Rottweiler with bone cancer? This dog was in severe pain from his disease, and his owner was not willing to use proven medicines to relieve this pain both because of her fears of these medicines and also because of her belief that the homeopathic remedies she was using were really helping Titan. Such beliefs, even when false, can be very strong and can lead users of homeopathy to reject scientific medical treatment.

Hahnemann himself clearly indicated he did not believe homeopathy should be used along with conventional medicine. And the Academy of Veterinary Homeopathy, the leading organization of veterinary homeopaths in the United States, continues to recommend this in their standards of practice today, though they make a few exceptions for obviously life-threatening illnesses. Many homeopaths do not accept the scientific explanations for disease, such as the concept that microorganisms like bacteria and viruses cause infections. These practitioners often discourage their patients or clients from using conventional medicine, including such common and clearly effective methods as vaccines and antibiotics. In humans, there have been tragic cases of people harmed by the use of homeopathy in place of scientific medicine.

Gloria Sam was a healthy baby when she was born near the end of 2001. Unfortunately, when she was only a few months old she developed eczema, an inflammatory skin condition. Symptoms of eczema can vary from mild to extremely painful with serious secondary infections. While it is not curable, eczema in young children often goes away or becomes less severe as they grow older, and it can be effectively controlled with medication. However, Gloria's parents did not choose to treat her with these medications. Her father was a homeopath, and he followed the strict rules of classical homeopathy, including avoiding conventional therapy. Despite the recommendations, and eventually desperate pleas of Gloria's doctors, her parents persisted in believing homeopathy would cure her

Gloria's disease progressed until she was eating poorly, not gaining weight and, according to the reports of her doctors and others who saw her, in severe pain and crying almost constantly. She eventually developed a secondary bacterial infection, and on May 8, 2002, little Gloria died. She was nine months old and weighed as much as a healthy three-month old baby. Ultimately, her parents were convicted and imprisoned for their fatal neglect of their daughter's health problem.[68]

So did homeopathy harm Gloria Sam? Well, not directly. The remedies her father gave her most likely did nothing at all. But her parents' belief in homeopathy did harm her. Despite not only the implausibility and clinical evidence against homeopathy in general but also the clear failure of homeopathic treatment to help Gloria, her parents persisted in believing in the approach and in refusing effective conventional treatments. Even after she died and her parents were convicted of neglect, her father continued to maintain that he had treated her appropriately. Such is the power of belief, and such is the kind of tragedy that can come from an unfounded confidence in homeopathy, even if the remedies themselves are harmless.

BOTTOM LINE

Homeopathy is based on ideas that are not compatible with well-established scientific principles of chemistry and biology, including the notion that "like cures like" and that diluting and shaking a substance strengthens its medicinal properties. The practices of homeopathy involve primarily subjective and intuitive judgments and have not been validated by objective research.

Clinical trials in homeopathy do not support the practice as an effective treatment for any condition. Though some positive studies can be found, these are usually methodologically flawed or subject to various sources of bias and error. Objective reviews of the total body of evidence, even by homeopaths who are absolutely convinced homeopathy works, fail to find compelling, consistent evidence to support this belief.

Homeopathic remedies themselves are harmless as they usually contain no active ingredients. However, improperly diluted preparations can contain chemical substances that can be directly toxic or can cause harm through allergic reactions or interactions with other medications. The real risk of homeopathic treatment, however, is when it is substituted for effective medical care. Adding homeopathy to conventional therapy is unlikely to be harmful (though it is contrary to the principles of homeopathy), but it is also unlikely to add any benefit.

[Homeopathy] is a subject which makes me more wrath, even than does clairvoyance: clairvoyance so transcends belief, that one's ordinary faculties are put out of question, but in homœopathy common sense & common observation come into play, & both these

Brennen McKenzie

must go to the Dogs, if the infinetesimal doses have any effect
whatever.

- Charles Darwin

[1] Collaboration N. NHS Homeopathy: 20 Years of Decline. https://www.nightingale-collaboration.org/news/190-nhs-homeopathy-20-years-of-decline.html. Published 2016. Accessed November 11, 2018.

[2] Dossett ML, Davis RB, Kaptchuk TJ, Yeh GY. Homeopathy use by US adults: Results of a national survey. *Am J Public Health*. 2016;106(4):743-745. doi:10.2105/AJPH.2015.303025

[3] Su S, Li L. Trends in the use of complementary and alternative medicine in the United States: 2002-2007. *J Health Care Poor Underserved*. 2011;22(1):296-310. doi:10.1353/hpu.2011.0002

[4] Relton C, Cooper K, Viksveen P, Fibert P, Thomas K. Prevalence of homeopathy use by the general population worldwide: a systematic review. *Homeopathy*. 2017;106(2):69-78. doi:10.1016/j.homp.2017.03.002

[5] Loudon I. A brief history of homeopathy. *J R Soc Med*. 2006;99(12):607-610. doi:10.1258/jrsm.99.12.607

[6] Hahnemann, S. *Organon of Medicine*. Kunzli J, Naude A, Pendleton P, trans. Los Angeles, CA: Houghton Mifflin Co.; 1982.

[7] Bradford TL. *The Life and Letters of Dr. Samuel Hahnemann*. Philadelphia, PA: Boericke & Tafel; 1895.

[8] Hahnemann S. *Materia Medica Pura*. (Hempel CJ, ed.). New York, NY: William Radde; 1846.

[9] Homeopathy A of V. AVH Standards of Practice. https://theavh.org/standards-of-practice/. Accessed December 11, 2018.

[10] Frazer JG. *The Golden Bough: A Study in Magic and Religion*. Abridged. New York, NY: The Macmillan Company; 1922.

[11] Gachelin G, Garner P, Ferroni E, Tröhler U, Chalmers I. Evaluating *Cinchona* bark and quinine for treating and preventing malaria. *J R Soc Med*. 2017;110(1):31-40. doi:10.1177/0141076816681421

[12] Grimes DR. Proposed mechanisms for homeopathy are physically impossible. *Focus Altern Complement Ther*. 2012;17(3):149-155. doi:10.1111/j.2042-7166.2012.01162.x

[13] Chaplin MF. The Memory of Water: an overview. *Homeopathy*. 2007;96(3):143-150. doi:10.1016/j.homp.2007.05.006

[14] Thomas Y. The history of the Memory of Water. *Homeopathy*. 2007;96(3):151-157. doi:10.1016/j.homp.2007.03.006

[15] Teixeira J. Can water possibly have a memory? A sceptical view. *Homeopathy*. 2007;96(3):158-162. doi:10.1016/j.homp.2007.05.001

[16] Jackson T. TV: Horizon—Homeopathy: The Test. *BMJ Br Med J*. 2002;325(7376):1367.

[17] Bell IR, Koithan M. A model for homeopathic remedy effects: low dose nanoparticles, allostatic cross-adaptation, and time-dependent sensitization in a complex adaptive system. *BMC Complement Altern Med*. 2012;12:191. doi:10.1186/1472-6882-12-191

[18] Anick DJ. High sensitivity 1H-NMR spectroscopy of homeopathic remedies made in water. *BMC Complement Altern Med*. 2004;4(1):15. doi:10.1186/1472-6882-4-15

[19] Moffett JR, Arun P, Namboodiri MAA. Laboratory research in homeopathy: con. *Integr Cancer Ther*. 2006;5(4):333-342. doi:10.1177/1534735406294795

[20] Vickers A, McCarney R, Fisher P, van Haselen R. Can homeopaths detect homeopathic medicines? A pilot study for a randomised, double-blind, placebo controlled investigation of the proving hypothesis. *Br Homeopath J*. 2001;90(3):126-130. doi:10.1038/sj/bhj/5800475

[21] Morrell P. Triumph of the light--isopathy and the rise of transcendental homeopathy, 1830-1920. *Med Humanit*. 2003;29(1):22-32. doi:10.1136/mh.29.1.22

[22] McCarney R, Fisher P, Spink F, Flint G, van Haselen R. Can homeopaths detect homeopathic medicines by dowsing? A randomized, double-blind, placebo-controlled trial. *J R Soc Med*. 2002;95(4):189-191..

[23] Becker-Witt C, Weißhuhn TER, Lüdtke R, Willich SN. Quality assessment of physical research in homeopathy. *J Altern Complement Med*. 2003;9(1):113-132. doi:10.1089/107555303321222991

[24] Vickers a, Goyal N, Harland R, Rees R. Do certain countries produce only positive results? A systematic review of controlled trials. *Control Clin Trials*. 1998;19(2):159-166.

[25] Holmes OW. *Homeopathy and Its Kindred Delusions: Two Lectures Delivered before the Boston Society for the Diffusion of Useful Knowledge*. Boston, MA: William D. Ticknor; 1842.

[26] Walach H, Köster H, Hennig T, Haag G. The effects of homeopathic belladonna 30CH in healthy volunteers -- a randomized, double-blind experiment. *J Psychosom Res*. 2001;50(3):155-160.

[27] Brien S, Prescott P, Owen D, Lewith G. How do homeopaths make decisions? An exploratory study of inter-rater reliability and intuition in the decision making process. *Homeopathy*. 2004;93(3):125-131.

[28] Fisher P, Dantas F. Homeopathic pathogenetic trials of Acidum malicum and Acidum ascorbicum. *Br Homeopath J*. 2001;90(3):118-125. doi:10.1038/sj/bhj/5800476

[29] Dantas F, Fisher P, Walach H, et al. A systematic review of the quality of homeopathic pathogenetic trials published from 1945 to 1995. *Homeopathy*. 2007;96(1):4-16. doi:10.1016/j.homp.2006.11.005

[30] Goodyear K, Lewith G, Low JL. Randomized double-blind placebo-controlled trial of homoeopathic "proving" for Belladonna C30. *J R Soc Med*. 1998;91(11):579-582.

[31] Prousky JE. Repositioning individualized homeopathy as a psychotherapeutic technique with resolvable ethical dilemmas. *J Evidence-based Integr Med.* 2018;23;1-4. doi: 10.1177/2515690X18794379

[32] Ennis M. Basophil models of homeopathy: a sceptical view. *Homeopathy.* 2010;99(1):51-56. doi:10.1016/j.homp.2009.11.005

[33] Ovelgönne JH, Bol AW, Hop WC, van Wijk R. Mechanical agitation of very dilute antiserum against IgE has no effect on basophil staining properties. *Experientia.* 1992;48(5):504-508.

[34] Brien S, Lewith G, Bryant T. Ultramolecular homeopathy has no observable clinical effects. A randomized, double-blind, placebo-controlled proving trial of Belladonna 30C. *Br J Clin Pharmacol.* 2003;56(5):562-568. doi:10.1046/J.1365-2125.2003.01900.X

[35] Vickers AJ. Independent replication of pre-clinical research in homeopathy: a systematic review. *Forsch Komplementarmed.* 1999;6(6):311-320. doi:10.1159/000021286

[36] Endler P, Thieves K, Reich C, et al. Repetitions of fundamental research models for homeopathically prepared dilutions beyond 10(-23): a bibliometric study. *Homeopathy.* 2010;99(1):25-36. doi:10.1016/j.homp.2009.11.008

[37] Maddox J, Randi J, Stewart WW. "High-dilution" experiments a delusion. *Nature.* 1988;334(6180):287-290. doi:10.1038/334287a0

[38] Hirst SJ, Hayes NA, Burridge J, Pearce FL, Foreman JC. Human basophil degranulation is not triggered by very dilute antiserum against human IgE. *Nature.* 1993;366(6455):525-527. doi:10.1038/366525a0

[39] Lytsy P. Creating falseness-How to establish statistical evidence of the untrue. *J Eval Clin Pract.* 2017;23(5):923-927. doi:10.1111/jep.12823

[40] Banerjee K, Mathie RT, Costelloe C, Howick J. Homeopathy for allergic rhinitis: A systematic review. *J Altern Complement Med.* 2017;23(6):426-444. doi:10.1089/acm.2016.0310

[41] Linde K, Scholz M, Ramirez G, Clausius N, Melchart D, Jonas WB. Impact of study quality on outcome in placebo-controlled trials of homeopathy. *J Clin Epidemiol.* 1999;52(7):631-636.

[42] Linde K, Clausius N, Ramirez G, et al. Are the clinical effects of homeopathy placebo effects? A meta-analysis of placebo-controlled trials. *Lancet.* 1997;350(9081):834-843.

[43] Linde K, Melchart D. Randomized controlled trials of individualized homeopathy: a state-of-the-art review. *Altern Complement Ther.* 1998;4(6):371-373. doi:10.1089/act.1998.4.371

[44] Mathie RT, Frye J, Fisher P. Homeopathic Oscillococcinum ® for preventing and treating influenza and influenza-like illness. *Cochrane Database Syst Rev.* 2015;1:CD001957. doi:10.1002/14651858.CD001957.pub6

[45] Mathie RT. Controlled clinical studies of homeopathy. *Homeopathy.* 2015;104(4):328-332. doi:10.1016/j.homp.2015.05.003

[46] Shang A, Huwiler-Müntener K, Nartey L, et al. Are the clinical effects of homoeopathy placebo effects? Comparative study of placebo-controlled trials of homoeopathy and allopathy. *Lancet*. 2005;366(9487):726-732. doi:10.1016/S0140-6736(05)67177-2

[47] Barnes J, Resch KL, Ernst E. Homeopathy for postoperative ileus? A meta-analysis. *J Clin Gastroenterol*. 1997;25(4):628-633..

[48] Cucherat M, Haugh MC, Gooch M, Boissel JP. Evidence of clinical efficacy of homeopathy. A meta-analysis of clinical trials. HMRAG. Homeopathic Medicines Research Advisory Group. *Eur J Clin Pharmacol*. 2000;56(1):27-33..

[49] Ernst E. A systematic review of systematic reviews of homeopathy. *Br J Clin Pharmacol*. 2002;54(6):577-582..

[50] Ernst E. Classical homoeopathy versus conventional treatments: a systematic review. 1999..

[51] Ernst E, Pittler MH. Re-analysis of previous meta-analysis of clinical trials of homeopathy. *J Clin Epidemiol*. 2000;53(11):1188.

[52] Ernst E, Pittler MH. Efficacy of homeopathic arnica: a systematic review of placebo-controlled clinical trials. *Arch Surg*. 1998;133(11):1187-1190.

[53] Ernst E, Barnes J. Are homoeopathic remedies effective for delayed-onset muscle soreness: a systematic review of placebo-controlled trials. *Perfusion*. 1998;11:4-8.

[54] Long L, Ernst E. Homeopathic remedies for the treatment of osteoarthritis: a systematic review. *Br Homeopath J*. 2001;90(1):37-43.

[55] Mathie RT, Clausen J. Veterinary homeopathy: meta-analysis of randomised placebo-controlled trials. *Homeopathy*. 2015;104(1):3-8. doi:10.1016/j.homp.2014.11.001

[56] Mathie RT, Clausen J. Veterinary homeopathy: Systematic review of medical conditions studied by randomised trials controlled by other than placebo. *BMC Vet Res*. 2015;11(1):236. doi:10.1186/s12917-015-0542-2

[57] Mathie RT, Clausen J. Veterinary homeopathy: systematic review of medical conditions studied by randomised placebo-controlled trials. 2014;175(15). doi:10.1136/vr.101767

[58] Lees P, Pelligand L, Whiting M, Chambers D, Toutain P-L, Whitehead ML. Comparison of veterinary drugs and veterinary homeopathy: part 1. *Vet Rec*. 2017;181. http://www.ncbi.nlm.nih.gov/pubmed/28801498. Accessed November 12, 2018.

[59] Lees P, Pelligand L, Whiting M, Chambers D, Toutain P-L, Whitehead ML. Comparison of veterinary drugs and veterinary homeopathy: part 2. *Vet Rec*. 2017;181(8):198-207. doi:10.1136/vr.104279

[60] Harris G. F.D.A. Warns Against Use of Popular Cold Remedy. *New York Times*.https://www.nytimes.com/2009/06/17/health/policy/17nasal.html. Published June 16, 2009.

[61] Consumer Updates - Hyland's Homeopathic Teething Tablets: Questions and Answers. https://www.fda.gov/forConsumers/ConsumerUpdates/ucm230762.htm. Accessed November 12, 2018.

[62] Chen L, Yeung JC, Anderson DR. Anisocoria secondary to anticholinergic mydriasis from homeopathic pink eye relief drops. *Clin Med Res*. 2017;15(3-4):93-95. doi:10.3121/cmr.2017.1356

[63] Krzyzak M, Regina A, Jesin RC, Deeb L, Steinberg E, Majlesi N. Anticholinergic toxicity secondary to overuse of topricin ream, a homeopathic medication. *Cureus*. 2018;10(3):e2273. doi:10.7759/cureus.2273

[64] Glatstein M, Danino D, Wolyniez I, Scolnik D. Seizures caused by ingestion of atropa belladonna in a homeopathic medicine in a previously well infant. *Am J Ther*. 2014;21(6):e196-e198. doi:10.1097/MJT.0b013e3182785eb7

[65] Posadzki P, Alotaibi A, Ernst E. Adverse effects of homeopathy: a systematic review of published case reports and case series. *Int J Clin Pract*. 2012;66(12):1178-1188. doi:10.1111/ijcp.12026

[66] Freckelton I. Death by homeopathy: issues for civil, criminal and coronial law and for health service policy. *J Law Med*. 2012;19(3):454-478.

[67] Shaw DM. Homeopathy is where the harm is: five unethical effects of funding unscientific "remedies". *J Med Ethics*. 2010;36(3):130-131. doi:10.1136/jme.2009.034959

[68] Alexander H. Parents guilty of manslaughter over daughter's eczema death. *Sydney Morning Herald*. https://www.smh.com.au/national/parents-guilty-of-manslaughter-over-daughters-eczema-death-20090605-bxvx.html. Published June 5, 2009.

4|
ACUPUNCTURE

There must be something to acupuncture -- you never see any sick

porcupines.

- Bob Goddard

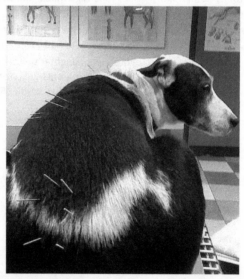

Acupuncture in a dog 2008 by Ziv Pugatch under Creative Commons license by SA 2.0

ACUPUNCTURE. WHAT'S THE POINT?

As an example of an alternative medicine practice, acupuncture differs from homeopathy in a number of important and illustrative ways. Rather than being the discrete invention of one man, acupuncture is a varied collection of theories and techniques and belief systems, some in clear conflict with others. And while some varieties of acupuncture focus on spiritual forces and mysterious "energies," as homeopathy does, others invoke plausible scientific theories to explain the potential effects of acupuncture treatment. Unlike the relatively new practice of homeopathy, acupuncture has a long history in human medicine, though much of this history, including that related to acupuncture in animals, is frequently misrepresented by promoters of the practice. And finally, while homeopathy can be pretty confidently dismissed as useless at every level, from basic theory to clinical trial research, the evaluation of acupuncture is quite a bit more complex and nuanced.

I will begin by admitting that I am certified in veterinary medical acupuncture and have treated patients with needling. Whether this information should influence how my conclusions about acupuncture are judged is something I will leave to you, the reader. However, I have made an exhaustive study, both informally and as part of my acupuncture training, of the theory and evidence concerning this practice, so at the least my assessment is well informed. I do, of course, have personal experiences with acupuncture that might also be considered relevant. However, as I made a great effort to point out in the beginning of this book, such experiences are the weakest kind of evidence when evaluating a medical therapy, so as with all other practices I discuss, I will endeavor to evaluate acupuncture primarily in terms of the available scientific evidence.

Brennen McKenzie

WHAT IS IT?

Defining acupuncture is complicated by the variety of theories and practices that use the label. In the broadest sense, acupuncture is the practice of inserting small needles into the body in order to have some beneficial effect. Such a definition is so vague as to be close to meaningless, but anything more specific will exclude at least some of the methods routinely identified as acupuncture. Hopefully, a brief description of the major acupuncture schools of thought and the most common techniques will be sufficient to define the practice for the purposes of our other two general questions: Does It Work? Is It Safe?

Traditional Chinese Medicine and Acupuncture

The largest group of acupuncturists, in both human and veterinary medicine, are those that adhere to the general approach known as Traditional Chinese Medicine (TCM, or TCVM for the veterinary variety). This is a bit of a misnomer since it implies a body of ideas and techniques with a long and established history. Some of the practices incorporated in TCM have been in use for centuries, such as the use of small needles for therapeutic purposes in humans (though even this doesn't go back the 3,000-4,000 years proponents often claim). Even these practices, however, have undergone radical changes in theory and technique over this time, so that much of what a modern acupuncturist does would likely not be recognized or supported by a practitioner of Chinese folk medicine a thousand years ago.[1,2]

Other aspects of TCM, however, have a much more modern origin. A hodgepodge of herbal remedies, needling techniques, dietary and massage practices, and a variety of theoretical structures to guide all of these, were

Placebos for Pets?

selected and cobbled together at the instigation of Chairman Mao Zedong in the 1950s for primarily political purposes. While the communist leader preferred conventional scientific medicine for himself, the destruction of the intelligentsia during the Cultural Revolution, including the killing or suppression of most scientifically trained doctors, left little in the way of a healthcare system for the people. And the conventional medical practices of the time were largely imported from more economically developed Western countries (and are still often erroneously referred to as "Western Medicine" despite the universal use by patients and the contributions of scientists and doctors from all over the world to science-based medicine). Therefore, conventional medicine was seen as ideologically "tainted," and an indigenous alternative was seen as politically useful.[3,4]

Even though I believe we should promote Chinese medicine, I personally do not believe in it. I do not take Chinese medicine.

- Mao Zedong

So a variety of disparate theories and practices were cobbled together and made to appear as a unified and ancient system of medicine. It would not, of course, say anything useful about the safety or effectiveness of acupuncture or other TCM practices even if TCM was a consistent and ancient system. After all, humoral medicine, with its bloodletting and purging, was a pretty old and consistent system of medicine, and it has been shown to be dangerous nonsense and has been properly abandoned. Nevertheless, Mao's intent in creating the TCM narrative was to suggest a time-honored and coherent set of theories and treatments because that generates greater confidence in patients and doctors. Since this confidence is misplaced, however, the truth is worth disclosing.

In terms of the application of TCM and acupuncture to animal patients, this is also falsely presented as an ancient practice. The reality is that most modern TCVM acupuncture is simply the haphazard extrapolation of techniques used in humans to animal patients by vets in the 1970s. Acupuncture was not generally applied to animals by the ancient Chinese. There were many reasons for this, but a significant one was the concept that many of the philosophical foundations of TCM acupuncture involve, once again, the manipulation of spiritual forces or energies. The ancient Chinese saw animals as objects, not living beings in the sense humans are, so they would not have applied such spiritual healing methods to them. Most of the claims that acupuncture was used in animals centuries ago turn out, when the texts are properly examined and translated, to be mischaracterizations of what were actually bloodletting techniques.[5,6]

So the dominant variety of acupuncture used on animals, the TCVM approach, is a recent adaptation of practices applied to humans. These practices, in turn, are a modern syncretism of disparate historical practices and theories repackaged to look like a unified traditional system of medicine. While this doesn't directly answer the more important questions of whether acupuncture is safe and effective, it is important to recognize that much of what proponents say about the history and origins of veterinary acupuncture is more marketing than genuine history.

In terms of the specific theories behind TCVM, these are complex, and entire books have been written about them.[7,8,9] There is some variation, but in general TCVM is based on elements of Daoist metaphysics and folk cosmology. The fundamental nature of the universe and everything in it is conceived as a condition of balance between opposing aspects of existence known as Yin and Yang. Cold and heat, dark and light, old and young, and so on are seen as examples of this balance between opposites, and all diseases are believed to arise from a disharmony or loss of balance between Yin and Yang. Infectious organisms, toxins, trauma, and other causes of illness recognized by scientific medicine are not considered as true causes in the TCM paradigm, but as manifestations of disharmony. According to one leading figure in veterinary TCM in the United States "No disease occurs if Yin and Yang maintain a relative balance."[10]

Yin and Yang are also identified with particular temperaments, organs of the body, seasons, and other features of living organisms and the environment, and this is taken to illustrate the centrality of these concepts and the balance between them to all features of the universe. This notion of balance between forces represented by the five elements (earth, air, fire, water, and wood) or bodily fluids bears a strong resemblance to the humoral medicine theories of ancient Greece and Rome, which I discussed in Chapter 2.[2,10] Humorism, practiced in the West until the twentieth century, identified imbalance in humors (blood/air, yellow bile/fire, black bile/earth, and phlegm/water) as the cause of all disease and associated these humors with pairs of opposites such as heat and cold, winter and summer, and so on. Practitioners of humorism attempted to maintain and restore health by restoring balance among the humors, much as TCM practitioners attempt to rebalance Yin and Yang. This was accomplished through bloodletting, herbal remedies, cauterization, and many other practices common to historical and contemporary TCM. This humorist model and the associated practices were abandoned in the West with the advent of modern scientific medicine.

The concept of Yin and Yang is applied to health through an intricate system that varies significantly between individual doctors who employ TCM. In general, practitioners evaluate the appearance of the tongue, the pulse, and a host of other characteristics of individual patients to categorize the problem in terms of excess or deficiency of Yin and Yang and the Five Elements. Individual treatments are assigned as promoting or reducing Yin and Yang or other metaphorical forces, so the remedies are chosen based on the categorization of the problem. Egg and banana, for example, are cooling foods, while garlic and ginger are warming foods. Herbs, acupuncture points, and other treatments are assigned in the same way by tradition, taste, or other criteria.

The names of internal organs are used in categorizing a disorder according to the TCM system, but it is important to note that this is a metaphorical use of these names, associating Yin or Yang with certain organs, somewhat like the metaphorical use of the heart as a symbol for strong emotions (as in "he followed his heart") and the association of bile, found primarily in the gallbladder, with a bitter or hostile temperament (as in "you've got a lot of gall!"). These names do not imply the anatomical or physiological relationships understood in scientific medicine. This makes it possible, for example, to adjust the Gallbladder Channel in a species like the horse, which doesn't actually have a gallbladder.

TCVM also emphasizes the importance of a type of spiritual force or energy called Qi. This, like the "Vital Force" of homeopathy, is a nonphysical substance or energy that is believed to animate living things. TCVM practitioners describe this Qi as moving along channels around the body, and these movements are believed to be associated with health and disease. Locations for acupuncture are selected based partly on the perception of the practitioner concerning where the patient's Qi is located, where it may be excessive or deficient, and needling is believed to shift or move Qi in a way that restores balance or harmony, thus protecting or restoring health.

Western Medical Acupuncture

TCVM is not the only approach to acupuncture in veterinary medicine. The variety I was trained in is known as Medical Acupuncture (or sometimes Western Medical Acupuncture, though again that is misleading both in implying that the scientific emphasis of this approach is somehow a product of Western culture, and in ignoring the reality that most of the details of medical acupuncture practice are borrowed from TCM or otherwise originate in East Asian countries, such as China and Japan). Essentially, medical acupuncture begins with the idea that inserting needles into nerves, muscles, and other body tissues may have measurable physiologic effects than can be studied and described in conventional scientific ways. These effects, then, can be evaluated scientifically to see if they are truly beneficial to patients. If so, then acupuncture can be treated like any other scientific medical practice, keeping effective practices and discarding ineffective or unsafe ones based entirely on scientific principles and research. The spiritual and metaphysical dimensions of TCM acupuncture can be ignored, and the conflicts between

105

these ideas and scientific knowledge will no longer undermine the study and use of acupuncture.[11,12]

This is a laudable and sound approach in many ways. As I have emphasized repeatedly, all the treatments we use on our animal companions should be expected to meet the same standards of testing for safety and efficacy, and these standards should be those of science. If there is real benefit to be found in acupuncture, the medical acupuncture approach is the most reliable way to find it. Whether or not this is actually the case, of course, is the focus of our second question.

Does It Work?

This is a far more complex question than it sounds, largely because it is so general. In science, it is most useful to ask narrow, specific questions that research can potentially answer. If I ask, for example, "Do antibiotics work?" the answer will always be "It depends." They can't cure viral infections or depression. But they most certainly do have tremendous benefits, including curing infections and saving lives, when the appropriate medication is used in the right circumstance. So while "Does it work?" is an important general issue to consider in evaluating any medical therapy, the answer is often going to be complex and nuanced. For some therapies, like homeopathy, there is sufficient evidence at all levels to say definitively and in broad terms "No, it doesn't work." But for many CAM practices, the answer is not as simple.

In order to get to more useful, specific questions about acupuncture (and other interventions I will discuss), I will talk about the evidence at several levels. This is a reflection of how medical therapies in general are best evaluated. I introduced these levels briefly in Chapter 1.

106

Biologic Plausibility

This means, is there a theory for how a treatment might work, and is this theory consistent with established scientific knowledge? Homeopathy, again, is the perfect example of a practice with an implausible theory that can only be true if much of the established basic science and medical knowledge is wrong.

Having a plausible theory does not, of course, mean a treatment actually works in the real world. Most new drugs and therapies in scientific medicine start with a plausible theory but fail to make it into clinical practice because they don't turn out to be sufficiently safe or effective in real patients. And since scientific knowledge does change and grow, seemingly implausible ideas sometimes turn out to be true (though not as often as promoters of such ideas would like us to believe). So plausibility is not the last word on whether a treatment works or not, it is simply one key piece of information to help us decide.

Preclinical Research Evidence

We generally do not take every new idea in medicine and start using it to treat patients immediately. That would be quite a reckless approach! Most new treatments are studied in *in vitro* systems, such as cells in a Petri dish, or in laboratory animals first. This helps us to see what effects the treatment might have that could be either beneficial or harmful to patients. Such research is a necessary precursor to trying treatments out in actual patients. It can often help us avoid unnecessary risk or the wasted time and expense of clinical trials for treatments that are unlikely to work. In fact, it is an accepted

principle of medical ethics and law that we should not conduct clinical studies of a treatment in real patients until we have good preclinical evidence
showing the treatment might be effective and does not seem to have any
unacceptable risks. Skipping this step is both dangerous and unethical.

Preclinical research, however, cannot by itself determine that a treatment is safe and effective in real patients. Rats are not the same as humans
or dogs, and isolated cancer cells in a Petri dish are very different from a
cancerous tumor in a living animal. A common mistake made in alternative
medicine is relying only on preclinical research and claiming that a treatment
which works in the lab must also work in patients. Bleach works great at
killing cancer cells in a test tube, but it is not something we should inject
into cancer patients to treat their disease! Like biologic plausibility, preclinical research is a necessary, but not a sufficient, step in deciding whether and
treatment is worth using or not.

Clinical Trials

The best evidence for whether a treatment is safe and effective comes from
testing it in real patients in a way that controls for all the sorts of biases and
errors I've talked about previously. Once the basic theory is worked out and
the preclinical evidence suggests a therapy might be worthwhile, then controlled clinical testing is the strongest form of evidence for exactly what that
therapy can and cannot do for patients.

However, even this is not as simple as it sounds. Clinical trials in humans, for example, are often very useful for veterinarians evaluating a possible treatment for their patients. Yet humans are clearly quite different from
cats, dogs, rabbits, and other veterinary patients, and studies in people don't

always accurately predict how treatments will work in the veterinary setting. There are also many different ways clinical trials can be designed and carried out, and some produce better evidence than others. So while clinical trial research in general is the best single piece of evidence for evaluating a specific treatment for a particular clinical problem, even clinical trials alone can fail to give us a clear answer to the question "Does it work?" In the worst case, poor quality clinical trials can actually mislead us!

In evaluating whether or not acupuncture has a place in veterinary medicine, I will try to look at all three of these kinds of evidence and be as specific as possible. While this is a lot more work (for me and for you!), it is the only way to give an honest, useful answer to the question.

Biologic Plausibility

Is there a theory for how acupuncture might work that we can evaluate in terms of existing scientific knowledge? Yes. In fact, there are several different theories given different emphasis in various schools of acupuncture. I talked about these a bit earlier, and I tried to give a brief sketch of the theoretical bases for both TCVM acupuncture and Medical Acupuncture. I will now look at these rationales from the perspective of biologic plausibility, that is how consistent they are with established scientific knowledge.

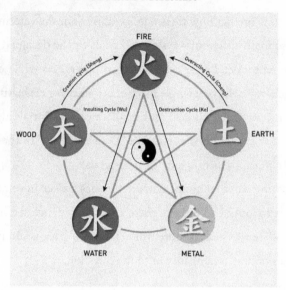

Five-Element Cycles 2018 by Yulicachen under Creative Commons license by SA 4.0

TCVM is fundamentally a vitalist practice, relying on belief in spiritual or nonphysical energies like Qi or metaphorical concepts such as Yin and Yang representing a particular philosophical belief in the balance of opposites as a fundamental feature of the universe. It is deeply rooted in Daoist and other historic Chinese religious and philosophical systems. As such, it is part of a view of the world that predates the scientific view, and it shares little in common with it. It is always difficult to evaluate ideas which are fundamentally religious in nature from a scientific perspective since science typically limits itself to the natural world, to phenomena which operate on the basis of consistent, predictable rules of "laws of nature" which can be discovered through observation and experimentation.

Placebos for Pets?

Qi and Yin and Yang cannot be directly observed, measured, or otherwise experimentally studied. They are believed to exhibit some regular, predictable properties, but they do not operate under the constraints of the laws of physics, chemistry, and biology that science uses to describe and predict the behavior of natural, physical phenomena. Therefore, while science has never found any direct evidence that Qi exists or that the natural world does operate on the principle of balance between opposing forces, it also cannot directly disprove these concepts since they are defined in terms that put them outside of the bounds of the physical reality scientific research concerns itself with.

Ultimately, the theoretical foundations for TCVM cannot be directly evaluated scientifically but must be accepted or rejected on faith, by personal belief alone. This raises the issue I discussed in Chapter 2, which is whether it is appropriate or useful for medical therapies to be based on untestable beliefs. The problem with such faith-based claims is that one has complete freedom to claim absolutely anything, and there is no way any claim can be disproven. Everything must be allowed to be true if one believes it, in which case the distinction between truth and falsehood becomes meaningless. Clients and patients are totally at the mercy of individual practitioner's personal beliefs and practices, since there is no objective basis on which to judge their claims or actions. Such reliance on the untestable beliefs of individuals or groups has been a tremendous impediment to real knowledge and progress in the history of medicine. Religion has never made effective medicine, and the emphasis in science on material, physical reality has led to tremendous improvements in our health and well-being.

It also seems that there are ethical problems with presenting personal spiritual beliefs as medical practices. Science is widely understood to be the most effective and appropriate basis for medicine. This is explicitly acknowledged in many of the laws that govern veterinary practice. Veterinarians are granted exclusive rights to practice veterinary medicine based on the understanding that they will not only have recognized scientific medical training, but that they will use this training as the basis for the care they provide. While pet owners are free to choose the type of care they want their pets to receive, they must also have a right to know when they are working with a doctor who employs a faith-based approach to medicine that essentially rejects the basic foundations of science and modern healthcare. Presenting untestable spiritual beliefs as systems of medicine denies pet owners the clear and accurate information they need to make choices about the care their pets receive.

Returning, then, to the plausibility of TCVM-based acupuncture, the most that can be said is that the approach is founded on a system of beliefs that cannot be definitively proven or disproven scientifically. Science has so far failed to find any evidence that these beliefs about Qi, meridians, Yin and Yang, and so on are true, but by their nature they are inconsistent with the scientific approach to understanding the world. Given how successful that approach has been in so many different areas, including medicine, this inconsistency suggests we should be skeptical of practices based on such beliefs.

The primary alternative to TCVM-based acupuncture, often called Medical Acupuncture, fares a bit better in terms of biologic plausibility. By definition, this approach to acupuncture begins by assuming that the scientific understandings of anatomy and physiology are the most reliable basis for any attempt to influence health and disease through needling.[11,13,14] The nervous system, the musculoskeletal system, and all the organs of the body are connected in an elegant and bewildering variety of ways. There are direct and indirect anatomical connections between nerves, blood vessels, muscles, and organs all over the body. And there are complex systems of chemical messages circulating through the body. All of these are plausible mechanisms by which needling, electroacupuncture, and related techniques might influence bodily functions and health.

The devil is, of course, always in the details. The idea that sticking needles or passing electricity through structures in the body might have beneficial local and distant effects is plausible if one sticks to rationales involving established anatomy and physiology. But whether this plausible idea is actually true, requires consideration of other types of evidence.

Preclinical Research Evidence

There is an enormous amount of research in laboratory animals and human subjects on the effects of various acupuncture practices, including needling at the innumerable points all the different acupuncture schools consider useful, putting pressure on such points through massage or devices of various kinds, injecting solutions or passing electricity through such points, and even shining low-level laser light on purported acupuncture points. This evidence varies in quality and reliability, and it concerns a wide variety of species and techniques and theoretical systems. This makes broad generalizations about preclinical evidence challenging. However, there are a few key issues related to the potential usefulness of acupuncture that can be addressed using the preclinical studies done on acupuncture. The first is the question of acupuncture points.[15]

A key element to acupuncture generally is the idea that inserting needles, and employing all the other related techniques, at specific points on the body has predictable, consistent effects. Whether one relies on movement of Qi or on stimulation of nerves and release of endorphins as the basis for needling, almost all acupuncturists argue that it makes a difference where one puts the needles. Acupuncture can hardly be said to exist at all if needling is equally effective (or ineffective) anywhere on the body and if it is not possible to predict the specific effects of inserting needles at particular locations.

These locations are typically known as "acupuncture points," and they are organized in a systematic way that depends on the particular acupuncture school. TCVM-based acupuncture uses a set of meridians or channels through which Qi is supposed to pass and locates acupuncture points at particular places along these channels. The locations of the channels and the points are derived from a hodgepodge of sources. Some correspond to points described in old books of Chinese folk medicine. Others are based on the compromises between competing Chinese folk medicine systems imposed by Mao when the modern style of TCM was codified. And, of course, in veterinary medicine points on animals are extrapolated from those used for humans.[13]

This process of extrapolation leads to some pretty odd results. There is, for example, a Gallbladder Channel that is commonly used in the horse despite the fact that the horse, unlike humans, has no gallbladder. And points that are located on the hand in humans are often relocated somewhat arbitrarily to parts of the leg in horses and other hoofed animals, which of course don't have the same number of digits we do.

But even in the nominally traditional schools of acupuncture, there are differences of opinion on the locations of many acupuncture points. Some schools locate points all over the body, using complex charts to identify point and meridian locations. However, studies have shown that individual acupuncturists vary dramatically in where exactly they put the needles when they are supposedly using the same point. For example,

This study took the approach of testing whether properly trained and experienced acupuncturists could consistently identify commonly used acupuncture points on a single patient. Twenty-three common points were selected and identified by the 71 test subjects. The area within which specific points were identified by 95% of the acupuncturists ranged from 2.7cm in diameter to 41.4cm in diameter.[16]

If an acupuncture point is really an acupuncture "zone" that can be anywhere from 3cm to 42cm in diameter depending on which acupuncturist is locating it, then how meaningful is the designation of such a point in the first place?

There are also schools of acupuncture that restrict themselves to points in one part of the body, with the belief that all body functions can be influenced from this area. Some use only points on the ear,[17] while others only needle the hand.[18] So there is no agreement or consistency about acupuncture point locations even among those convinced acupuncture is a real and powerful therapy.

The more science-based approaches to acupuncture do try to create a more consistent and rational system for choosing where to put needles. Medical acupuncturists generally begin with traditional acupuncture maps based on TCM and then tend to try to rationalize the use of these by identifying measurable anatomic or functional features to the points chosen. They frequently claim that such points and channels can be consistently associated with nerves, locations where nerves divide or emerge from channels in bones, blood vessels and their associated innervation, tendons and ligaments, and the connective tissue planes that separate muscles and other structures. They may also claim that there are special features of the tissue in the region of acupuncture points identifiable with biopsy, with equipment testing electrical conductivity, or by other means.[19] Some also claim that acupuncture points often correspond to "trigger points," areas of pain or sensitivity which are themselves somewhat uncertain in definition. Stimulation of these sorts of structures could plausibly have physiological and even clinically beneficial effects since there are functionally important means of communication between different parts of the nervous system, and between nerves and other anatomic structures and organs.

There is no question that if you take a particular channel or set of points from any acupuncture map and look at the anatomy underlying it, you can find all sorts of structures that could possibly respond to needling in potentially beneficial ways. But there are a number of problems with this strategy. One is the vagueness and inconsistency of point locations in these traditional systems that I have already discussed.

Given the vague nature of points and channels, and the fact that structures which might respond to needling are densely packed in nearly every part of the body, it is inevitable that any map at all is likely to overlie some structure that could be claimed to be the intended target of stimulation. It would be like dropping a large net on a sidewalk in central London and then claiming that the location chosen was exactly the right one because some people were caught in the net. The same outcome would have happened wherever you dropped the net. Ultimately, trying to rationalize scientifically the use of acupuncture points after the fact when these points are originally based on spiritual and philosophical beliefs is a questionable strategy.

While it makes sense that needling nerves, tendons, and other such structures could have beneficial effects, the evidence that traditional acupuncture maps have a meaningful or predictable relationship to these structures is weak. The associations claimed between acupuncture channels and points and identifiable anatomic structures seem more likely to be rationalizations after the fact for locations originally chosen without any actual understanding of, or relationship to, functional anatomy and retained as historical holdovers.

In addition, there is much research that shows that the apparent effects of acupuncture seem to be the same regardless of the location chosen for needling.[20,21] Indeed, even some prominent acupuncturists have claimed that the location for needling is irrelevant, or that even needling non-acupuncture points has beneficial effects roughly equivalent to needling where the various theoretical systems indicate you should.[22]

If this is true, however, then it again raises the question of whether one can say acupuncture even exists as a distinct medical therapy. If we cannot consistently predict the effects of needling a given location, or needling anywhere is as good as somewhere in particular, then how is acupuncture a system of medicine at all? Shouldn't a system of medicine require a rational theory and set of techniques that one must learn and that have consistent, generally predictable results? If needling location doesn't matter, then we could all needle our pets anywhere we like for any problem and expect results just as good as those we could expect from a trained acupuncturist.

Overall then, the preclinical research does not strongly support the existence of discrete acupuncture points that can be readily located and reliably stimulated to achieve desired results.[15,16,20,21] This is a significant problem for the treatment claims made by acupuncturists.

There is, however, some evidence that stimulating particular nerves or other structures, especially using electrical current, does have consistent effects, both locally and elsewhere in the body. A number of good-quality preclinical studies show, for example, that electroacupuncture at the point often labeled Stomach 36, or Zusanli, which sits in the general vicinity of the tibial nerve, has objective and potentially useful effects on the function of the stomach and other parts of the gastrointestinal tract and possibly blood pressure.[23,24] This suggests that sometimes needling could have meaningful effects, and this possibility is worth investigating at the level of clinical trials (which has been done, and we will look at the results in a moment).

However, if clinical research does find some real effects to needling a few specific nerves or other structures, this may well be a case of even a broken clock being right twice a day. If some of the hundreds of traditional acupuncture points fall close to peripheral nerves or other anatomic structures we might reasonably want to use as targets for medical treatment, this doesn't show that the overall pattern of channels and points used, even if acupuncturists could agree on only one, is a rational or scientific schema.

And even if electrical stimulation of specific nerves using needles, or potentially needling in some locations without electrical stimulation, turns out to have consistent and objective clinical effects, this doesn't make any and all claims made for acupuncture plausible or sound any more than the efficacy of one antibiotic for one type of infection validates the use of all antibiotics or even all drugs. Specific treatments, whether conventional or alternative, must be carefully and rigorously evaluated individually. That has been a key component to the great success of scientific medical research. And the best tool for doing this is the clinical trial.

Clinical Trials

As I have previously discussed, clinical trials are the best form of evidence we have for deciding if a medical treatment works or not. They are the most effective tools available for controlling the myriad sources of bias and error that can mislead us. I will try to summarize the often vast and contradictory clinical trial literature concerning acupuncture and give you a general sense of the conclusions that can most reasonably be drawn from it.

In addition to their other limitations, clinical trials are expensive and time-consuming to conduct. As a result, in veterinary medicine we usually have far fewer of them than we would like, and those we have are often not the best quality. In the case of acupuncture, there are very few studies, and none of high quality. Most of the evidence we must rely on, then, for evaluating acupuncture as a treatment for veterinary patients comes from clinical trials in humans. Such extrapolation is common in veterinary medicine since there is nearly always more clinical trial evidence in humans than in our patients. However, even though we must make use of it, we can never forget that there are often important differences between humans and other animals, and we cannot always trust that what works in people will work in dogs or cats or other companion animal species.

In acupuncture research, one particular problem is that it is difficult to accomplish one of the most important aspects of an effective clinical trial, creating a placebo treatment that can fool the patients and the investigators so that no one knowns who is getting the real treatment and who is not. Such a placebo control is vital to reducing the impact of bias and other placebo effects on the results, especially when the measures one is using to see if a therapy is working are inherently subjective symptoms, such as pain and nausea. I discussed placebo effects earlier, and they can easily and quickly lead us far astray if we don't have good controls in place in our clinical studies to account for them.

With acupuncture, it is difficult to keep patients unaware of whether they are getting the acupuncture treatment being tested or a placebo treatment. Partly this is because one almost always knows whether one has actually been stuck with a needle or not. And partly this is because of the vague and ill-defined nature of acupuncture points. If one sticks a needle a few centimeters away from a designated treatment point and it has the same apparent effect as the treatment being tested, is this because the effects for both were placebo effects or because the control point chosen was just as effective as the "real" acupuncture point?

Even more concerning, it is essentially impossible to blind investigators to whether they are giving a real or sham acupuncture treatment. Unlike a clinical trial for a drug, in which the placebo tablet and the real tablet are indistinguishable to everyone, in an acupuncture study the acupuncturist always knows whether or not they are giving real or sham treatments. This is important because there is research showing that the attitude and demeanor of the acupuncturist has a tremendous effect on the extent to which patients report successful results after a treatment.

In one study, for example, patients were given a real or sham electroacupuncture treatment or no treatment at all. Patients were also given different expectations for how likely their treatment was to help them. Some were told the treatment was very likely to help, and others were told the effects were uncertain or variable. The results clearly found that the expectations generated by the therapists predicted how likely the patients were to feel better after treatment far better than what treatment these patients actually received.[25] Other studies also show that patient beliefs and expectations account for a significant proportion of the perceived effects of acupuncture treatment.[26]

Because expectations and the attitude of the acupuncturist greatly influence the perceptions of patients (or, in veterinary medicine, the patients' caretakers) about whether or not the treatment works, the inability to effectively blind therapists and most patients to the treatment they are given creates a huge opportunity for bias to influence clinical trial results.

There are many hundreds of clinical trials in humans of all the different treatments that are commonly called acupuncture. No brief summary can completely capture the complexity of this vast literature. However, a few clear patterns do emerge.

One is that in the very best acupuncture studies, which use a sham treatment that fools most patients and even the investigators, the fake acupuncture usually works as well as the "real" acupuncture treatment being tested. It has proven impossible to convincingly and consistently show that real acupuncture is more effective than sham acupuncture.[27,28] Needling in locations not believed to be acupuncture points, retractable needles that don't actually penetrate the skin, and even light pressure against the skin with toothpicks have all performed as well as real acupuncture in quite a few studies. While there are exceptions, and the clinical trial literature for acupuncture is nothing if not inconsistent and contradictory, overall the highest quality studies that control most effectively for placebo effects and other sources of error find no difference between sham and real acupuncture treatment.

The most obvious interpretation of this result, of course, is that acupuncture is simply a potent placebo therapy.[29] Not surprisingly, acupuncturists rarely accept this interpretation. Some have come to argue that sham treatment works as well as real acupuncture because specific points don't matter or because pressure at these is as good as actually inserting needles. If this is true, then of course it again raises the question of what is acupuncture and how is it a consistent and predictable therapy if the core idea of needling at specific locations isn't valid?

Another approach to coping with the lack of difference between real acupuncture and placebo controls is to suggest that placebo effects are actually powerful and beneficial effects on disease. This "mind over matter" approach suggests that people feel better when treated with a placebo because they are actually making themselves better with the power of their belief.

The problem with this is that there is a great discrepancy between the influence of placebo treatments on subjective symptoms, such as pain, and objective disease outcomes such as measures of organ function or death.[30,31]

One acupuncture study makes this point especially starkly.[32] Patients with asthma were randomly assigned to receive no treatment, treatment with an inhaled medication to open up the airways constricted by their asthma, a placebo identical to the inhaled treatment, and sham acupuncture presented as a real acupuncture treatment (with the purpose of generating an expectation of benefit in the patients). All patients were rotated through all the treatments and assessed after each, and the patients and investigators were blinded to the treatments insofar as possible. Obviously, patients and researchers could tell the difference between no treatment, an inhaler, and acupuncture. And as is always the case in studies of acupuncture, the acupuncturist undoubtedly knew that they weren't providing what they would call genuine acupuncture treatment.

The patients were evaluated both in terms of their own perceptions of any improvement in their symptoms as well as an objective measure of their respiratory function. When given no treatment at all, patients reported an improvement in their symptoms of 21%. This likely represents a variety of effects, such as the natural change in symptoms with time and the general tendency of patients to get better overall care and to feel better when in a clinical trial.

There was no difference in the improvement perceived by patients regardless of which of the other treatments they received. Between 45-50% improvement was reported after treatment with the inhaled medication, the placebo inhaler, and sham acupuncture. So patients experienced nearly twice as much benefit from some treatment as from no treatment, but it made no difference whether the treatment was real or inert. This would seem to suggest that the placebo is a potent therapy and as good as a physiologically active medicine. After all, asthma symptoms are quite recognizable and uncomfortable, so it seems unlikely that such high rates of improvement would be only a function of the patients' imagination.

Fortunately, the study did something else which helps clarify that these placebo effects actually aren't as good as the effects of real medicine. In addition to asking the patients how they felt after each treatment, the investigators also measured their lung function, using an instrument that records, among other things, how much air the patients could force out of their lungs in a given period of time. It turns out that this objective measure showed a 20% improvement with the inhaled medication, but a significantly lower 7% improvement with the fake therapies or no treatment at all. So while the patients couldn't tell the difference between real and fake therapies, their lungs certainly could!

If these patients used these sham therapies themselves, they likely would feel they had found an effective treatment. Over time, though, the lack of a real effect on their lungs could lead to chronic loss of lung function or even death during a severe asthma attack. There is a danger in trusting that placebo effects are a sign of real improvement.

This is a key point about the placebo effect that is worth repeating: It can make us feel better without actually affecting our physical health. In any discussion of the placebo effect, we must bear this fact in mind. There is no magical power of mind over body involved. Placebo treatments affect our perceptions of our symptoms, but they do not improve our underlying medical condition.[33]

While it is a desirable and appropriate for doctors to make their patients feel better, and for veterinarians to make their clients happy, it is not enough to do so only in ways that leave the physical health of the patient fundamentally unchanged. We owe it to our patients to apply rigorous scientific methods to investigating our therapies and to developing interventions which actually treat the cause of the symptoms, not just the patients' perceptions of them.

As a veterinarian, I have to be particularly careful about treatments that may make me or my clients believe our animal friends have been helped when they really have not. Using treatments that clearly work in humans only through belief and expectation is dangerous and unethical in veterinary medicine, since these are very likely to mislead owners into believing the therapy is working without actually benefitting the patient.[34,35]

Of course, even though the best acupuncture studies with good sham controls suggest acupuncture is primarily a placebo in humans, there are studies that appear to show objective benefits, and even some that claim real acupuncture to be better than sham acupuncture. There are a number of reasons to be skeptical of these studies. Most lack the rigorous design and controls for bias of the highest quality studies. This leaves them vulnerable to erroneous or misleading results.

And some sources of bias in clinical trials can be subtle and difficult to quantify. It is widely known, for example, that the source of funding for medical studies is often associated with the outcome. Studies funded by the pharmaceutical industry, for example, are more likely to find beneficial effects than those conducted independently. This funding bias appears to occur consistently even with some of the traditional clinical trial methods in place that are supposed to control for bias. It is not clear exactly how such subtle and insidious biases work. It is not a simple matter of fraud or deliberate falsification of results, which is extremely rare. However, there are a million decisions that have to be made at every point in the design, execution, analysis, and publication of medical research studies, and small biases at each step can accumulate and affect the overall results.

Similar types of bias appear to be a factor in the acupuncture literature. As an example, much of the research on acupuncture is conducted and published in China. However, Chinese journals rarely seem to publish studies that find acupuncture, or other treatments tested, failed to work. One review actually found that from 1966 to 1995, not a single medical research study published in China showed the treatment to be ineffective (as compared with England, for example, in which 25% of studies published reported the treatment tested didn't work).[36]

A more recent review from China published in 2014 found very similar results.[37] This review found 847 reported randomized clinical trials of acupuncture in Chinese journals. It found 99.8% of these reported positive results. Of those that compared acupuncture to conventional therapies, 88.3% found acupuncture superior, and 11.7% found it as good as conventional treatments. Very few of the studies properly reported important markers of quality and control for bias and error.

So there appears to be a powerful cultural bias against publishing negative study results in China. This doesn't mean that the Chinese acupuncture literature can be ignored, any more than we can ignore the majority of drug research simply because it is funded by pharmaceutical companies. It is the richest source of evidence on the subject we have. But we do have to consider this potential bias in our evaluation of this and all information sources.

Overall, the clinical trial literature for acupuncture is complex and inconsistent. There are many, many studies of acupuncture, most of pretty poor quality or high risk for bias. When these are aggregated and assessed for quality, generally there is no consistent difference between real and sham acupuncture, though both do better in terms of subjective outcomes like pain than no treatment at all or less dramatic ineffective therapies.[38] This evidence is most consistent with acupuncture being mostly a placebo therapy, with perhaps some small effects on pain and other symptoms via non-specific mechanisms.[29,39,40]

Unfortunately, the clinical trial literature on acupuncture in animals is extremely limited and mostly poor quality. The handful of studies in dogs, cats, and other veterinary species are small and have significant weaknesses, so no firm conclusion can be drawn from them. Just as most acupuncture techniques used in animals are extrapolated from the human acupuncture field, so most claims about animal acupuncture are supported by extrapolation from studies in people.

The best evidence for objective effects from acupuncture come from studies looking at electrical stimulation of points that appear to be close to specific anatomical structures, such as nerves. There is overlap between this electroacupuncture literature and research on the conventional practices of percutaneous and transcutaneous electrical nerve stimulation. While there is decent evidence that such electrical nerve stimulation has real clinical benefits, it is more difficult to say whether this has anything much to do with the larger question of whether acupuncture works.

IS IT SAFE?

There are undoubtedly risks with acupuncture.[41] In humans relatively mild adverse effects are commonly reported, such as dizziness or fainting, and pain where the needles are inserted. Some of these may be real physiologic effects. And while adverse effects from medical treatment are always undesirable, in a strange way it is encouraging when they are seen for the simple reason that it means the therapy is doing something. Remember McKenzie's Law!

However, the kind of mild, subjective negative effects often reported by acupuncture patients may also be an example of a nocebo effect.[42] The nocebo effect is the evil twin of the placebo, an unpleasant or undesirable effect of a medical treatment created by the expectations or beliefs of patients or other factors but not directly caused by the treatment.

More serious complications have also been seen with acupuncture.[41, 43,44,45] Inserting needles into the body can cause direct injury and introduce infectious organisms that lead to serious illness. Needles can break and become lodged in the body at the insertion site. Sometimes, these needle fragments can migrate and cause injury or infection elsewhere. In 2011, for example, the former president of South Korea had to have surgery to remove an acupuncture needle that had somehow been left in his body and migrated into his lung.[46]

Potentially fatal infections, such as HIV and drug-resistant bacteria have resulted from acupuncture treatment. People have experienced severe bleeding, collapsed lungs, organ puncture, and other serious injuries. Deaths attributable to acupuncture treatment have also occurred.[41,43–45]

As is commonly the case, there is little evidence concerning the risks of acupuncture in veterinary patients. Anecdotes of some injuries similar to those seen in humans are sometimes reported, but there is no systematic research or reporting of such events.

Overall, the evidence suggests that serious harm from acupuncture is rare. However, the key to benefitting our pets is making sure the benefits exceed the risks for the treatments we give them. The risks for acupuncture are likely quite small, but it also appears to have few confirmed benefits, which should make us more cautious about what risks we take when using it.

MY ACUPUNCTURE EXPERIENCE

I have made a clear and consistent point of emphasizing that personal experience is not a very reliable way to judge the safety or effectiveness of medical treatments, due to all of the biases and sources of error in human observation and judgement I have discussed. However, our own personal experiences are still quite compelling for each of us, and personal anecdotes from others can be persuasive despite their deep unreliability. As a firm believer in science-based medicine who also uses acupuncture in my patients, I am often asked for my own experiences and impressions even after I have explained why they don't matter much compared to better evidence.

When discussing acupuncture with clients, I begin with an abbreviated version of what I have just discussed here. I talk about the various theories and why I don't find the TCVM approach plausible or reliable. I also explain the limitations and inconsistencies in the acupuncture research and the dearth of evidence in veterinary species. In order to give informed consent to acupuncture treatment, my clients must understand that there is very little evidence to support meaningful benefits, and that there are real risks.

Because the risks are real, though likely small, and the benefits are uncertain, I do not offer acupuncture unless my patients' caregivers are already employing all of the scientific medical therapies available that have better evidence, including medicines for pain, weight loss, and other conventional treatments. Acupuncture should never be seen as a substitute for proven pain control, sedation or anesthesia, or other conventional methods shown to be truly effective.

In the few cases where all these conditions are met and the client still has an interest in acupuncture, I have done both dry needling and electrical stimulation, mostly for patients with chronic pain or neurologic dysfunction due to arthritis or other degenerative diseases. I typically bribe my patients with food, and most seem to enjoy the bribe and pay little attention to the treatment. Despite the legitimate doubt about the effectiveness of acupuncture in animals, I think characterizations of it by skeptics as cruel or "torture" are histrionic and unrealistic.

Invariably, despite all of the other information I provide, people than ask me to tell them, based on my personal experience, "Does it work?" Of course, by now you know that the answer must be "I don't know," because such experience alone is not a sufficient or reliable way to make such a judge-ment, even *my own* experience.

Nearly all of my clients believe acupuncture has helped reduced their pets' pain. However, this is what we would expect from the caregiver placebo effect. And the progressive loss of function that always occurs with such con-ditions is not stopped or reversed. Is it slower than it would be without acu-puncture? Who knows? Is the absence of dramatic and definitive cures in my patients evidence acupuncture doesn't work, or evidence that I'm not doing it right because I don't use TCVM principles to guide me?

Ultimately, most of what I have learned from my experience offering acupuncture is not about the treatment itself, but about how vets and pet owners think about such treatments. I would very much like to accept the credit I am given when happy clients tell me how much better their pets feel after acupuncture treatment. Even though I know how unreliable such sub-jective observations are, naturally I want to help my patients, make my cli-ents happy, and feel like I am an effective caregiver. Such emotions are a powerful incentive to believe what we see and want to believe, even for those of us who should know better.

Similarly, I have learned that my clients generally see the treatment and the results in the most hopeful, positive terms possible. Even when I see little evidence of significant change, clients often have the sense that their pets feel better. The love we have for our pets motivates us to do everything we can to alleviate their suffering, and that is a good thing. However, this same drive can push us to see what we want and hope for rather than what is. I have had clients give glowing reports of improvement in mobility and func-tion at home, only to have the pet brought in for treatment by another family member who gives a much less positive description of how the animal is doing.

My own experiences with acupuncture don't prove anything about whether or not the treatment works. They do, however, illustrate for me just how easy it is to be misled by our experiences, and how problematic it is that we find them, and the stories other people tell us about their experiences, so moving and persuasive.

BOTTOM LINE

Even this quite long summary cannot really do full justice to the complexity of the issues and the evidence concerning acupuncture. It is even difficult to clearly and consistently define the practice, which is necessary for an effective evaluation. The theories underlying acupuncture in animals vary, but the most common system of thought, that of Traditional Chinese Veterinary Medicine, is ultimately a spiritual and philosophical belief system rather than a field of medicine. Science cannot effectively evaluate the principles of this system other than to say that it is largely inconsistent with the scientific understanding of nature.

The conventional approach of Medical Acupuncture makes more plausible hypotheses about how needling might have beneficial effects on patients. However, a thorough and critical look at the research evidence best supports the view that while needling has physiological effects, it has not been convincingly demonstrated that these are predictable, repeatable, and controllable to achieve beneficial clinical outcomes. It also seems unlikely that acupuncture points or channels exist as a consistent network of identifiable anatomical structures that can be predictably identified and manipulated to achieve a desired clinical goal.

Most acupuncture clinical trials cannot be viewed as very reliable. The best controlled studies suggest that acupuncture affects subjective symptoms and perceptions more than objectively measurable indicators of disease. This is most consistent with a placebo effect.

There is some room for rational uncertainty about the extent to which acupuncture might have small benefits in terms of pain, nausea, and a couple of other clinical symptoms. Conclusions in science are always provisional and proportional to the available evidence. However, there is an enormous amount of evidence regarding acupuncture, and the powerful, reliable benefits so often claimed for it should not be as elusive as they appear to be based on this research so far. It really shouldn't be so hard to prove it works if it works as well as its advocates claim.

There are definitely risks associated with acupuncture. Infections and injuries from needles, some serious or even fatal, have been reported. Overall, however, serious adverse effects seem to be quite rare when experienced, formally trained acupuncturists are providing the treatment.

My own experiences with acupuncture haven't altered my view that acupuncture is mostly a placebo. However, I also know that personal experience, even my own, shouldn't be viewed as proving or disproving the safety and efficacy of medical treatments unless no better evidence is available. The reliance of acupuncturists on anecdotal evidence as probative is one of the greatest reasons to be skeptical about the practice, especially when controlled research hasn't been able to confirm these experiences. I have seen firsthand how easily and naturally both vets and pet owners can be led into an unjustified confidence in our treatments based more on what we want them to do than what we can prove they actually accomplish.

Since it has proved impossible to find consistent evidence after more than 3000 trials, it is time to give up. The outcome of this research...is that the benefits of acupuncture are likely nonexistent, or at best are too small and too transient to be of any clinical significance. It seems that acupuncture is little or no more than a theatrical placebo.

- Steven Novella and David Colquhoun

Placebos for Pets?

[1] Lehmann H. Acupuncture in ancient China: How important was it really? *J Integr Med*. 2013;11(1):45-53. doi:10.3736/jintegrmed2013008

[2] Buell PD, May T, Ramey D. Greek and Chinese horse medicine: déjà vu all over again. *Sudhoffs Arch*. 2010;94(1):31-56.

[3] Levinovitz A. Chairman Mao Invented Traditional Chinese Medicine. *Slate*. October . https://slate.com/technology/2013/10/traditional-chinese-medicine-origins-mao-invented-it-but-didnt-believe-in-it.html.

[4] Taylor K. *Chinese Medicine in Early Communist China, 1945-1963: A Medicine of Revolution (Needham Research Institute Series)*. 1st ed. New York, NY: RoutledgeCurzon; 2005.

[5] Buell PD, May T, Ramey D. Greek and Chinese horse medicine: déjà vu all over again. *Sudhoffs Arch*. 2010;94(1):31-56.

[6] Ramey DW, Rollin BE, eds. *Complementary and Alternative Veterinary Medicine Considered*. Ames, Iowa, USA: Iowa State Press; 2003. doi:10.1002/9780470344897

[7] Xie HP. *Xie's Veterinary Acupuncture (1st Edition)*. Hoboken: John Wiley; 2013.

[8] Matern C. *Acupuncture for Dogs and Cats : A Pocket Atlas*. Stuttgart ;;New York: Thieme; 2012.

[9] Schoen AM, Wynn SG. *Complementary and Alternative Veterinary Medicine :* Principles and Practice. 1 ed. St.Louis (Misuri): Mosby; 1998.

10 Xie H. Traditional Chinese Veterinary Medicine : Fundamental Principles. Reddick Fla.: Chi Institute; 2007.

[11] White A, Editorial Board of Acupuncture in Medicine. Western medical acupuncture: a definition. Acupunct Med. 2009;27(1):33-35. doi:10.1136/aim.2008.000372

[12] Robinson N. Why we need minimum basic requirements in science for acupuncture education. Medicines. 2016;3(3):21. doi:10.3390/medicines3030021

[13] Robinson NG. One Medicine, One Acupuncture. Animals. 2012;2(3):395-414. doi:10.3390/ani2030395

[14] Robinson NG. *Interactive Medical Acupuncture Anatomy*. Jackson, WY; Teton New Media; 2016.

[15] Ramey DW. A Review of the Evidence for the Existence of Acupuncture Points and Meridians. In: *Proceedings of the Annual Convention of the American Association of Equine Practitioners*; 2000:220-224.

[16] Molsberger AF, Manickavasagan J, Abholz HH, Maixner WB, Endres HG. Acupuncture points are large fields: The fuzziness of acupuncture point localization by doctors in practice. Eur J Pain. 2012;16(9):1264-1270. doi:10.1002/j.1532-2149.2012.00145.x

[17] Gori L, Firenzuoli F. Ear acupuncture in European traditional medicine. *Evid Based Complement Alternat Med*. 2007;4(Suppl 1):13-16. doi:10.1093/ecam/nem106

[18] Magovern P. Koryo Hand Acupuncture: a Versatile and Potent Acupuncture Microsystem. *Acupunct Med*. 1995;13(1):10-14.

[19] Zhou F, Huang D, YingXia. Neuroanatomic Basis of Acupuncture Points. In: *Acupuncture Therapy for Neurological Diseases*. Berlin, Heidelberg: Springer Berlin Heidelberg; 2010:32-80. doi:10.1007/978-3-642-10857-0_2

[20] Moffet HH. Sham Acupuncture May Be as Efficacious as True Acupuncture: A Systematic Review of Clinical Trials. *J Altern Complement Med*. 2009;15(3):213-216. doi:10.1089/acm.2008.0356

[21] Zhang H, Bian Z, Lin Z. Are acupoints specific for diseases? A systematic review of the randomized controlled trials with sham acupuncture controls. *Chin Med*. 2010;5(1):1. doi:10.1186/1749-8546-5-1

[22] Mann F. *Reinventing Acupuncture: A New Concept of Ancient Medicine*. 2nd ed. London: Butterworth-Heinemann; 2000.

[23] Suo X-Y, Du Z-H, Wang H-S, et al. The effects of stimulation at acupoint ST36 points against hemorrhagic shock in dogs. *Am J Emerg Med*. 2011;29(9):1188-1193. doi:10.1016/j.ajem.2010.07.009

[24] Yang Q, Xie Y-D, Zhang M, et al. Effect of electroacupuncture stimulation at Zusanli acupoint (ST36) on gastric motility: possible through PKC and MAPK signal transduction pathways. *BMC Complement Altern Med*. 2014;14(1):137. doi:10.1186/1472-6882-14-137

[25] Suarez-Almazor ME, Looney C, Liu Y, et al. A randomized controlled trial of acupuncture for osteoarthritis of the knee: Effects of patient-provider communication. *Arthritis Care Res (Hoboken)*. 2010;62(9):1229-1236. doi:10.1002/acr.20225

[26] Colagiuri B, Smith CA. A systematic review of the effect of expectancy on treatment responses to acupuncture. *Evid Based Complement Alternat Med*. 2012;2012:857804. doi:10.1155/2012/857804

[27] MacPherson H, Maschino AC, Lewith G, et al. Characteristics of acupuncture treatment associated with outcome: An individual patient meta-analysis of 17,922 patients with chronic pain in randomised controlled trials. Eldabe S, ed. PLoS One. 2013;8(10):e77438. doi:10.1371/journal.pone.0077438

[28] Gorski DH. Integrative oncology: really the best of both worlds? *Nat Rev Cancer*. 2014;14(10):692-700. doi:10.1038/nrc3822

[29] Colquhoun D, Novella SP. Acupuncture is theatrical placebo. *Anesth Analg*. 2013;116(6):1360-1363. doi:10.1213/ANE.0b013e31828f2d5e

[30] Hróbjartsson A, Gøtzsche PC. Is the placebo powerless? *N Engl J Med*. 2001;344(21):1594-1602. doi:10.1056/NEJM200105243442106

[31] Hrobjartsson A, Gotzsche PC. Is the placebo powerless? Update of a systematic review with 52 new randomized trials comparing placebo with no treatment. *J Intern Med*. 2004;256(2):91-100. doi:10.1111/j.1365-2796.2004.01355.x

[32] Wechsler ME, Kelley JM, Boyd IOE, et al. Active albuterol or placebo, sham acupuncture, or no intervention in asthma. *N Engl J Med*. 2011;35(2):119-126. doi:10.1056/NEJMoa1103319

[33] Kienle GS, Kiene H. The powerful placebo effect: fact or fiction? *J Clin Epidemiol.* 1997;50(12):1311-1318.

[34] Conzemius MG, Evans RB. Caregiver placebo effect for dogs with lameness from osteoarthritis. *J Am Vet Med Assoc.* 2012;241(10):1314-1319. doi:10.2460/javma.241.10.1314

[35] Gruen ME, Dorman DC, Lascelles BDX. Caregiver placebo effect in analgesic clinical trials for cats with naturally occurring degenerative joint disease-associated pain. *Vet Rec.* 2017;180(19):473-473. doi:10.1136/vr.104168

[36] Vickers a, Goyal N, Harland R, Rees R. Do certain countries produce only positive results? A systematic review of controlled trials. *Control Clin Trials.* 1998;19(2):159-166.

[37] Wang Y, Wang L, Chai Q, Liu J. Positive results in randomized controlled trials on acupuncture published in chinese journals: a systematic literature review. *J Altern Complement Med.* 2014;20(5):A129.

[38] Jiao S, Tsutani K, Haga N. Review of Cochrane reviews on acupuncture: how Chinese resources contribute to Cochrane reviews. *J Altern Complement Med.* 2013;19(7):613-621. doi:10.1089/acm.2012.0113

[39] Derry CJ, Derry S, McQuay HJ, Moore RA. Systematic review of systematic reviews of acupuncture published 1996-2005. *Clin Med.* 6(4):381-386..

[40] Ernst E. Acupuncture - a critical analysis. *J Intern Med.* 2006;259(2):125-137. doi:10.1111/j.1365-2796.2005.01584.x

[41] Chan MWC, Wu XY, Wu JCY, Wong SYS, Chung VCH. Safety of Acupuncture: Overview of Systematic Reviews. *Sci Rep.* 2017;7(1):3369. doi:10.1038/s41598-017-03272-0

[42] Koog YH, Lee JS, Wi H. Clinically meaningful nocebo effect occurs in acupuncture treatment: a systematic review. *J Clin Epidemiol.* 2014;67(8):858-869. doi:10.1016/j.jclinepi.2014.02.021

[43] Ernst E. Acupuncture - a treatment to die for? *J R Soc Med.* 2010;103(10):384-385. doi:10.1258/jrsm.2010.100181

[44] Zhang J, Shang H, Gao X, Ernst E. Acupuncture-related adverse events: a systematic review of the Chinese literature. *Bull World Health Organ.* 2010;88(12):915-921. doi:10.2471/BLT.10.076737

[45] Ernst E. Deaths after acupuncture: A systematic review. *Int J Risk Saf Med.* 2010;22(3):131-136. doi:10.3233/JRS-2010-0503

[46] NewsCore. Needle found in leader's lung. *The Courier Mail.* https://www.couriermail.com.au/ipad/mystery-needle-found-in-lung/news-story/8bb443b8468ca7d1b005f43f4a1cdc49?sv=5945c6eff67b3b154aebe49f42812f34 Published May 12, 2011.

5 |
MANUAL THERAPIES

Nature needs no help, just no interference...Healing is a process
afforded you by your Creator and is above and beyond the control of
man... INNATE is God in human beings...Your Chiropractor
does everything possible to help INNATE heal...When the right
adjustment is made, INNATE goes to work. You feel the results
when dis-ease turns to ease.

- BJ Palmer

HANDS-ON TREATMENT: CHIROPRACTIC, MASSAGE, AND PHYSIOTHERAPY

There is a great variety of techniques for putting hands on a patient to alleviate suffering and disease. Chiropractic, massage, osteopathy, physical therapy, therapeutic touch, and many other practices fall under the heading of manual therapies. About the only thing they have in common is the use of the therapist's hands touching the patient to exert some effect. Otherwise, these therapies vary greatly in their theoretical rationales and the specific form and placement of touch they employ.

Manual therapies from the mystical to the mechanical, the spiritual to the scientific, have been widely employed in human patients as far back in history as we can tell. We are a tactile species. We often seek and enjoy the touch of other people, and we frequently imbue it with comforting, even healing properties. And wherever non-human animals are kept as companions, this love of touch is applied to them. We pet and stroke and thump our animal companions affectionately, and we take pleasure in doing so. Some research suggests that touching animals has measurable physiologic effects on us, such as lowering blood pressure and heart rate and releasing the hormone oxytocin, which has uplifting effects on mood.[1,2]

Any of us who spend time with companion animals cannot help but feel they enjoy our touch as well. With a few exceptions (generally the non-mammalian varieties, such as reptiles, amphibians, spiders, and so on), the species we have domesticated and turned into companions are themselves species which seek the touch of their own kind. And just as we take these animals into our homes and lives as family members, friends, and surrogate children, so they seem to view us as members of their community or family. I think our dogs, cats, horses, and such understand that we are not of their kind, but they accept us and react to us as one of their own in a way they don't treat other animal species.

Dogs, in particular, actively and persistently seek our touch, sometimes even when they are frightened and in pain and might otherwise shy away from physical contact. And dogs, as well as horses and some other domesticated animals (yes, even cats!), exhibit the same kinds of physiologic effects from human touch as we experience from touching them, such as decreased heart rate, blood pressure, and stress hormone levels.[3-8]

Since humans and their animal companions appear to enjoy each other's touch, it is reasonable to ask whether touch can have health benefits, and if so whether the type or location of touch is important in determining the results. While there are, as I mentioned, many manual therapies based on the idea that touch can have health benefits, I will focus on three of the most popular and researched practices: chiropractic, massage, and the broad field of physical therapy (known, for bureaucratic reasons, as "rehabilitation" when applied to veterinary patients).

CHIROPRACTIC

What is it?

Chiropractic is primarily the manipulation of bones in the spine in an effort to treat or prevent disease or to reduce discomfort. Though therapeutic manipulation of bones in the spine has a long history, chiropractic as it is understood today was invented in the late nineteenth century by Daniel David Palmer. He conceived the notion that all disease results from vertebrae in the spine being out of place (so-called "subluxations"), and that forceful manipulation of the vertebrae (an "adjustment") can prevent or treat disease. He gave varying explanations for this idea over time, often claiming that nerves carried a spiritual energy, called "innate intelligence," and that obstruction of the flow of this energy by vertebral subluxations caused medical symptoms. This is a classic vitalist concept similar to those we have already seen in homeopathy and acupuncture, and it is at the core of many prescientific healing practices.[9,10]

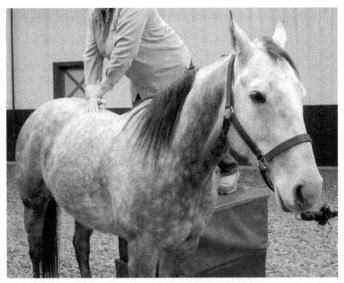

Chiropractic Treatment of a Horse by Dennis Eschbach under Creative Commons SA 3.0

Few chiropractors today still adhere to the notion of a mystical energy such as innate intelligence as the source of disease or the focus of chiropractic treatment. However, there is a split in the field with respect to the subluxation concept. [11,12] Most traditionalist chiropractors still view the subluxation, or the Vertebral Subluxation Complex (VSC), as a real entity that causes illness and can be corrected by chiropractic manipulation. These practitioners also often reject modern scientific explanations of illness sometimes denying that infectious organisms, such as bacteria and viruses, cause disease, and recommending their patients avoid accepted medical prevention or treatment, such as vaccination.[13–16]

Other chiropractors have rejected the subluxation idea and have tried to find alternative rationales for how spinal manipulation might treat disease. This group tends to be less inclined to reject science-based medical theory and practice. However, they have not had great success in influencing the chiropractic profession as a whole, which still tends to focus primarily on the VSC as both the cause of most disorders and the target of chiropractic therapy.[12,16]

For the most part, the principles and practices of animal chiropractic are extrapolated and adapted from those applied to humans, despite the obvious anatomic differences between bipedal humans and our four-legged veterinary patients. As in human chiropractic, the core concept behind chiropractic for animals is the VSC. For example, the American Veterinary Chiropractic Association (AVCA) criteria for certification includes familiarity with "the anatomical, biomechanical and physiological consequences of the Vertebral Subluxation Complex."[17] The British Veterinary Chiropractic Association (BVCA) also identifies the VSC as central to chiropractic treatment of animals.[18] Veterinary journal articles about chiropractic often emphasize that the subluxation "is at the core of chiropractic theory, and its detection and correction are central to chiropractic practice."[19]

Technically, in most jurisdictions chiropractic is defined in terms of treatment of humans, and chiropractors are thereby licensed only to treat humans. However, there are a variety of ways for people to obtain chiropractic treatment for their animals. Some chiropractors will simply treat animals and ignore the fact that it isn't technically legal for them to do so. Alternatively, veterinarians can take one of the many training courses available in animal chiropractic and then employ it as part of their practice of veterinary medicine. There is, however, a tremendous lack of consistency or rigorously scientific content in most of these courses. [20]

The national regulatory body in the UK, the Royal College of Veterinary Surgeons (RCVS), allows chiropractic treatment of animals so long as it is under the direction and supervision of a qualified veterinarian.[21] In the US, where veterinarians are licensed separately in each state, veterinary practice acts will sometimes create legal space for animal chiropractic under another name, which avoids the jurisdictional problem of calling it chiropractic when that term is usually legally defined in reference to humans. In California, for example, the practice of "musculoskeletal manipulation" on animals must meet certain requirements specific to the state veterinary practice act.[22]

A veterinarian must examine the animal, determine that musculoskeletal manipulation (MSM) is appropriate and safe, and take official responsibility for supervising the treatment.

Then the owner is supposed to sign a form: "The veterinarian shall obtain as part of the patient's permanent record, a signed acknowledgment from the owner of the patient or his or her authorized representative that MSM is considered to be an alternative (nonstandard) veterinary therapy."

Then a licensed chiropractor can examine the pet, determine that MSM is appropriate, and then consult with the supervising vet before performing treatment.

I know of many chiropractors treating animals in this state, with and without veterinary supervision, and unfortunately I have never seen anyone follow all of these rules. In reality, there is often little oversight of chiropractors who employ their techniques on veterinary patients.

There are a number of professional veterinary chiropractic organizations that promote and defend the use of chiropractic in animals. The

AVCA, for example, offers a certification program which allows either chiropractors or veterinarians to claim to be board-certified in animal chiropractic, though this is a bit misleading since the official organization which establishes and regulates veterinary specialties, the American Board of Veterinary Specialties (ABVS), does not recognize this certification.

The International Veterinary Chiropractic Association (IVCA), based in Europe, is largely indistinguishable from the AVCA in terms of the content and general approach to promoting animal chiropractic and certifying chiropractors, including the lack of recognition of their specialty certification by the European Board of Veterinary Specialisation (EBVS).

These groups are not to be confused with the International Association of Veterinary Chiropractitioners (IAVC), a group of veterinarians, chiropractors, and others who apparently treat subluxations with methods difficult to distinguish from chiropractic but who claim to be practicing an entirely original form of therapy called Veterinary Orthopedic Manipulation (VOM) and who prefer to be referred to by the proprietary term "chiropractitioner." This is just one example of the many schisms that have occurred in chiropractic, homeopathy, acupuncture, and other CAVM disciplines and which can make a consistent, universal definition of these practices difficult to find.

While the very definition of chiropractic, and the theories and practices the term encompasses, is contested even among those who promote and use these techniques, the predominant theoretical concept remains the VSC. And the dominant treatment concept is the "chiropractic adjustment." Generally, this involves locating a VSC, by touch or utilizing X-rays, and then applying some kind of force to the area of the spine in which the VSC is found to resolve it and relieve its harmful effects. Most often, this force is applied by the hands, utilizing a high-velocity, low-amplitude thrust, meaning a short, hard push or twist of the bones in the spine to cause a small movement of the vertebral bones and joints. This is often accompanied by a loud popping or a sound similar to cracking one's knuckles.

Some chiropractors prefer to use a mechanical device to adjust a VSC. Hammers, mallets, and hydraulic devices of various kinds are often employed, especially in large animals such as the horse. It is also quite common for chiropractors to employ a variety of other alternative therapies, including acupuncture, herbal remedies, unusual diets, and more.

Most chiropractors tend to focus primarily on treating musculoskeletal problems, such as pain or lameness, or enhancing and maintaining athletic performance. However, some believe that the VSC is the cause of a much broader range of health problems, from allergies to ear infections, colic to seizures. These practitioners claim that because the nervous system is connected to every organ in the body, and the VSC interferes with normal nervous system function, chiropractic can potentially treat almost any ailment.

Chiropractic is one of the most widely used and familiar alternative therapies for humans. Treatment is frequently covered by health insurance, and despite resistance and objections from mainstream medicine, it has become a routine therapy for millions of people. Chiropractic is less commonly used in veterinary patients, and it is more popular among horse owners than among dog and cat owners. Nevertheless, because people are often acquainted with the practice and may feel it has benefitted them, they are sometimes interested in the potential benefits of chiropractic treatment for their animal companions.

Does It Work?

The Vertebral Subluxation

The first place to start, as always, is by evaluating the underlying theoretical principles behind chiropractic. Unfortunately, the core theoretical construct of the Vertebral Subluxation Complex hasn't fared well when investigated scientifically.

Historically, chiropractors defined the subluxation as an interruption in the flow of "innate intelligence," a spiritual force responsible for normal health. Of course, no scientific evaluation of such a supernatural force is possible, and I've already discussed the problems with untestable vitalist notions as the basis of medical therapies. Because the problematic nature of such beliefs is widely recognized, and they tend to carry little weight with healthcare professionals and patients, most chiropractors have gradually moved away from this concept. It is now more commonly argued that the misalignment of vertebrae damages health by impinging on nerves leaving the spine. This theory makes some sense when used to explain musculoskeletal pain, though it is less plausible when used to justify chiropractic as a treatment for ear infections, asthma, allergies, or many other complaints.

As it turns out, however, chiropractors have never been able to convincingly demonstrate that the bones they are adjusting into proper position are actually out of position in the first place.[23] It doesn't seem to be possible to consistently and predictably locate a vertebral subluxation. Chiropractors employ various methods to find subluxations, from feeling a patient's spine to using X-rays or other technological tools. Studies of these methods have generally not found very good agreement between different chiropractors in terms of where these lesions are in a given patient.[24,25] Unlike a broken bone or dislocated shoulder, a vertebral subluxation cannot be convincingly demonstrated on X-rays or other imaging methods. After more than a century of study, the vertebral subluxation has still failed to meet even the basic criteria for determining that it exists and causes disease.[23,24,25]

In response to this failure, some chiropractors further modify the definition of the VSC, describing the subluxation not as a misalignment of bones but "a complex of functional and/or structural and/or pathological articular changes that compromise neural integrity and may influence organ function and general health."[26] Unfortunately, that's vague enough to make the concept as unverifiable as innate intelligence. If a VSC cannot be seen or measured or identified in any way other than the subjective impression of a chiropractor during an examination, then is it still an appropriate basis for an entire specialized system of medical treatment?

Because proof of the very existence of a VSC has proven elusive, some chiropractors have come to see it as an outdated metaphor rather than a real physical problem. Those who wish to see their profession taken seriously as a scientific medical practice have had to largely abandon the subluxation concept. A number of schools of chiropractic have even taken the concept out of their training curricula except as a historical curiosity. Unfortunately, there are still plenty of chiropractors, practicing on humans and on animals, who base their treatment on this hypothetical, and likely imaginary, abnormality.[11,19]

Of course, if we acknowledge that the subluxation, as defined in various ways within the chiropractic profession, likely does not exist, this leaves the profession without a compelling justification for the particular treatment method that distinguishes it from other manual therapies. If chiropractic is not the correction of a subluxation but simply the manipulation of bone and muscle tissue, how is it different from massage or conventional physical therapy? Just as the vision of acupuncture as a distinct and coherent system of treatment becomes fuzzy and unreliable if the location of needle placement doesn't matter, so the very concept of chiropractic as a distinct method of treatment becomes questionable if there is no specific and validated rationale behind it.

Research on Chiropractic Treatment

Jumping right to testing a treatment before we have a clear and demonstrable theory for how it might work can cause serious problems. Even most treatments that start out with a plausible, promising hypothesis fail to work as hoped once they are tested under the complex conditions of clinical trials in real patients. And with all the ways that our observations, and even our scientific research can mislead us into seeing effects that aren't there, applying a treatment to patients without a good idea of how it might work is a recipe for false results. There is an important connection between having a scientifically coherent explanation for a therapy and developing convincing evidence for its effects in actual patients, and neither pure theory nor testing without a strong theoretical rationale works very well to show us the true effects of our treatments.

Nevertheless, since chiropractic became a popular treatment before it was realized that the underlying concept of the vertebral subluxation was more metaphor than reality, there have been quite a few clinical studies of the effects of chiropractic manipulation on human patients, and we must still consider the meaning of this evidence.

Placebos for Pets?

As always, the good-quality scientific studies require blinding, meaning that the patients and researchers do not know whether each subject is getting the real treatment or a fake (placebo) treatment. This can be difficult with chiropractic since a patient familiar with the practice may be able to tell which treatment they are getting, and it is impossible to blind the person giving the treatment. Many other factors complicate interpretation of human clinical trials, so confidence in the results can only come from consistent, repeatable outcomes of numerous well-designed trials conducted by different investigators.

When the best quality studies, with reasonable numbers of subjects and good controls for bias, are reviewed they find spinal manipulation to be ineffective for almost all conditions in which it has been tested. It is at least quite clear that the claims chiropractic is an effective treatment for non-musculoskeletal disorders, are almost certainly untrue. There is some evidence that spinal manipulation provides mild relief for back pain, but this evidence is weak and inconsistent.[27-33]

The best we can say for spinal manipulation in humans, then, is that it might have a small, short-term impact on back pain, though possibly not enough to matter to many patients and no better than conventional therapy.[28,29,33] After more than a hundred years of research since chiropractic was invented, this is not a particularly impressive showing.

As we have already seen is often the case with alternative and conventional therapies, there is no high-quality research on chiropractic in animals. Only anecdotal evidence and small studies with poor methodology and a high risk of bias have been published.[19,34-39] Reviews of the veterinary chiropractic literature by chiropractors themselves acknowledge that rigorous

149

scientific evidence is lacking in veterinary patients, and the best they can do is rely on anecdotes or extrapolate from the evidence in humans.

A major problem with this, of course, is that there are significant anatomical differences between humans and other mammals. A therapy useful only for lower back pain in humans is unlikely to be relevant to many other problems in our four-legged veterinary patients. And there is reason to question how effective the mainstay of chiropractic treatment, the low-velocity, high-amplitude thrust, is in larger animals. Horses are one of the species most commonly treated with spinal manipulation, and chiropractors have claimed to be able to effectively treat even much larger creatures, such as elephants and giraffes. Can the force applied by hand or with other instruments impact the large and robust bones and muscles of these animals? Or conversely, could the forces applied to the human spine be more likely to cause injury in smaller and more delicate species? This leads us to the crucial question of safety.

Is it Safe?

Though adverse effects of chiropractic treatment are probably under-reported,[40] there is still strong evidence that both minor and serious harm can occur with chiropractic manipulation.[41-52] Mild side effects, such as headache, soreness, dizziness, and numbness occur in roughly half of human chiropractic patients. Much less common, but also much more serious events have been reported. Tears in vertebral arteries can occur following manipulation of the neck, and these have led to stroke and permanent disability or death in some patients. Fractures of the vertebrae and ruptures of intervertebral disks have also been reported. Because evidence of benefits in people are so tenuous, vigorous adjustments of the neck should be avoided.

Many chiropractors make extensive use of X-rays despite the lack of any evidence that such imaging methods can identify subluxations or other lesions amenable to chiropractic treatment. Though the danger of a single X-ray is minimal, repeated X-rays can increase cancer risk.

No reliable research exists on the safety of chiropractic treatment for veterinary patients. Injuries to horses from chiropractic manipulations have occasionally been reported. It is likely that the risk of vertebral artery tears would be lower in this species given the differences in anatomy of the spine. The risks in smaller animals or animals with ruptured intervertebral disks, fractures, tumors, or other serious spinal problems may well be higher, but unfortunately this has not been studied.

While direct risks, other than possibly for neck manipulation in people, appear to be small, there are indirect risks of chiropractic therapy that come from some of the views often held by chiropractors. Chiropractors treating humans, for example, sometimes recommend against vaccination,[15,53,54,55] and it is not uncommon for them to employ a variety of therapies besides musculoskeletal manipulation, including colon cleansing, untested herbal remedies, homeopathy, and so on. Chiropractors also frequently make claims about their treatments that are not supported by scientific evidence.[56]

Chiropractors practicing on animals have also been known to stir up irrational fear of vaccination, claim toxins in pet food are common causes of cancer, and otherwise express disdain for science-based veterinary medicine. Even a small real benefit from manual treatment may not be worth it if the practitioner discourages safe and effective conventional treatment for the patient. This sort of indirect risk is a common problem associated with CAVM therapies even when the treatments themselves pose little risk of direct injury to patients.

I have had a direct experience with this approach to chiropractic care which illustrates the risk to patients. I was once asked to examine a rabbit that had come to my hospital to be treated by a chiropractor, at the advice of the veterinarian who had seen the patient at another hospital. The rabbit had been anesthetized for treatment of dental disease earlier in the day and upon waking was paralyzed in its hind legs. It is a well-known issue in rabbit medicine that when frightened or disoriented, these delicate creatures can sometimes kick their powerful hind legs uncontrollably and actually fracture their own spine.

In this case, the rabbit had the typical symptoms associated with a spinal cord injury in the lower back. The process of locating a lesion in the nervous system is a well-established part of the basic training that veterinarians, and supposedly chiropractors, receive in conducting a physical examination. The history and physical exam findings made a broken back almost the only possible diagnosis in this rabbit.

The chiropractor, however, examined the rabbit and concluded it had a subluxation in its neck. He recommended giving a chiropractic adjustment to the neck and sending the pet home, with additional adjustments likely necessary in the following days or weeks. When I asked how he reconciled his diagnosis with the symptoms and history, which fit the classic pattern associated with a spinal cord injury in the lower back, the chiropractor informed me that he was familiar with conventional neurology theory and training but had chosen to ignore them because they were not consistent with his daily experience in practice.

This is an example of a truly alternative approach to medicine, in which even well-established scientific knowledge is ignored in favor of unproven alternative theories and personal experience and belief. While there are absolutely chiropractors who genuinely try to adhere to scientific principles and practices, this sort of preference for private belief over scientific fact is all too common in the profession.

The client permitted me to take an X-ray which confirmed a traumatic lumbar vertebral fracture and severe spinal cord trauma. The patient was humanely euthanized in light of the severe symptoms and poor prognosis. Though this was sad, I consider it a better outcome for the animal than having its neck manipulated and being sent home paralyzed and with a fractured spine but without any pain control, as the chiropractor had recommended. Of course, this story doesn't directly prove anything about the safety or efficacy of animal chiropractic therapy, but it is illustrative of the risks of substituting a belief system for science-based medicine.

Bottom Line

Traditional chiropractic is based on the idea of fixing an imaginary problem, the vertebral subluxation. A minority of chiropractors are trying to move beyond this concept, as well as the vitalism and resistance to mainstream science that still dominates the profession. So far, however, there is not a cogent explanation for how or why chiropractic might be helpful, to animals or people.

There is also very little good research evidence to show chiropractic actually is helpful, despite many studies over decades. The best that can be said in humans is that it might provide some relief to people with back pain and other musculoskeletal complaints, similar to physical therapy and other manual treatments. Even this has not been shown in veterinary species, and the little research that exists does not convincingly show chiropractic to be worthwhile.

In humans, the most serious direct risks of chiropractic come from forceful manipulations of the neck in adults or of any part of the body in infants and children. Major harm appears to be uncommon, while minor discomfort occurs more frequently. The lack of good-quality research makes it impossible to accurately assess the direct risks of chiropractic treatment in animals.

As is true for many CAM therapies, the most serious danger of chiropractic is the delay or avoidance of truly safe and effective medical treatment. To the extent that some chiropractors discourage science-based treatment and offer unproven alternative therapies besides musculoskeletal manipulation, they can do significant harm to their animal patients even when their ministrations are not causing any direct injury. Anyone seeking chiropractic care for their animals should certainly consult with a veterinarian and make sure that such care is gentle and appropriate and does not interfere with other, more science-based treatments.

MASSAGE

What Is It?

Most people find a massage feels pleasant and relaxing. A gentle or vigorous massage, depending on your tastes, can leave you feeling more comfortable and rejuvenated. And if this is your goal, then having a massage isn't really a medical treatment, and there is little need for scientific research or discussions about evidence.

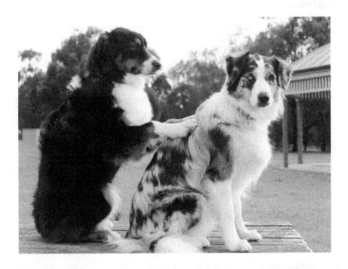

However, massage is sometimes presented as far more than simply a relaxing experience. Practitioners may claim benefits ranging from better athletic performance and healing of injuries to treatment of serious neuromuscular conditions or other diseases. These do count as medical claims, and they should be evaluated scientifically just like those for any other medical treatment. It may seem obvious that massage is safe and makes you feel better, but the obvious turns out not to be true surprisingly often, for all the reasons I talked about in Chapter 2, and it is important to check our feelings and intuitions against reliable research evidence.

Unlike most chiropractors, many animal massage therapists acknowledge that massage should not be represented as a medical treatment. The National Board of Certification for Animal Acupressure and Massage (NBCAAM) states that massage and acupressure are "never a substitute for veterinary medicine,"[57] and the International Association of Animal Massage Therapists (IAAMT) includes in its code of ethics "the injunction against diagnosing any medical illness of condition."[58]

However, other advocates of massage do claim medical benefits. The Ch'i Institute, which teaches Tui Na as part of its Chinese Medicine courses, refers to massage as "healing with hands" and claims it can treat and prevent serious disease.[59] Individual massage therapists sometimes go even farther, claiming massage can substitute for science-based medical treatment or cure serious illnesses.

Like chiropractic, and many other alternative medical disciplines, there isn't a single agreed-upon definition for massage therapy. In general, it involves varying degrees of pressure applied in different ways by the hands or other body parts to the skin, muscles, and connective tissues of patients. How's that for vague?! As far back as we can tell from historical records and oral tradition, people have been rubbing, tapping, kneading, and otherwise touching each other with the goal of improving health and comfort. There is an astonishingly varied array of ways to do this, all of which arguably fit under the catchall term of "massage."[60]

The most familiar type of massage therapy in Europe and North America is Swedish or Classical massage, which includes a specific set of named and defined manual techniques. Other schools use the feet, elbows, and other parts of the body to provide massage.[61] Some use instruments, from simple stones to complicated mechanical and electrical devices. And every school focuses on different types of movement, degrees of pressure, and parts of the body. Clearly, even defining massage clearly for the purposes of studying its effects is quite a challenge!

The theories behind massage therapy are also highly varied. Some approaches claim specific physiological effects, such as improvements in blood and lymph flow, reduction of inflammation, or mechanical breakdown of scar tissue.[62] Other advocates of massage therapy claim more general and less clearly defined effects, such as "restoring balance" and "eliminating toxins." Still others characterize massage as manipulating spiritual energy forces, not only the physical body. Acupressure and Tui Na, for example, are massage practices associated with Traditional Chinese Medicine, and they incorporate many of the alternative theories that characterize that approach, such as manipulating Qi, Wind, Heat, Damp, Yin, Yang, and so on.[63] Ayurvedic massage uses both manual stimulation and combinations of oils and herbs to manipulate and balance the three doshas, energies or forces associated with the elements (Air, Space, Water, Fire, and Earth).[64]

The three Doshas and five Great Elements of Ayurvedic Medicine

One of the more common modern theoretical concepts in massage therapy is the myofascial trigger point (MTrP). Myofascial trigger points are supposed to be focal areas of tension or contraction in muscles which are irritable and contribute to chronic refractory pain. The theory is that these develop in response to local injury, to certain postural or activity patterns, or even to diseases in internal organs or the nervous system. Practitioners who treat such trigger points claim to be able to detect them as knots or taut bands within muscles. Such trigger points are treated primarily by "releasing" them via some kind of stimulus, such as needling, electrical stimulation, massage, laser therapy, and so on.[65,66]

Massage Training and Regulation

There are many organizations which offer training and certification in massage therapy for animals. Like those associated with animal chiropractic, these organizations are generally not recognized or endorsed by the American Board of Veterinary Specialties (ABVS), so their claims to expert status are not officially recognized.

The National Board of Certification for Animal Acupressure and Massage (NBCAAM), the International Association of Animal Bodywork and Massage (IAAMB), and the International Association of Animal Massage Therapists (IAAMT) are a few of the industry groups that promulgate codes of practice, ethics, and training for those providing massage therapy to animal patients.

There are dozens, perhaps hundreds, of organizations offering training in all varieties of veterinary massage therapy. The standards and details of the curriculum are established entirely by the training schools themselves, and there is no universal standard for what constitutes animal massage therapy or how it should be taught and regulated. While massage therapists practicing on humans must often meet requirements of national, state, and local governments for training and supervision to be licensed and legally allowed to practice, this is not typically the case for providing therapeutic massage to animals.

In the United States, for example, individual states vary in how they regulate massage therapy. Some consider it part of the practice of veterinary medicine and allow only veterinarians to offer it, with or without a requirement for specific training in massage. Other states exempt massage therapy from regulation under laws governing veterinary medicine, though they may or may not require therapists to have some form of formal training in massage or to work under veterinary supervision.[58]

In contrast, in the United Kingdom, massage therapy, like chiropractic, is considered a form of "physiotherapy," and it can be provided by anyone over the age of eighteen so long as a qualified veterinary surgeon has evaluated the patient and prescribed the therapy.[21]

Does It Work?

Theories

Due to the variety of techniques and theories involved, implementing a clear and focused scientific study of the health effects of massage in animals is very difficult. Vitalist theories, which underlie many massage practices, aren't really amenable to scientific. These ideas tend to be accepted or rejected as part of larger belief systems rather than specific research evidence. From the perspective of science, we can evaluate whether massage reduces pain and shortens the time to normal function after a muscle tear, and whether it does this by increasing blood flow or reducing inflammation. There is no way to study whether massage heals the body by balancing spiritual energies or flushing out imaginary toxins when these things cannot be clearly defined, identified, and measured.

More scientific theoretical concepts for how massage might work, however, can be studied. The concept of the MTrP is pretty widely accepted in the conventional medical community, and it is also one of the principles behind Western Medical Acupuncture, the variety of acupuncture in which I am certified. However, there is significant and growing controversy about the existence of this theoretical construct.[65,67–70]

Placebos for Pets?

A research review challenging this concept was published in 2015, and the authors were quite confident in their conclusions:

We have critically examined the evidence for the existence of MTrPs…and for the vicious cycles that are said to maintain them. We find that both are inventions that have no scientific basis…Therefore, the theory of MPS caused by MTrPs has been refuted.[66]

This strong claim is based on several problems that have emerged from the relevant research. These are problems that will look familiar to you as they closely resemble those found in studying acupuncture points and vertebral subluxations.

The first is the problem with consistent identification of trigger points. Several studies involving experts who treat MTrP looked at whether these experts could agree on where such points were located. These experts were asked to examine the same patients and give independent assessments of where trigger points were found. In these studies, the practitioners claimed to locate trigger points in different places and did not agree with each other to any significant extent unless they were first told what the underlying diagnosis was. This suggests that without knowing what is wrong with the patient in advance, massage experts cannot reliably detect trigger points on physical exam. They unconsciously base their identification of such points primarily on what they expect to find when they already know the diagnosis, rather than on what they actually feel when doing a physical exam.[67-71]

This is a pretty serious problem given that physical examination is supposed to be the main way trigger points are located. If this inability to locate trigger points is a repeatable finding in multiple studies, it would strongly suggest that such points are not objective structures which can be detected by physical examination, which would undermine the idea that they exist at all or are a major source of clinical symptoms.

The authors also reviewed other ways of identifying and characterizing trigger points, including biopsies and measurement of the electrical activity in muscles, and they concluded that the evidence is unclear. It doesn't seem possible to consistently determine whether there is a single, common lesion that can be identified and associated with clinical disease and which we can call a myofascial trigger point.[66,70]

I am concerned by the inherent subjectivity in the detection of trigger points and assessment of how patients respond to treating them. As both a vet who has practiced for many years and someone with a prior career studying animal behavior, I know how easy it is to project our own expectations onto the behavior of other animals. If I expect to find pain in a certain spot and initially don't, it is easy to press just a little harder until I get the reaction I expect, often without even realizing I am doing so. The lack of an objective method for locating trigger points and assessing their resolution with massage is a significant problem for the use of massage therapy in veterinary medicine.

There are other purported explanations for how massage might affect health and disease besides the MTrP, and reviewing all of them and the associated evidence would be sufficient material for an entire book. Overall, there is some evidence to support most theories but no single, definitive or clearly proven concept that validates the general idea that rubbing, pressing, tapping, or otherwise manipulating tissues has meaningful benefits beyond feeling pleasant for some patients. The lack of such a theory does not, of course, mean massage doesn't have such benefits, only that we don't yet have a clear and convincing reason why it should. In the meantime, what does the evidence say about the actual effects of massage on patients? Let's have a look.

Massage Research

Besides the lack of a precise definition of massage and the multiplicity of practices and theories, there are other difficulties with studying massage that are similar to those involved in studying other CAM methods, such as acupuncture and chiropractic. It is very difficult to develop an effective placebo or sham therapy against which to compare massage. Whether real or sham treatment is given can also not be effectively concealed from patients or therapists in most cases. This introduces significant bias, especially if care is not taken to evaluate only objective measures of response to treatment and to ensure the people doing the evaluation are unaware of which treatment each patient receives in a study.

The evidence in humans for both the narrow and broad claims concerning massage therapy is mixed and inconsistent. There are hundreds of reviews of clinical trials, but clear, unequivocal evidence of significant objective benefits seems hard to find. Studies do show that people often feel more comfortable and relaxed after massage therapy, and they may report less pain. However, placebo effects are very difficult to control in such studies, and there is a lack of strong evidence supporting specific improvements in muscle function, healing, or athletic performance. There is certainly no good evidence to suggest massage is a powerful treatment or a cure for serious illnesses. Overall, massage seems a reasonable choice for musculoskeletal pain or discomfort in humans, though it is unclear how much of the benefits are due to real physiologic changes and how much are psychological.[72-80]

As is all too often the case, there is no high-quality research on massage therapy in veterinary patients. The most recent review of massage therapy in small animals states that "techniques described in this article were originally intended for use in humans and scientific data supporting anecdotal, beneficial effects in domestic animals are still lacking."[81]

Another review of massage therapy in animals has said much the same thing, but with a different emphasis: "Massage is gaining recognition as a beneficial modality for the treatment of many ailments due to recent scientific research in humans. We can infer that these benefits apply to dogs and cats due to their similar physiology and anatomy."[82] The two main problems with this idea that we can extrapolate the benefits of massage in humans to our animals are that: 1) there isn't much evidence for most benefits claimed in humans, beyond some possible reduction in pain with certain conditions, and 2) extrapolating from one species to another in medicine can get us in serious trouble.

While humans share many features of our anatomy and physiology with dogs and cats, there are also some important differences, and these sometimes mean that what is safe and beneficial for one species may not be effective, or may even cause harm, in another. Most of us have found ibuprofen or paracetamol helpful on many occasions, but both can be deadly to our dogs and cats. And while our cats can happily thrive on a diet of raw mice, I wouldn't recommend it for those of you reading this book!

There is some very limited research evidence regarding massage in veterinary species, but it doesn't add up to any kind of clear or reliable conclusion. One small study of sled dogs found no effect of pre-race massage on the level of creatinine phosphokinase in the blood after exercise (a measure of muscle injury).[83] A few studies in horses have found possible effects in reducing the sensitivity of nerves to painful stimuli in normal horses and making the horses more relaxed.[37,84]

With such limited research evidence, nearly every claim for the benefits of massage in veterinary patients is based on theoretical reasoning, anecdotal observations, extrapolation from research in humans, and lab animal studies. While all of these are useful and important sources of information, none can reliably tell us what kind of massage might benefit our pets and patients, for which conditions or how significant such benefits might actually be. This requires the kind of clinical studies that haven't yet been done.

Is It Safe?

In humans, minor adverse effects from massage are quite common. Soreness and fatigue, especially following more forceful forms of massage therapy, are quite common. More serious, even life-threatening injuries and complications have been reported, but these are extremely rare.[85,86] It is generally recommended to avoid massage in people with certain conditions, such as bleeding or clotting disorders, fractures or very brittle bones (osteoporosis), burns or healing wounds, some tumors, and possibly pregnancy. With these basic precautions, however, massage therapy in humans is very safe.

The risks of massage therapy in animal patients are unknown. Certainly, the same sort of conditions in which massage is inappropriate for humans would likely make it a bad idea for veterinary patients. In addition, animals who are fearful or in pain are unlikely to benefit. Serious direct risks seem unlikely if common sense is used. And the indirect risks of massage are likely much the same as those for chiropractic and other alternative therapies. Any use of massage in place of proper diagnosis and treatment is likely to do more harm than good.

Bottom Line

The concepts behind massage therapy are diverse and mostly unproven. Humans often find massage pleasant, and there is evidence it may relieve pain in some people. Most domesticated animals also find human touch enjoyable, or at least not objectionable, so it may be that these animals will find massage to be pleasant as well. Of course, we all know animals who do not particularly enjoy being touched or who are fearful of strangers, and the stress of human contact may negate any enjoyment from a massage in these individuals.

Since there is not yet any evidence to show massage has significant health benefits in veterinary patients, it should be viewed only as a complementary therapy, perhaps worth trying if there is no obvious reason to avoid it, such as fear, uncontrolled pain, injuries that might be exacerbated by handling, and so on. Hopefully, the necessary studies will eventually be done and we can start confidently employing massage for conditions it might improve. Until then, however, it should be employed sensibly and cautiously and not used to replace treatments with better evidence for their benefits.

PHYSIOTHERAPY, PHYSICAL THERAPY, AND REHABILITATION

What is It?

Unlike massage and chiropractic, physical therapy (also called physiotherapy and rehabilitation, depending on where you live) is a conventional, broadly evidence-based therapeutic system. While there are undoubtedly unproven or ineffective practices in the field, as there are in all areas of medicine since our understanding and the evidence are always developing and improving, there are also thousands of studies demonstrating clear benefits from specific physical therapy treatments for particular ailments in humans. When I dislocated my shoulder in martial arts, there was clear and compelling evidence to show that I shouldn't hurry to have surgery and that prolonged immobilization was not a great idea. When I had to stop running due to Achilles tendon pain, I was able to look to clinical trial evidence to support specific exercises that got me back out on the road.

Given the mainstream, science-based nature of physical therapy in human medicine, you may be wondering why the subject comes up in a book examining mostly alternative medicine practices. As it happens, the discipline is an excellent illustration of the confusing and potentially dangerous chimera known as "integrative medicine." I mentioned this concept briefly in Chapter 1, and veterinary physical therapy or rehabilitation provides an opportunity to explore it in more detail.

Essentially, integrative medicine is the idea that both standard, science-based treatments and unproven alternative therapies with theories that don't rely on scientific principles should be viewed as tools in a medical toolbox, and that practitioners should choose whichever tool seems appropriate for a particular problem without prejudice or distinction between conventional and alternative methods. This sounds like a marvelously pragmatic and fair-minded approach. However, it ignores the crucial fact that treatments founded in established scientific knowledge and tested by scientific methods are much more likely to actually be safe and effective than methods based on unscientific theories or historical tradition and validated primarily by anecdote or personal experience. Mixing the two together as if they were equally useful ignores all the reasons, which I discussed in the first two chapters, why we should have more confidence in science-based medicine than in alternative therapies.

My favorite metaphor for the failings of the integrative medicine concept comes from the sharp wit of infectious disease specialist Mark Crislip: "If you integrate fantasy with reality, you do not instantiate reality. If you mix cow pie with apple pie, it does not make the cow pie taste better; it makes the apple pie worse."[87] Until alternative therapies are shown to be safe and effective by reliable testing, mixing them with science-based therapies cannot be trusted to make healthcare more effective, and it is very likely to make it less so.

Veterinary physical therapy and rehabilitation medicine is in its infancy. There is very little research testing specific treatments on veterinary patients.[88] Professional organizations of veterinarians specializing in rehabilitation recommend a vast array of therapies, including: therapeutic exercise, orthotic devices, stretching and range-of-motion activities, low-level laser therapy, electromagnetic therapies, stem cell therapy, massage, chiropractic, acupuncture, homeopathy, and many others. The best of these have been demonstrated as effective for certain conditions in humans, with minimal research for veterinary applications. The worst, such as homeopathy, are clearly ineffective in any species. Many others are dubious at best. The field is a mélange of different treatments with wildly different theoretical foundations and levels of supporting evidence, and specialists in the area seem to make little distinction between the apples and the other ingredients in this pie.

Unlike the other fields I have discussed, there is a recognized board specialty in veterinary physical therapy. In the United States, the American College of Veterinary Sports Medicine and Rehabilitation (ACVSMR) is the official specialty college for the discipline. In Europe, specialists are members of the European College of Veterinary Sports Medicine and Rehabilitation (ECVSMR).

According to the American Board of Veterinary Specialties (ABVS), which establishes medical specialties in the US, a specialty college is supposed to "represent a distinct and identifiable specialty of veterinary medicine, one that is supported by a base of scientific knowledge and practice that is acceptable to the profession and the public."[89] While much of the information the ACVSMR requires diplomates to master for certification meets the criterion of having "a base of scientific knowledge," up to 6% of the material prospective specialists are tested on includes alternative therapies, such as homeopathy, acupuncture, chiropractic, and herbal medicine.[90] Physical therapy specialists are also supposed to be knowledgeable about massage, which we have already discussed, and nutraceuticals, which will be addressed in a later chapter. Both of these approaches have questionable scientific support.

Even many of the scientifically plausible methods widely accepted in veterinary physical therapy actually have little compelling evidence that they really work, including low-level laser therapy, hyperbaric oxygen therapy, electromagnetic treatments, and stem cell therapy. While these at least have a basis in theories compatible with established science, and often some lab animal evidence suggesting they might be useful, none have clearly proven their worth in studies of real patients.

Overall, veterinary physical therapy is a discipline which freely mixes scientific and CAM treatments in a manner that is potentially misleading to pet owners. The official recognition of the field as a whole, and the use of established scientific treatments alongside untested, implausible, and even disproven methods creates a misleading sense of scientific legitimacy for all of the components of the physical therapy discipline, including those that don't merit it.

As with so many fields I have already talked about, the variety of treatments and the individual differences in what individual physiotherapy specialists offer makes a clear definition of the discipline challenging. The American Association of Rehabilitation Veterinarians (AARV) defines it this way:

Physical rehabilitation is the diagnosis and management of patients with painful or functionally limiting conditions, particularly those with injury or illness related to the neurologic and musculoskeletal systems.[91]

The ECVSMR uses this definition:

Veterinary sports medicine and rehabilitation is defined as a multidisciplinary specialty that encompasses the in-depth physical and clinical examination, diagnosis, treatment and prevention of sport and work-related injuries/disorders and rehabilitation of animals' health through a holistic approach at the core of which is controlled exercise, functional training manual therapy techniques, therapeutic exercises and physical modalities.[92]

Under these definitions, animal physiotherapy seems to adhere pretty closely to the concept of integrative medicine, focusing on achieving the goals of decreasing pain and improving function without making much distinction between the widely varied tools in the physiotherapy toolbox or the scientific merits of each. While this appears at first to be a sensible approach, it does lead us into trouble if we ignore the very real possibility that many of our "tools" don't work.

It is clearly not practical for me to evaluate the scientific merits of the entire field of veterinary physiotherapy, or of all the possible treatments that practitioners in this area might choose to use. I will, however, try to look at what science says about some of the most prominent tools in the rehabilitation toolbox, from the most science-based to those with a more alternative medicine orientation.

Does It Work?

As I said at the beginning of this section, physical therapy is an established discipline in human medicine, and there is abundant evidence to support many of the treatments employed. As always in science and medicine, the devil is in the details. Very specific exercises may be proven effective for particular conditions, but that doesn't necessarily generalize to the entire field of physiotherapy. For example, the heel-drop exercise that helped me rehabilitate my Achilles tendon has been demonstrated to be effective in humans in multiple clinical studies.[93,94,95] That doesn't mean, of course, that we can assume joint mobilization is an effective therapy for ligament injury in the knee of a dog. Even more drastic extrapolations are even less justifiable. Suggesting that massage or acupuncture will reduce arthritis pain in horses simply because it is a form of "physical therapy" just like my Achilles exercises is not a sound way to approach evaluating medical therapies. Each treatment needs to be studied properly for each particular use. This is laborious and expensive and not always possible, but it is necessary before we can confidently declare that we know which treatments work and which don't.

As a brief and practical way of looking at what science has to tell us about veterinary rehabilitation generally, I will look at a few of the commonly employed treatments in the field representing both the most and the least scientifically supported. The same method should, of course, be applied to any other therapies claimed to be useful as physiotherapy.

Science-based Physiotherapy: Therapeutic Exercises

This is the element of physical therapy that most of us probably think of first when we hear the term. Therapeutic exercises are some of the most well-supported physical therapy treatments in humans. There have been a number of studies showing that various exercises have benefits for veterinary patients as well. For example, dogs who have experienced a rupture of the cruciate ligament in the knee and have undergone surgical treatment recovered faster with a program of swimming and passive range of motion activities than with exercise restriction.[96] Other studies using different exercise protocols have also found benefits from post-surgical physical therapy in such dogs.[88]

These studies are small and have significant limitations, and a recent review concluded that we cannot make strong claims about the value of post-operative exercises in dogs with cruciate ligament disease.[97] However, the existing evidence is encouraging and consistent with the much stronger evidence in humans that therapeutic exercise after knee surgery can improve recovery.

There is some evidence for various types of therapeutic exercise in dogs with arthritis and neurologic disorders as well.[88,98,99] Of course, there are also some studies that show no benefits to particular exercise regimes for specific conditions, even in the very sparse research literature we have now. As always, we cannot safely assume what works in one species or for one medical condition will be effective in another. Even for a treatment as well-supported in humans as therapeutic exercise, there is currently very little evidence to help us distinguish what works and what doesn't in animal patients.

Because therapeutic exercise is based on well-established knowledge about how injury and healing of animal tissues occur, and because there are many examples of clearly effective exercise treatments for humans, it is reasonable to expect the general category of treatment will be helpful to our pets. However, it is still necessary to show that individual treatments work for specific problems in the species in which we plan to use them. It is also important that pet owners be told about the limited evidence for these treatments so they can give properly informed consent. This is how science-based medicine is supposed to work, and in this case veterinary physiotherapy is an example of a science-based practice. Unfortunately, not all aspects of the field are as well-justified as therapeutic exercises.

PLAUSIBLE BUT UNPROVEN PHYSIOTHERAPY

There are a number of treatments used widely in veterinary rehabilitation which are based on conventional, scientific theoretical principles like those underlying therapeutic exercise. However, most of these have yet to be clearly validated for use in humans, and most have very little research evidence showing they work for veterinary patients. While scientific in principle, these therapies are employed largely on the basis of anecdote and personal experience, and they are much like many alternative therapies in this respect.

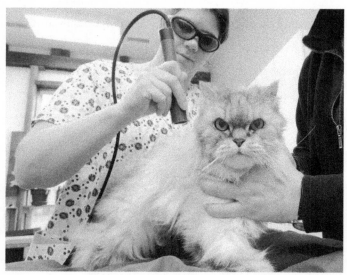

Cat Undergoing Cold Laser Therapy

Cold Laser Therapy

Cold laser or low-level laser therapy is one example (I review this practice in more detail in Chapter 9, so I will skip the usual three questions here). There is good evidence in test tubes and lab animals that laser light of certain wavelengths can affect the metabolism and functioning of animal cells. Some of these effects might be useful in actual patients, but even in humans there is not yet much evidence for this.

The most common recommended uses of low-level laser therapy are to facilitate wound healing, reduce inflammation, and treat musculoskeletal pain. However, proponents of laser therapy, and companies selling lasers, often suggest that this tool can treat many other medical conditions. Lasers have been promoted for specific problems (e.g. allergic skin disease, gingivitis, bacterial and viral infections, envenomation), vaguely defined general health improvement (e.g. enhancing immune function, normalizing metabolic function), and unscientific nonsense (e.g. fixing "Qi-stagnation" and "energizing" cells). This tool is ubiquitous in veterinary physiotherapy, but does it actually work?

There are hundreds of systematic reviews of laser therapy available for specific conditions in humans. Often, there are several different reviews of the same set of clinical studies. Unfortunately, there is great inconsistency in the results. Many reviews conclude that the evidence is not strong enough to support definitive statements about efficacy. Some reviews do show results supporting benefit for particular conditions, though in some cases other reviews of the same evidence reach different conclusions.[100,101,102]

Unsurprisingly, there are no systematic reviews of clinical studies available in veterinary medicine for low-level laser therapy because there have been only a handful of studies done. However, the sparse clinical trial literature in veterinary species has shown some positive effects, but no consistent pattern of meaningful clinical benefit has yet emerged.[103,104]

Cold laser is an example of a therapy based on scientific principles but used in a way more typical of an alternative treatment. Despite limited evidence in humans and even less in veterinary patients, it is widely used in physiotherapy practice. The popularity of lasers is based largely on anecdotal evidence and economic factors. Laser units are being aggressively marketed to veterinarians, often using unsubstantiated claims of clinical benefits. Laser therapy represents a potential source of income for practitioners and for laser device manufacturers. It is possible that this profit potential contributes to an enthusiasm for laser therapy not matched by the quality of scientific evidence for its benefits to patients.

Hopefully, future research will clarify the benefits of laser therapy, identifying which techniques are useful for which conditions and in what circumstances laser treatment is not beneficial. Right now, the horse is well out in front of the cart, with acceptance of the method greatly exceeding anything justified by the available evidence. Even if evidence emerges that laser therapy is not actually useful for most patients, it may still persist as a truly alternative therapy since the confidence most clinicians have in its effects is based on anecdote more than science.

Stem Cell Therapy

Stem cell therapy is another example of a practice used in veterinary physiotherapy which, like low-level laser, has some foundation in scientific principles but which is mostly employed on the basis of anecdote and personal experience without much scientific evidence. In stem cell therapy, cells derived from the patient or a donor are injected into animals with the idea of repairing tissue or easing pain. This is a promising avenue of research, and there are hundreds of systematic reviews of clinical studies in humans, yet these treatments are still illegal in many countries due to insufficient evidence of safety.[105,106] Some human patients travel to countries with more lax regulatory oversight to try these treatments, and there have been at least a few examples of serious harm from this practice.[107,108,109] While stem cell therapy might someday be the revolution in medicine it is often billed to be, there is not yet sufficient evidence to justify widespread use, and such use in humans is widely prohibited.

However, regulations for treatment of animals are typically much less stringent. This is partly due to the lesser value society places on the welfare of animals compared to humans, reflected in lesser legal protections. It is also a recognition of the reality that veterinarians have to treat our patients as best we can even when there is less evidence than we would like, because this is almost always the case. Without more flexibility than our counterparts in human medicine have, we would have very few tools available to us. This sad reality, however, doesn't change the fact that without adequate evidence, we are often rolling the dice in our use of inadequately tested treatments, and this is certainly the case with stem cell therapies.

There are few high-quality research studies to support the use of stem cells in veterinary physiotherapy.[110,111,112] The same is true for hyperbaric oxygen therapy[113] and many other examples of theoretically science-based treatments that haven't yet completed the necessary testing to show they are truly safe and beneficial to our pets. Using such treatments is often an unfortunate necessity in veterinary medicine, but we must always be open and honest with our clients that we lack the level of evidence needed to have strong confidence in such methods. If we are not careful about how we promote such treatments, and if we give our experiences and anecdotes more faith than they merit, we run the risk of practicing in a manner more consistent with alternative medicine than truly science-based medicine, even if our treatments have their roots in scientific knowledge and reasoning.

SCIENTIFICALLY DUBIOUS PHYSIOTHERAPY

Finally, there are plenty of CAVM methods employed in veterinary rehabilitation practice alongside the proven and the promising-but-unproven treatments. Apart from those I've already discussed, such as homeopathy, acupuncture, chiropractic, and massage, there is a widespread use of supplements, nutraceuticals, and dietary therapies. These are subjects I will cover in much more detail in upcoming chapters. While some dietary and supplement therapies are in the intermediate zone occupied by laser and stem cell treatment, based on science but not yet fully evaluated, others are clearly unscientific and either untested or demonstrably ineffective.

Perhaps the most widely used veterinary supplement of all is glucosamine and chondroitin, a combination used for decades to prevent and treat arthritis. Despite this widespread use, considerable research in humans and animals has failed to generate convincing evidence of any meaningful benefit. While science can't ever prove a negative to a degree of 100% confidence, there is a point where failure to find a benefit for a treatment justifies giving up and moving on to more productive hypotheses. Glucosamine and chondroitin are, at this point, so unlikely to have significant benefits that using them is the medical equivalent of tossing spilled salt over your shoulder—it's not likely to do any harm, but there's not much reason to believe it does anything useful either.[114]

The case is not so dire for all supplements and dietary therapies, though many are used without any compelling scientific evidence they work, which is a hallmark of the integrative medicine approach that dominates much of veterinary physiotherapy. Unfortunately, the case is even more dire for some of the treatments recommended by reputable, established organizations in veterinary rehabilitation.

For example, the American Association of Rehabilitation Veterinarians (AARV) still endorses the use of elastic tape to prevent or treat muscle injuries, a practice invented by a Japanese chiropractor and made popular by the endorsement of some high-profile human athletes. This fad has begun to fade in human sports medicine as the evidence mounts that it is a useless practice, and it has never been shown effective for animal patients.[115,116,117] The use of homeopathy, cupping, herbal remedies, and other alternative methods is all too common in veterinary rehabilitation, illustrating the problematic nature of the integrative medicine approach and how easy it is to drift away from reliable science-based medical principles in the direction of less reliable, unscientific practices.

BOTTOM LINE

Physiotherapy is a well-established, largely science-based discipline in human medicine. Specific treatments range from well-supported to plausible but insufficiently tested, but the field as a whole has moved in the direction of evidence-based medicine. Veterinary rehabilitation or physiotherapy, in contrast, is just beginning as a discipline, and it is a hodgepodge of various attitudes and practices. Some veterinary physiotherapists follow evidence-based medicine principles and aim to emulate the standards of physical therapy for humans. Even though it is necessary to utilize treatments not yet fully tested in veterinary patients, this can be completely ethical and consistent with evidence-based medicine if we are careful to proportion our claims and our confidence to the level of evidence available and if we are clear with our clients about the uncertainty involved.

Unfortunately, there is also a tendency towards an integrative medicine approach in this emerging field. Confident claims about plausible but untested therapies are common, and the use of unscientific or even clearly ineffective alternative practices is widespread. In the absence of pressure from government regulation and other external forces, pet owners and veterinarians bear the responsibility for encouraging a sound, science-based approach to physical therapy. As veterinarians, we can be clear and honest with clients about the rationale and evidence behind the treatments we offer. As pet owners, we can demand such disclosure and choose to avoid treatments that do not have a solid footing in science. The promise of veterinary physiotherapy to improve the lives of our animal companions is great, but it will only be realized if we recognize the pitfalls of the integrative medicine approach and insist on rigorous and reliable scientific evaluation of physiotherapy treatments.

HANDLING MANUAL THERAPIES FOR PETS

As veterinarians and other caregivers for animals, our hands are a primary tool. There are many ways we can offer comfort and even effective treatment with our hands. But like any tool in medicine, manual therapies need to be critically and scientifically evaluated to separate what works from what doesn't and to avoid harming our pets and patients. There is a tremendous variety of manual therapy approaches, and they differ dramatically in the plausibility of their theoretical foundations and in the evidence for their effects.

Chiropractic is a widely used CAM practice born out of the intuition and spiritual views of one person. It has proven very difficult to find real benefits in humans, and there is no compelling reason to believe chiropractic does anything of value for our animal patients. Similarly, while a massage might feel good for some, there is little reason to believe it is much more than a weird kind of petting for most animals, likely harmless but unlikely to have much real impact on health.

Veterinary rehabilitation or physiotherapy is a discipline that frequently utilizes an integrative medicine approach. Some rehabilitation practices are plausible but unproven in animals. Others are dubious or have failed to prove their value in humans. Veterinary physiotherapy is at a critical, early stage of development, and it remains to be seen whether it will evolve into a truly science-based medical specialty or retain the less reliable ethos of integrative medicine.

Though manual therapies may seem very different from surgery or pharmaceutical medicines, if they are characterized and used as a means for preventing or treating disease, then they are a form of medical therapy, and they should be evaluated as such. Critical thinking, scientific research, and all of the lessons of history I discussed in Chapter 2 must be applied to hands-on treatments if we want to know we are truly helping our animal companions and our patients.

Science, my lad, is made up of mistakes, but they are mistakes which it is useful to make, because they lead little by little to the truth.

- Jules Vern

Placebos for Pets?

[1] Beetz A, Uvnäs-Moberg K, Julius H, Kotrschal K. Psychosocial and psychophysiological effects of human-animal interactions: the possible role of oxytocin. *Front Psychol.* 2012;3:234. doi:10.3389/fpsyg.2012.00234

[2] Vormbrock JK, Grossberg JM. Cardiovascular effects of human-pet dog interactions. *J Behav Med.* 1988;11(5):509-517..

[3] Dudley ES, Schiml PA, Hennessy MB. Effects of repeated petting sessions on leukocyte counts, intestinal parasite prevalence, and plasma cortisol concentration of dogs housed in a county animal shelter. *J Am Vet Med Assoc.* 2015;247(11):1289-1298. doi:10.2460/javma.247.11.1289

[4] Mariti C, Carlone B, Protti M, Diverio S, Gazzano A. Effects of petting before a brief separation from the owner on dog behavior and physiology: A pilot study. *J Vet Behav.* 2018;27:41-46. doi:10.1016/j.jveb.2018.07.003

[5] Shiverdecker MD, Schiml PA, Hennessy MB. Human interaction moderates plasma cortisol and behavioral responses of dogs to shelter housing. *Physiol Behav.* 2013;109:75-79. doi:10.1016/j.physbeh.2012.12.002

[6] Hama H, Yogo M, Matsuyama Y. Effects of stroking horses on both humans' and horses' heart rate responses. *Jpn Psychol Res.* 1996;38(2):66-73. doi:10.1111/j.1468-5884.1996.tb00009.x

[7] Lynch JJ, Fregin GF, Mackie JB, Monroe RR. Heart rate changes in the horse to human contact. *Psychophysiology.* 1974;11(4):472-478..

[8] Vitale Shreve KR, Mehrkam LR. Social interaction, food, scent or toys? A formal assessment of domestic pet and shelter cat (Felis silvestris catus) preferences. *Behav Processes.* 2017;141:322-328. doi:10.1016/J.BEPROC.2017.03.016

[9] Palmer DD. *Textbook of the Science, Art, and Philosophy of Chiropractic for Students and Practitioners.* Portland, OR: Portland Printing House Company; 1910.

[10] Singh S, Ernst E (Edzard). *Trick or Treatment? : Alternative Medicine on Trial.* London: Corgi; 2009.

[11] Good CJ. The great subluxation debate: a centrist's perspective. *J Chiropr Humanit.* 2010;17(1):33-39. doi:10.1016/j.echu.2010.07.002

[12] Vernon H. Historical overview and update on subluxation theories(). *J Chiropr Humanit.* 2010;17(1):22-32. doi:10.1016/j.echu.2010.07.001

[13] Wiese G. Chiropractic's tension with the germ theory of disease. *Chiropr Hist.* 1996;16(1):72-87.

[14] Jones RB, Mormann DN, Durtsche TB. Fluoridation referendum in La Crosse, Wisconsin: contributing factors to success. *Am J Public Health.* 1989;79(10):1405-1408.

[15] Busse JW, Morgan L, Campbell JB. Chiropractic antivaccination arguments. *J Manipulative Physiol Ther.* 2005;28(5):367-373. doi:10.1016/j.jmpt.2005.04.011

[16] Smith M, Carber LA. Survey of US Chiropractor Attitudes and Behaviors about Subluxation. *J Chiropr Humanit.* 2008;15:19-26. doi:10.1016/S1556-3499(13)60166-7

[17] AVCA Certification Application. http://avcaexam.regstep.com/. Accessed November 17, 2018.

[18] Veterinary Chiropractic – BVCA. http://bvca-uk.org/veterinary-chiropractic/. Accessed November 17, 2018.

[19] Maler MM. Overview of Veterinary Chiropractic and Its Use in Pediatric Exotic Patients. *Vet Clin North Am Exot Anim Pract*. 2012;15(2):299-310. doi:10.1016/j.cvex.2012.03.001

[20] Kjellin RE, Kjellin O. An appraisal of courses in veterinary chiropractic. *Sven Veterinärtidning*. 2010;62(6):19-24.

[21] Surgeons RC of V. *Code of Professional Conduct for Veterinary Surgeons: Supporting Guidance*. United Kingdom; 2018.

[22] 16 C.C.R. § 2038 *Musculoskeletal Manipulation*.

[23] Mirtz TA, Morgan L, Wyatt LH, Greene L. An epidemiological examination of the subluxation construct using Hill's criteria of causation. *Chiropr Osteopat*. 2009;17(1):13. doi:10.1186/1746-1340-17-13

[24] Hestbaek L, Leboeuf-Yde C. Are chiropractic tests for the lumbo-pelvic spine reliable and valid? A systematic critical literature review. *J Manipulative Physiol Ther*. 2000;23(4):258-275..

[25] French SD, Green S, Forbes A. Reliability of chiropractic methods commonly used to detect manipulable lesions in patients with chronic low-back pain. *J Manipulative Physiol Ther*. 2000;23(4):231-238.

[26] Association of Chiropractic Colleges. Chiropractic Paradigm/Scope & Practice. http://www.chirocolleges.org/resources/chiropractic-paradigm-scope-practice/. Accessed November 18, 2018.

[27] Gross A, Langevin P, Burnie SJ, et al. Manipulation and mobilisation for neck pain contrasted against an inactive control or another active treatment. *Cochrane Database Syst Rev*. September 2015. doi:10.1002/14651858.CD004249.pub4

[28] Rubinstein SM, Terwee CB, Assendelft WJ, de Boer MR, van Tulder MW. Spinal manipulative therapy for acute low-back pain. *Cochrane Database Syst Rev*. September 2012. doi:10.1002/14651858.CD008880.pub2

[29] Rubinstein SM, van Middelkoop M, Assendelft WJ, de Boer MR, van Tulder MW. Spinal manipulative therapy for chronic low-back pain. *Cochrane Database Syst Rev*. February 2011. doi:10.1002/14651858.CD008112.pub2

[30] Proctor M, Hing W, Johnson TC, Murphy PA, Brown J. Spinal manipulation for dysmenorrhoea. *Cochrane Database Syst Rev*. July 2006. doi:10.1002/14651858.CD002119.pub3

[31] Posadzki P, Ernst E. Spinal manipulation: an update of a systematic review of systematic reviews. *N Z Med J*. 2011;124(1340):55-71.

[32] Ernst E, Canter PH. A systematic review of systematic reviews of spinal manipulation. *J R Soc Med*. 2006;99(4):192-196. doi:10.1258/jrsm.99.4.192

[33] Posadzki P. Is spinal manipulation effective for pain? An overview of systematic reviews. *Pain Med*. 2012;13(6):754-761. doi:10.1111/j.1526-4637.2012.01397.x

[34] Haussler KK, Bertram JE, Gellman K, Bertram EA, Gellman K. In Vivo Segmental Kinematics of the Thoracolumbar Spinal Region in Horses and Effects of Chiropractic Manipulations.*Journal of Equine Veterinary Sciences*; 1999:327-329..

[35] Haussler KK, Erb HN. *Pressure Algometry:Objective Assessment of Back Pain and Effects of Chiropractic Treatment (21-Nov-2003)*. www.ivis.org. Accessed November 18, 2018.

[36] Haussler KK. The Role of Manual Therapies in Equine Pain Management. *Vet Clin North Am Equine Pract*. 2010;26(3):579-601. doi:10.1016/J.CVEQ.2010.07.006

[37] Sullivan KA, Hill AE, Hausler KK. The effects of chiropractic, massage and phenylbutazone on spinal mechanical nociceptive thresholds in horses without clinical signs. *Equine Vet J*. 2008;40(1):14-20. doi:10.2746/042516407X240456

[38] Alvarez CBG, L'ami JJ, Moffatt D, Back W, Weeren PR. Effect of chiropractic manipulations on the kinematics of back and limbs in horses with clinically diagnosed back problems. *Equine Vet J*. 2008;40(2):153-159. doi:10.2746/042516408X250292

[39] Rome, PL, McKibbin M. Review of chiropractic veterinary science: An emerging profession with somatic and somatovisceral anecdotal histories. *Chiropr J Aust*. 2011;41(4):127-139.

[40] Gorrell LM, Engel RM, Brown B, Lystad RP. The reporting of adverse events following spinal manipulation in randomized clinical trials—a systematic review. *Spine J*. 2016;16(9):1143-1151. doi:10.1016/j.spinee.2016.05.018

[41] Nielsen SM, Tarp S, Christensen R, Bliddal H, Klokker L, Henriksen M. The risk associated with spinal manipulation: an overview of reviews. *Syst Rev*. 2017;6(1):64. doi:10.1186/s13643-017-0458-y

[42] Stevinson C, Ernst E. Risks associated with spinal manipulation. *Am J Med*. 2002;112(7):566-571.

[43] Ernst E. Chiropractic: A Critical Evaluation. J Pain Symptom Manage. 2008;35(5):544-562. doi:10.1016/j.jpainsymman.2007.07.004

[44] Ernst E. Deaths after chiropractic: a review of published cases. Int J Clin Pract. 2010;64(8):1162-1165. doi:10.1111/j.1742-1241.2010.02352.x

[45] Ernst E. Adverse effects of spinal manipulation: a systematic review. J R Soc Med. 2007;100(7):330-338. doi:10.1177/014107680710000716

[46] Ernst E. Prospective investigations into the safety of spinal manipulation. J Pain Symptom Manage. 2001;21(3):238-242.

[47] Puentedura EJ, O'Grady WH. Safety of thrust joint manipulation in the thoracic spine: a systematic review. J Man Manip Ther. 2015;23(3):154-161. doi:10.1179/2042618615Y.0000000012

[48] Swait G, Finch R. What are the risks of manual treatment of the spine? A scoping review for clinicians. Chiropr Man Therap. 2017;25(1):37. doi:10.1186/s12998-017-0168-5

[49] Todd AJ, Carroll MT, Robinson A, Mitchell EKL. Adverse events due to chiropractic and other manual therapies for infants and children: A review of the literature. J Manipulative Physiol Ther. 2015;38(9):699-712. doi:10.1016/j.jmpt.2014.09.008

[50] Gouveia LO, Castanho P, Ferreira JJ. Safety of chiropractic interventions. *Spine (Phila Pa 1976)*. 2009;34(11):E405-E413. doi:10.1097/BRS.0b013e3181a16d63

[51] Wynd S, Westaway M, Vohra S, Kawchuk G. The quality of reports on cervical arterial dissection following cervical spinal manipulation. *PLoS One*. 2013;8(3):e59170. doi:10.1371/journal.pone.0059170

[52] Vohra S, Johnston BC, Cramer K, Humphreys K. Adverse events associated with pediatric spinal manipulation: A systematic review. Pediatrics. 2007;119(1):e275-e283. doi:10.1542/peds.2006-1392

[53] Gleberzon B, Lameris M, Schmidt C, Ogrady J. On vaccination & chiropractic: When ideology, history, perception, politics and jurisprudence collide. J Can Chiropr Assoc. 2013;57(3):205-213..

[54] Campbell JB, Busse JW, Injeyan HS. Chiropractors and vaccination: A historical perspective. Pediatrics. 2000;105(4):E43.

[55] Busse JW, Wilson K, Campbell JB. Attitudes towards vaccination among chiropractic and naturopathic students. Vaccine. 2008;26(49):6237-6243. doi:10.1016/j.vaccine.2008.07.020

[56] Ernst E, Gilbey A. Chiropractic claims in the english-speaking world. J New Zealand Med Assoc; 2010;123(1312);36-44.

[57] National Board of Certification for Animal Acupressure and Massage. http://www.nbcaam.org/. Accessed November 20, 2018.

[58] International Association of Animal Massage & Bodywork / Association of Canine Water Therapy. Laws By State. https://iaamb.org/resources/laws-by-state/. Accessed November 20, 2018.

[59] Veterinary Tui-na | Chi Institute of Chinese Medicine. Veterinary Tui Na. http://www.tcvm.com/CECourses/AdvancedCECourses/VeterinaryTuiNa.aspx. Accessed November 20, 2018.

[60] Kennedy AB, Cambron JA, Sharpe PA, Travillian RS, Saunders RP. Clarifying definitions for the massage therapy profession: The results of the best practices symposium. Int J Ther Massage Bodywork. 2016;9(3):15-26..

[61] Sherman KJ, Dixon MW, Thompson D, Cherkin DC. Development of a taxonomy to describe massage treatments for musculoskeletal pain. BMC Complement Altern Med. 2006;6:24. doi:10.1186/1472-6882-6-24

[62] Weerapong P, Hume PA, Kolt GS. The mechanisms of massage and effects on performance, muscle recovery and injury revention. Sport Med. 2005;35(3):235-256. doi:10.2165/00007256-200535030-00004

[63] Xie H. Traditional Chinese Veterinary Medicine : Fundamental Principles. Reddick Fla.: Chi Institute; 2007.

[64] Schoen AM, Wynn SG. *Complementary and Alternative Veterinary Medicine : Principles and Practice.* 1 ed. St.Louis (Misuri): Mosby; 1998.

[65] Shah JP, Thaker N, Heimur J, Aredo J V., Sikdar S, Gerber L. Myofascial Trigger Points Then and Now: A Historical and Scientific Perspective. PM&R. 2015;7(7):746-761. doi:10.1016/j.pmrj.2015.01.024

[66] Quintner JL, Bove GM, Cohen ML. A critical evaluation of the trigger point phenomenon. Rheumatology. 2015;54(3):392-399. doi:10.1093/rheumatology/keu471

[67] Hsieh CY, Hong CZ, Adams AH, et al. Interexaminer reliability of the palpation of trigger points in the trunk and lower limb muscles. Arch Phys Med Rehabil. 2000;81(3):258-264.

[68] Myburgh C, Larsen AH, Hartvigsen J. A systematic, critical review of manual palpation for identifying myofascial trigger points: Evidence and clinical significance. Arch Phys Med Rehabil. 2008;89(6):1169-1176. doi:10.1016/j.apmr.2007.12.033

[69] Lew PC, Lewis J, Story I. Inter-therapist reliability in locating latent myofascial trigger points using palpation. Man Ther. 1997;2(2):87-90. doi:10.1054/math.1997.0289

[70] Rathbone ATL, Grosman-Rimon L, Kumbhare DA. Interrater Agreement of Manual Palpation for Identification of Myofascial Trigger Points. Clin J Pain. 2017;33(8):715-729. doi:10.1097/AJP.0000000000000459

[71] Rathbone ATL, Grosman-Rimon L, Kumbhare DA. Interrater Agreement of Manual Palpation for Identification of Myofascial Trigger Points. Clin J Pain. 2017;33(8):715-729. doi:10.1097/AJP.0000000000000459

[72] Kumar S, Beaton K, Hughes T. The effectiveness of massage therapy for the treatment of nonspecific low back pain: a systematic review of systematic reviews. Int J Gen Med. 2013;6:733. doi:10.2147/IJGM.S50243

[73] Nelson NL, Churilla JR. Massage therapy for pain and function in patients with arthritis. Am J Phys Med Rehabil. 2017;96(9):665-672. doi:10.1097/PHM.0000000000000712

[74] Loew LM, Brosseau L, Tugwell P, et al. Deep transverse friction massage for treating lateral elbow or lateral knee tendinitis. Cochrane Database Syst Rev. 2014;(11). doi:10.1002/14651858.CD003528.pub2

[75] Hillier SL, Louw Q, Morris L, Uwimana J, Statham S. Massage therapy for people with HIV/AIDS. Cochrane Database Syst Rev. 2010;(1). doi:10.1002/14651858.CD007502.pub2

[76] Patel KC, Gross A, Graham N, et al. Massage for mechanical neck disorders. Cochrane Database Syst Rev. 2012;(9). doi:10.1002/14651858.CD004871.pub4

[77] Hansen NV, Jørgensen T, Ørtenblad L. Massage and touch for dementia. Cochrane Database Syst Rev. 2006;(4). doi:10.1002/14651858.CD004989.pub2

[78] Shin E-S, Seo K-H, Lee S-H, et al. Massage with or without aromatherapy for symptom relief in people with cancer. Cochrane Database Syst Rev. 2016;(6). doi:10.1002/14651858.CD009873.pub3

[79] Poppendieck W, Wegmann M, Ferrauti A, Kellmann M, Pfeiffer M, Meyer T. Massage and performance recovery: A meta-analytical review. Sport Med. 2016;46(2):183-204. doi:10.1007/s40279-015-0420-x

[80] Bervoets DC, Luijsterburg PA, Alessie JJ, Buijs MJ, Verhagen AP. Massage therapy has short-term benefits for people with common musculoskeletal disorders compared to no treatment: a systematic review. J Physiother. 2015;61(3):106-116. doi:10.1016/j.jphys.2015.05.018

[81] Formenton MR, Pereira MAA, Fantoni DT. Small animal massage therapy: A brief review and relevant observations. Top Companion Anim Med. 2017;32(4):139-145. doi:10.1053/j.tcam.2017.10.001

[82] Corti L. Massage therapy for dogs and cats. Top Companion Anim Med. 2014;29(2):54-57. doi:10.1053/j.tcam.2014.02.001

[83] Huneycutt HW, Davis MS. Effect of pre-exercise massage on exercise-induced muscle injury in sled dogs. Comp Exerc Physiol. 2015;11(4):245-248. doi:10.3920/CEP150034

[84] Kowalik S, Janczarek I, Kędzierski W, Stachurska A, Wilk I. The effect of relaxing massage on heart rate and heart rate variability in purebred Arabian racehorses. Anim Sci J. 2017;88(4):669-677. doi:10.1111/asj.12671

[85] Posadzki P, Ernst E. The safety of massage therapy: an update of a systematic review. Focus Altern Complement Ther. 2013;18(1):27-32. doi:10.1111/fct.12007

[86] Yin P, Gao N, Wu J, Litscher G, Xu S. Adverse events of massage therapy in pain-related conditions: a systematic review. Evid Based Complement Alternat Med. 2014;2014:480956. doi:10.1155/2014/480956

[87] Crislip M. Perpetual Motion: More on the Bravewell Report. Science-based Medicine Blog. February, 2012 Available at: https://sciencebasedmedicine.org/perpetual-motion-more-on-the-bravewell-report/. Accessed June 23, 2019

[88] Millis DL, Ciuperca IA. Evidence for Canine Rehabilitation and Physical Therapy. Vet Clin North Am Small Anim Pract. 2015;45(1):1-27. doi:10.1016/j.cvsm.2014.09.001

[89] American Board of Veterinary Specialties. Appendix 1 Standards for Recognized Veterinary Specialty Organizations (RVSOs) and Recognized Veterinary Specialties (RVSs). https://www.avma.org/ProfessionalDevelopment/Education/Specialties/Documents/ABVS-PP-Appendix-1.pdf. Accessed November 25, 2018.

[90] American College of Veterinary Sports Medicine and Rehabilitation. American College of Veterinary Sports Medicine and Rehabilitation Topic Rubric for the 2018 Core Knowledge Board-Certification Examination.; 2016. http://vsmr.org/_downloads/2018-Core-Rubric-Reading-List-080117.pdf. Accessed November 25, 2018.

[91] American Association of Rehabilitation Veterinarians. What Is Rehabilitation? http://www.rehabvets.org/what-is-rehab.lasso. Published 2009. Accessed November 25, 2018.

[92] European College of Veterinary Sports Medicine and Rehabilitation. Veterinary Sports Medicine and Rehabilitation. https://www.ecvsmr.org/. Accessed November 25, 2018.

[93] Krämer R, Lorenzen J, Vogt P, Knobloch K. Systematische Literaturanalyse über exzentrisches Training bei chronischer Mid-portion-Achillestendinopathie: Gibt es einen Standard? Sport · Sport. 2010;24(04):204-211. doi:10.1055/s-0029-1245820

[94] Kingma JJ, de Knikker R, Wittink HM, Takken T. Eccentric overload training in patients with chronic Achilles tendinopathy: a systematic review. Br J Sports Med. 2007;41(6):e3-e3. doi:10.1136/bjsm.2006.030916

[95] van der Plas A, de Jonge S, de Vos RJ, et al. A 5-year follow-up study of Alfredson's heel-drop exercise programme in chronic midportion Achilles tendinopathy. Br J Sports Med. 2012;46(3):214-218. doi:10.1136/bjsports-2011-090035

[96] Marsolais GS, Dvorak G, Conzemius MG. Effects of postoperative rehabilitation on limb function after cranial cruciate ligament repair in dogs. J Am Vet Med Assoc. 2002;220(9):1325-1330.

[97] Cartlidge H. Evidence for the use of post-operative physiotherapy after surgical repair of the cranial cruciate ligament in dogs. Vet Nurse. 2014;5(1):30-37. doi:10.12968/vetn.2014.5.1.30

[98] Sims C, Waldron R, Marcellin-Little DJ. Rehabilitation and physical therapy for the neurologic veterinary patient. Vet Clin North Am - Small Anim Pract. 2015;45(1):123-143. doi:10.1016/j.cvsm.2014.09.007

[99] Henderson AL, Latimer C, Millis DL. Rehabilitation and physical therapy for selected orthopedic conditions in veterinary patients. Vet Clin North Am Small Anim Pract. 2015;45(1):91-121. doi:10.1016/j.cvsm.2014.09.006

[100] Rayegani SM, Raeissadat SA, Heidari S, Moradi-Joo M. Safety and effectiveness of low-level laser therapy in patients with knee osteoarthritis: A systematic review and meta-analysis. J lasers Med Sci. 2017;8(Suppl 1):S12-S19. doi:10.15171/jlms.2017.s3

[101] Wyszyńska J, Bal-Bocheńska M. Efficacy of high-intensity aser therapy in treating knee osteoarthritis: A first systematic review. Photomed Laser Surg. 2018;36(7):343-353. doi:10.1089/pho.2017.4425

[102] Huang Z, Chen J, Ma J, Shen B, Pei F, Kraus VB. Effectiveness of low-level laser therapy in patients with knee osteoarthritis: a systematic review and meta-analysis. Osteoarthr Cartil. 2015;23(9):1437-1444. doi:10.1016/j.joca.2015.04.005

[103] McKenzie BA. Uses, Evidence, and Safety of Laser Therapy. Vet Pract News. August 2018:32-33.

[104] Millis DL, Francis D, Adamson C. Emerging modalities in veterinary rehabilitation. Vet Clin North Am Small Anim Pract. 2005;35(6):1335-1355. doi:10.1016/j.cvsm.2005.08.007

[105] Reisman M, Adams KT. Stem cell therapy: a look at current research, regulations, and remaining hurdles. P T. 2014;39(12):846-857.

[106] Board on Health Sciences Policy; Board on Life Sciences; Division on Earth and Life Studies; Institute of Medicine; National Academy of Sciences. Stem Cell Therapies: Opportunities for Ensuring the Quality and Safety of Clinical Offerings: Summary of a Joint Workshop. Washington, DC; National Academies Press. 2014.

[107] Berkowitz AL, Miller MB, Mir SA, et al. Glioproliferative Lesion of the Spinal Cord as a Complication of "Stem-Cell Tourism." N Engl J Med. 2016;375(2):196-198. doi:10.1056/NEJMc1600188

[108] Brown C. Stem cell tourism poses risks. CMAJ. 2012;184(2):E121-2. doi:10.1503/cmaj.109-4073

[109] Julian K, Yuhasz N, Hollingsworth E, Imitola J. The "growing" reality of the neurological complications of global "stem cell tourism." Semin Neurol. 2018;38(02):176-181. doi:10.1055/s-0038-1649338

[110] Devireddy LR, Boxer L, Myers MJ, Skasko M, Screven R. Questions and challenges in the development of mesenchymal stromal/stem cell-based therapies in veterinary medicine. Tissue Eng Part B Rev. 2017;23(5):462-470. doi:10.1089/ten.TEB.2016.0451

[111] Hoffman AM, Dow SW. Concise review: Stem cell trials using companion animal disease models. Stem Cells. 2016;34(7):1709-1729. doi:10.1002/stem.2377

[112] Whitworth DJ, Banks TA. Stem cell therapies for treating osteoarthritis: Prescient or premature? Vet J. 2014;202(3):416-424. doi:10.1016/j.tvjl.2014.09.024

[113] Hochman L, Shmalberg J. Veterinary hyperbaric oxygen therapy: A critical appraisal. Plumb Ther Br. 2017;(June):37-40..

[114] Bhathal A, Spryszak M, Louizos C, Frankel G. Glucosamine and chondroitin use in canines for osteoarthritis: A review. Open Vet J. 2017;7(1):36-49. doi:10.4314/ovj.v7i1.6

[115] Parreira P do CS, Costa L da CM, Hespanhol Junior LC, Lopes AD, Costa LOP. Current evidence does not support the use of Kinesio Taping in clinical practice: a systematic review. J Physiother. 2014;60(1):31-39. doi:10.1016/j.jphys.2013.12.008

[116] Nelson NL. Kinesio taping for chronic low back pain: A systematic review. J Bodyw Mov Ther. 2016;20(3):672-681. doi:10.1016/j.jbmt.2016.04.018

[117] Kalron A, Bar-Sela S. A systematic review of the effectiveness of Kinesio Taping--fact or fashion? Eur J Phys Rehabil Med. 2013;49(5):699-709.

6|
HERBAL MEDICINE

I know that most men, including those at ease with problems of the greatest complexity, can seldom accept even the simplest and most obvious truth if it be such as would oblige them to admit the falsity of conclusions which they have delighted in explaining to colleagues, which they have proudly taught to others, and which they have woven, thread by thread, into the fabric of their lives.

- Leo Tolstoy

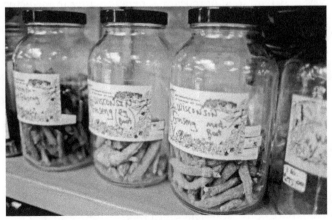

Bottled Ginseng Root

WHAT IS IT?

Herbal medicine is one of the most varied and challenging of alternative medicine practices to clearly define and evaluate. The use of plants as medicine can include anything from conventional scientific pharmacology to pure mysticism. Historical herbalism traditions have existed in nearly every culture we know about, and there are currently several major competing theoretical systems as well as innumerable local or regional herbal medicine traditions.

In trying to answer our standard first question "What Is It?" I will do my best to focus on general concepts and principles that illuminate the complex, varied domain of herbal medicine. Understanding the strengths and weaknesses of general concepts and approaches to herbal medicine can help us evaluate the plausibility of particular claims as well as guide us in the direction of the most promising route to identifying the true value of plant-based medicines.

However, as I am fond of repeating, details matter in medicine. When we get to the question of "Does It Work?" specific claims in herbal medicine have to be evaluated on their own merits, from the plausibility of the core hypothesis through lab studies and ultimately clinical trials in real patients. The general question of whether herbal medicine as a whole "works" is meaningless. The more meaningful question is whether particular herbal remedies or methods of selecting them is effective for addressing specific medical problems.

Of course, I can't evaluate every claim for every herbal remedy, and it would be pointless to try, especially since there is little evidence from which to draw solid conclusions about most specific herbal treatments. However, we can still use critical thinking and science to help us assess the risks and benefits of herbal therapies and which are most worth spending our scarce resources to research further.

In some ways, herbal remedies are among the most promising alternative therapies. There is no question that plants contain chemicals which can influence health. Plants such as hemlock, deadly nightshade, and wolfsbane have been used as poisons for centuries, and their effects on health are pretty clear! On the brighter side, important medicines have also been developed from plants, including digoxin, from foxglove, for treating heart failure and taxol, extracted and purified from the yew tree, for treating breast cancer. The process of pharmacognosy, developing useful drugs from plant compounds, is one of the richest sources of new and better medicines.

However, like most areas of alternative medicine, herbal medicine suffers from many unscientific, or even actively anti-science, ideas that limit its usefulness and create potential risks for patients. Many herbalists still rely on outdated, prescientific theories to characterize illness and choose herbal remedies. Vitalism, the notion that disease is due primarily to disorders of the spirit or mysterious energy forces rather than the physical body, still underlies many herbal medicine approaches, just as it is still one of the main principles behind homeopathy and many other CAM practices. There is also a dangerous tendency for people to believe that herbal remedies can only be helpful and cannot cause harm, despite abundant evidence to the contrary.

Herbal medicine has the potential to be a fully scientific practice that can identify and make use of the beneficial properties of plants and other natural products. To realize this potential, however, many unscientific folk medicine concepts must be shed and replaced with systematic, controlled scientific research. If we do this, then the truly useful elements of plant medicines can be identified and the ineffective or dangerous can be avoided.

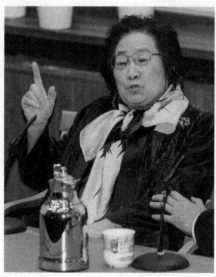

Youyou Tu, Nobel Laureate in medicine in Stockholm December 2015 by Bengt Nyman under Creative Commons license by SA 4.0

A perfect example of this is the work of Youyou Tu, a Chinese scientist who led the discovery of the compound artemisinin. Derived from a plant used in Traditional Chinese Medicine (TCM), artemisinin is an effective treatment for malaria. Dr. Tu was awarded the Nobel Prize in Medicine in 2015. This well-deserved honor is often cited as evidence that TCM herbalism is a validated medical practice. However, the true lesson of Dr. Tu's work is that science is much more effective at creating effective treatments for disease than the anecdotal, trial-and-error processes of folk medicine.[1,2]

Placebos for Pets?

In the 1960s and 70s, Dr. Tu evaluated about 2,000 Chinese herbal preparations, and found over 600 that had some effect on the malaria parasites in mice. Hundreds of specific chemical compounds were isolated from these preparations and evaluated. After many years of work one, artemisinin, was found to inhibit the growth of this parasite in a way that could be clinically useful.

However, the amount of artemisinin produced varies dramatically in different species of the *Artemisia* plant. There is too little present in most species to extract for medical use. Many different species of *Aretemisia* were tested, and the one with the highest quantity of artemisinin was used as a source for the compound, which was then extracted and purified for medical use.

Even more research and modification of the original remedy were then necessary to make an effective medicine. Artemisinin itself has pretty weak effects on the malarial parasite, so Dr. Tu also had to alter the compound chemically to make it more stable and more effective. And it turned out a capsule form allowed for much better absorption of the drug than a pill or the original plant material.

Ultimately, however, after decades of work, Dr. Tu had found an important, lifesaving medicine in a plant used by TCM. So isn't this evidence that TCM is a worthwhile medical approach which can sometimes accomplish things scientific medicine can't?

There are a number of reasons why this view of Dr. Tu's story doesn't hold up. For one thing, *Artemisia* wasn't used in TCM specifically to treat malaria, it was used to treat fevers of any kind. This is because TCM doesn't distinguish fevers caused by viral infections, bacterial infections, autoimmune diseases, or parasites such as the one that causes malaria. Without a scientific understanding of the different causes of these diseases, the potential value of *Artemisia* for malaria patients was unrecognized, and it was commonly used in many other patients for whom it would have no benefit. What is more, the raw plant itself would not be effective even for patients with malaria since, as I mentioned, there is not enough artemisinin in the plant tissues to effectively inhibit the parasite, and what is present is unstable and poorly absorbed when eaten whole or drunk in an infusion, as is usually done in TCM.

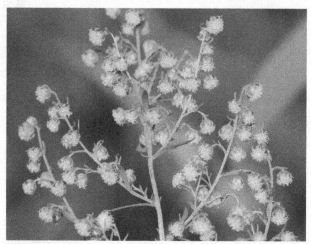

Artemesia annua by Kristian Peters under Creative Commons license by SA 3.0

Furthermore, to find this one medicine, Dr. Tu had to evaluate hundreds of compounds from thousands of herbal preparations in rigorous scientific studies, from mice in the laboratory to human patients in the field. The vast majority of the remedies and compounds she tested were not useful.

Despite thousands of years of trial and error with herbal remedies, TCM never properly identified the cause of malaria and never found an effective treatment for it even when it had such a treatment hidden in its collection of herbal remedies. Dr. Tu's research illustrates not only the power of science to find useful treatments for disease but the inability of haphazard folk medicine methods to do so.

COMMON CONCEPTS IN HERBAL MEDICINE

TCM is not, of course, the only system that uses herbal remedies. Discussing herbal medicine in general is challenging because the term encompasses many different theoretical and practical approaches using thousands of different plants in a multitude of ways. However, there are also many similarities to these systems, all of which ultimately derive from folk tradition or other prescientific ways of understanding health and disease. I will talk first about some of the common general principles that are found in herbal medicine systems, particularly those that can conflict with science and make it harder to identify those plant compounds with real medical value. I will then look at a few of the more important specific systems for using herbal remedies, such as TCM, the Indian system of Ayurvedic medicine, and the contemporary integrative herbal medicine approach.

Vitalism in Herbal Medicine

As I mentioned earlier, many practitioners who use herbal remedies to treat animal patients rely on the concept of vitalism. In the leading textbook on herbal medicine for veterinarians, comments like these appear frequently:

In many indigenous cultures, the process whereby the plant informs the healer is indeed a spiritual phenomenon that is treated with reverence. Is biochemical screening for biochemical activity more or less efficient than communing with a plant? Only time will tell.

Herbal medicine is empiricist, holistic, and vitalist in orientation, and some herbalists argue it should remain so, even as modern medicine tries to incorporate the use of herbs as 'drugs' seeking the 'active constituent.'

Whether or not the Vital Force exits from a scientific perspective the relative 'vitality' of the patient is important in prescribing.

By its very nature, herbalism is vitalistic and holistic in its approach.[3]

As I've discussed before, the belief that disease is not primarily a dysfunction in the physical body of the patient but an imbalance or disruption in some spiritual life force is not a reliable basis for making decisions about which medical treatments work and which are ineffective or unsafe. Beliefs founded in personal faith or revealed as part of a spiritual tradition cannot be demonstrated true or false objectively but must be simply accepted or rejected on the basis of faith alone. Vitalism makes any claim based on it immune to challenge and scientific evidence, and the persistence of vitalist views in herbal medicine interferes with the kind of robust scientific processes, such as those used by Dr. Tu, that we need to use to find the true medical potential of herbal products.

Detoxification

Herbalists also make frequent reference to the use of herbs to "detoxify" patients, by which they mean to remove supposedly toxic physical substances or to perform a spiritual or "energetic" cleansing. The notion of detoxification is based on the belief that our bodies accumulate harmful substances, either from the environment or from the waste products of our own normal metabolism, and that these need to be removed or neutralized by some therapeutic process in order to prevent or cure disease.[3,4,5]

This concept freely mixes bits of reality and science with unproven assumptions and outright myth to create a "toxic" brew that can mislead us into irrational or inappropriate use of herbal remedies. To begin with, what is a "toxin?" Most people understand it to be some kind of substance that causes harm when it gets into our body. But reality is a lot more complicated than this. Whether or not something that gets into your body causes harm depends on the nature of the substance itself, the amount you are exposed to, your own susceptibility, and many other factors.

Bee venom is a mild toxin which usually causes a brief unpleasant reaction at the site of a sting for most people. However, it can cause severe illness or even death in people who are allergic to it. Other toxins, such as botulinum, the chemical produced by certain bacteria that leads to the disease botulism, almost always cause severe illness even in very small amounts. Even this toxin, however, can be harmless or even beneficial if prepared and dosed properly. Science has found that botulinum toxin can actually be a useful treatment for chronic migraine headaches.

On the other hand, substances that are vital to life can be toxic, or even deadly, if the dose is large enough. Drinking too much water and breathing too high a concentration of oxygen can kill you even though you need both of these substances to live.[6,7]

All of these examples, I hasten to point out, are substances found in nature, not made by humans. As I discussed in Chapter 1, the term "natural" is often used in alternative medicine to suggest something is inherently safe or even beneficial, the pernicious and dangerous Appeal to Nature Fallacy. The term "toxin" is often used, by herbalists and others, primarily to suggest that man-made substances, including vaccines, medicines, and other tools of scientific healthcare, are inherently dangerous or must somehow be purged from our bodies. One of the marketing strategies for herbal medicine is to employ this notion to suggest herbal medicines can "detoxify" patients or have other benefits because they are "natural," which we now understand is not a valid argument.[8]

In any case, whether toxins are natural or manmade, their risks must be assessed in terms of their own properties, the dose, and the susceptibility of the individual exposed to it. Herbalists who promote detoxification rarely identify specific toxins or discuss these factors. Instead they tend to appeal to a vague, undefined collection of toxins that we are told we ought to fear. Herbal treatments are then offered to cleanse us of these toxins, without specific explanation of how either the toxins or the purification works. Such vagueness is a hallmark of unscientific approaches.

Herbal detoxification is a variant of ritual purification, which has been a part of religious and folk healing practices in many cultures. Humans have an innate emotion called disgust, which is a powerful, visceral fear of things that are perceived to be unclean or unhealthy. In most cultures, common triggers for this emotion include human waste and bodily fluids, as well as parasites, spoiled food, and others. Since most of these triggers have clear potential to cause disease, the value of having evolved such a reaction is obvious, though it is hard to prove that this is why we experience the emotion of disgust.[9-13]

However, humans also extend this emotion to other triggers which are learned and more culturally variable through the concept of contagion. Contaminating agents that are more culturally specific than the universal triggers of disgust include the body of a dead person, women who are menstruating, persons of a lower social caste, or the violation of some dietary or behavioral taboo.[9,11] We may also view the social, sexual, or religious practices of cultures outside our own with disgust and feel "contaminated" by exposure to them.

Many religions, as well as spiritual healing practices, incorporate purification rituals to help us shed the feeling of disgust elicited by illness of contact with something seen as a contaminating agent. These rituals often include herbal substances. For example, folk medicine systems as different as those of the Navajo of North American, the humoral medicine of Europe, Ayurvedic medicine in India, and others share the practice of using herbs to induce vomiting as part of a purification ceremony.[14,15]

The vague modern notion of a toxin employed in many CAM practices strongly resembles a learned trigger for the emotion of disgust. And the use of herbal detoxification treatments resembles a purification ritual more than the scientific medical treatment of poisoning or toxin exposure. This modern form of traditional purification practices is an example of how much modern herbal medicine retains concepts and treatments from its origins in folk medicine that are inconsistent with specific and focused approaches towards identifying and treating the immediately and underlying causes of disease that is employed by modern scientific medicine.

In general, there is no scientific evidence to support claims for herbal detoxification. There certainly are compounds produced by our bodies and present in the environment that can be harmful to our health. However, without evaluating specific compounds in terms of their dose and effects, the general idea that we can blame illness on these toxins or that we can prevent or treat illness by removing them is, at best, an unproven assumption. At worst, it is simply an invocation of the unscientific concepts of spiritual contamination and ritual purification.

There is also no evidence that herbal remedies actually help our bodies to eliminate toxic substances or that they benefit our health by doing so. We have many systems, in our liver and kidneys in particular, that render potentially dangerous chemicals harmless and eliminate them from the body. Herbal compounds might well help support these functions, and there is weak evidence for a couple of plant chemicals that might support and protect the liver in the face of a toxic challenge.[16] But the general concept of detoxification is too vague to be meaningful, and there is no good evidence to support it.

Many of the herbs used for supposed detoxification have not been studied scientifically, and their effects, for good or ill, aren't known. Others contain chemical compounds that function as emetics (to induce vomiting), laxatives and diuretics (to promote defecation and urination), or diaphoretics (to promote sweating). While these clearly induce the body to excrete, thus providing the sense that we have eliminated something unclean from our bodies, there is no evidence that this reduces any harm done by toxins or makes us healthier. Such substances are likely toxins in their own right or they would not trigger our bodies to reject them so dramatically!

Emetics and laxatives, along with bloodletting, were mainstays of the humoral medicine tradition I discussed in Chapter 1, based on the notion that encouraging excretion somehow eliminated unhealthy substances or brought the body into a healthier balance. These practices have been largely abandoned since the humoral approach proved to be both ineffective and inconsistent with scientific explanations of normal body function and of disease. The persistence of these practices in herbal medicine, under the label of detoxification, is yet another example of the retention of prescientific concepts which interfere with applying scientific methods to finding the real benefits likely hidden in the herbal pharmacopeia.

Individualization of Treatment

Like homeopathy and many other alternative therapies, herbal medicine makes much of the fact that it often lacks a standard, consistent treatment for particular diseases. It is said that each individual receives a personalized herbal prescription, and this is often contrasted with a characterization of scientific medicine as having a "cookie-cutter" approach, in which identical treatments are automatically given to all patients with the same general diagnosis. For example, one popular textbook on veterinary herbal medicine makes this claim:

> One of the key features of traditional systems of medicine that differentiates it from orthodox or conventional medicine is the method of matching a particular treatment to the constitution and auxiliary needs of the individual patient, rather than treating on the

basis of a single diagnosis...[and] prescribing identical treatments to individuals with the same diagnosis.

Herbalists are interested in the patient's unique signs as much as they are in the diagnosis...This picture can provide clues about the vitality and constitution of the patient...[and] direct us to the selection of herbs for an individualized formula to restore health.[3]

This certainly sounds like a great way to provide the best, most effective treatment. Each patient is undoubtedly different in many ways from all others, and providing a unique treatment matched to that particular patient's needs ought to be the best way to ensure safe, effective therapy. However, there are a number of problems with this intuitively appealing approach.

The first is that it mischaracterizes scientific medicine. It is true that diseases are identified and named using specific features, such as the cause (as in malaria, which is caused by an infestation of a specific parasite), the physiologic process that is disturbed (such as diabetes, which refers to a disorder in the regulation of blood sugar levels that can have a variety of specific causes), or the general mechanism (such as allergies, which is a catchall term for a variety of clinical problems caused by excessive and uncomfortable immune system reactions to substances in the environment). However, scientists and conventional doctors don't believe that all patients with a particular disease are identical or will respond to the exact same treatment. The individual variations in cause and symptoms, the presence of other health conditions, the age, sex, and lifestyle of the patient, and many other factors are incorporated into the approach to treating every single patient. Doctors would have long since been replaced by cheaper and more reliable computers if anyone actually believed individual differences didn't matter and no personal judgment was needed to select and implement an individual treatment regime.

When alternative medicine practitioners claim that formal scientific research and science-based medicine ignore individual variation, they are often referring to clinical trials, the practice of studying groups of patients under controlled conditions and then applying lessons learned from those studies to the care of individuals. They sometimes claim that since we are all utterly unique, what is learned from groups cannot tell us much that is useful about individual patients.

This argument fails most dramatically on the simple evidence of the tremendous effectiveness of science-based medicine. As I illustrated in Chapter 1, tens of thousands of years of looking at patients one by one and trying to figure out based on those experiences what to do for the next patient failed to control or eliminate any common diseases or meaningfully improve the length and quality of human life and health. Yet only a couple of centuries of relying more on formal scientific research has wiped out or dramatically reduced many common and deadly diseases, nearly doubled average life expectancy (at least for those who can afford to use science-based medicine), and in many other ways unequivocally improved our health. It requires deep self-delusion to deny that science works better than prescientific, unstructured ways of figuring out how to preserve and restore health.

On a more theoretical level, however, consider this. Statistics can indicate the probability of winning or losing a game of chance very precisely, on the group level. As an individual, of course, you can't know with certainty whether you will win or lose if you go to Las Vegas and play these games because these statistics only describe what happens over the course of many trials, that is, what will happen on average when large numbers of people play. They don't predict for you, as a unique individual, what your results at blackjack or roulette will be. This is very much like the situation in science, where controlled studies look at outcomes on the level of the group but can't precisely predict the results of a therapy in an individual patient.

And yet, casinos make enormous sums of money by playing the odds and expecting that most people will lose. This is a successful strategy for them. And many people lose, some with disastrous personal consequences, by imagining that they are exempt from the statistical rules that apply to groups and that some special individual factor will allow them to beat the odds. Choosing to believe that general statistical principles don't apply to them because they are special and unique ruins people's lives in Las Vegas, and in medicine. Choosing to play with or against the odds, as defined by formal research, is no guarantee, but it is much more likely to lead to a good outcome than imagining the odds don't matter because each of us is unique.

The other major problem with herbalists' claims to individualize treatments is that they essentially use the same general process for coming up with individual treatments that science uses, only they use a far less reliable version of it. If a series of controlled studies indicates that Treatment X is better than Treatment Y for a certain disease, and if I use this to support giving patients with that disease Treatment X most of the time, then I am applying information gained from population research to individuals. I am playing the odds. This is imperfect, and it still requires monitoring, feedback from the patient, and ongoing adjustment. But history shows this method works pretty well much of the time.

However, if a herbalist looks at a patient and evaluates their particular characteristics and then decides on a specific treatment, where do they come up with the connection between the patient's characteristics and the treatment? They typically use their personal experience, gained from seeing what happens with prior patients. If, for example, they have seen certain symptoms resolve when using a particular herbal remedy, then they are likely to use that same remedy in the future with patients who have similar symptoms. This is a rational approach but, as I discussed at the very beginning of this book, it is subject to all the errors and pitfalls of anecdote and personal observation.

Alternative therapists also often use rules laid down by other practitioners based on their own experiences. Just as homeopaths frequently rely on books written by Hahnemann or other homeopaths that indicate which remedies are useful for which symptoms, so herbalists may choose therapies based on the observations or experiences of other herbalists, whether historical figures, teachers and mentors, or contemporary colleagues. They specifically identify herbal medicine as a "traditional" therapy precisely because it often means relying on tradition, that is the use of particular plants for specific conditions or symptoms as dictated by the trial-and-error observations of past herbalists.

Herbalists and other alternative practitioners also commonly rely on general rules based on the theoretical ideas behind the approach they use to decide which therapies to employ for a particular patient. Beliefs about vital energies, seasonal symptom patterns, or clinical observations such as the color of the tongue, are used to guide the selection of treatments. Herbal recipes are "individualized" partly by using theoretical patterns of association described or invented by other herbalists based on their experiences with their own patients.

In all of these methods, however, the practitioners are extrapolating from observations made on other patients to the individual they are currently treating. This is exactly the same as what a science-based practitioner does with one important difference: the generalizations that scientific medicine applies to individual patients come from formal, controlled research designed to compensate for the unreliability of individual observations and judgments, whereas the generalizations used in alternative therapies come from informal, unstructured observations with no control for bias or the many common errors that mislead us when we study disease. Alternative practitioners, such as herbalists, are using generalizations based on the study of groups to decide how to treat each new case just like clinicians in scientific medicine do. They are just relying on poorer quality group evidence.

Pharmacognosy and Zoopharmacognosy

Herbalists often justify their practices, whether rooted in one of the popular folk traditions or ostensibly more scientific theories, by pointing out that many conventional medicines are derived from plants. This is somehow intended to justify the use of plants as medicine generally, but we have already seen, in the example of artemisinin, why this is mistaken.

The scientific practice of pharmacognosy (deriving medicines from natural substances) involves a time-consuming, rigorous process of identifying chemical compounds, evaluating their properties in light of all that is known about chemistry, physiology, and the specifics of particular diseases, and then testing the potential value of these compounds at every level, from the test tube and lab animal model through clinical trials in real patients.[17] This is the best method for finding the truly safe and effective medicines hidden in plants. It weeds out the majority of candidates, and most compounds fail to prove safe enough or useful enough to actually test in patients. As slow and frustrating as this process can be, it has been stunningly successful and led to much greater reduction in human and animal suffering than thousands of years of folk herbal medicine practices.

Veterinary herbalists will sometimes also make the claim that we should believe in the value of plant remedies without following the conventional scientific process because animals in nature use plants medicinally (a behavior called zoopharmacognosy). Evolution clearly would not have favored such a behavior if it wasn't effective, so we are encouraged to rely on this as a source of evidence for veterinary herbal medicine.

This is an appealing idea, but is it true? Do animals self-medicate? I would say the answer is a qualified "Yes." However, the leap from the few examples of animals selecting plants to eat that have some beneficial health effects to the idea that herbal medicine is a safe and reliable approach to therapy is a long one, and I wouldn't encourage you to take it.

There is good evidence that some animals have evolved adaptive behaviors which include selecting certain food sources preferentially when the individual has a medical problem which that particular food source can improve. Most of this comes from the study of relatively simple animals. Some butterflies, for example, choose to lay eggs on plants with different levels of certain chemicals depending on whether or not the butterflies are infested with a particular parasite.[18] This choice improves the survival of larvae infested with the parasite, so it is a kind of self-medication.

209

There is considerably less evidence that animals consistently make accurate choices about ingesting specific substances to treat or prevent specific medical conditions.[19] The numerous anecdotes of behaviors which appear to suggest this could easily be matched by anecdotes of behaviors which are clearly self-injurious. There is ample evidence that animals make maladaptive choices about food. Animals ingest poisons and inedible foreign objects readily, so we can't rely on what they choose to eat to indicate which plants might have medicinal value.

A common experience for many pet owners is seeing their dog or cat eat grass. Sometimes, these pets will vomit after eating grass, and many of my clients believe that their pets do this on purpose, that they eat grass intentionally to make themselves vomit because they need to expel something from their system. Other clients worry that plant eating in their pets indicates a nutritional deficiency or other health problem. Is this a case of zoopharmacognosy?

The evidence is limited, but it indicates that eating grass and other plants is a normal behavior for domestic cats and dogs and even for some wild carnivores.[20-24] Studies have not found any association between eating grass and illness, and most of the time cats and dogs don't vomit after eating plant material. In a beautiful illustration of the kind of cognitive bias I discussed in Chapter 1, we simply notice when our pets vomit after eating grass and fail to notice when they don't, which leaves us with the impression they must be eating grass to induce vomiting. It requires controlled studies to show that this normal behavior, whatever its cause or function, is not a response to sickness or an effort to purge something toxic from the body.

In any case, while some animals may have evolved to seek out plants or other substances with medicinal effects in some situations, this has little to do with the elaborate systems of theory and belief that underlie most herbal prescribing, and it doesn't validate the particular claims for specific herbal remedies.

VARIETIES OF HERBAL MEDICINE

Herbal medicine is a catchall term for any use of plants as remedies for illness. However, there are many different approaches to understanding disease and then selecting herbal remedies to prevent or treat it. While these different approaches often have a lot in common, such as some of the general concepts I have just discussed, they also have significant theoretical and practical differences. Interestingly, herbalists and other alternative practitioners don't often seem concerned about the fundamentally incompatible concepts that distinguish different approaches to herbal medicine or other alternative therapies.

If, for example, the principles of homeopathy I described earlier, such as the Law of Similars and the strengthening of remedies by dilution are true, then the principles behind most herbal medicine diagnosis and prescribing must be wrong since they are incompatible. Yet it is common for homeopaths to use herbal remedies and for herbalists to recommend treatments from homeopathy or acupuncture or other alternative approaches. And many herbalists subscribe to the integrative medicine concept, in which science-based and traditional folk remedies can be compatible or even synergistic despite being derived from completely different and contradictory understandings of health and disease.

Nevertheless, most herbalists will at least nominally follow one of the predominant approaches to herbal prescribing. These include the Traditional Chinese Medicine system, the Ayurvedic herbal practices of India, a variety of herbalism traditions originating in Europe or North America and collectively often referred to as Western Herbal Medicine, as well as the less common practice of using herbs based predominantly on conventional scientific diagnoses and the limited scientific research information available about herbal remedies.

Chinese Herbal Medicine

I discussed briefly the basic theoretical foundations of TCM in the earlier chapter on acupuncture. Though this is quite an extensive and complex set of theoretical principles, it is heavily rooted in Daoist philosophy and pre-scientific religious and folk beliefs. Disease is seen as an imbalance in largely metaphorical substances such as Heat and Cold, Wind and Damp, Yin and Yang, Qi of various kinds, and so on. Such imbalance is detected in the quality of the pulse, the color and texture of the tongue, and in patterns of symptoms, such as the season or time of day they appear to improve or worsen, their location in the body, subjective character, and many others.[25]

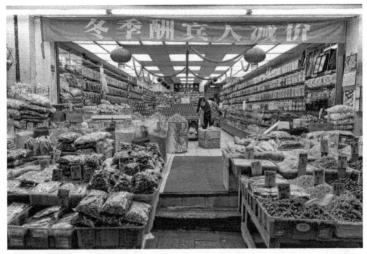

Chinese Medicine Shop 2016 by Edna Winti under Creative Commons by SA 2.0

While it is a very complex system, it is ultimately highly subjective. Both the interpretation of specific indicators, such as the quality of the pulse, and the relevance of historical details, such as the time of day the animal owner recalls the symptoms seeming better or worse, are subject to the whims of individual observation and memory. This subjectivity is seen as part of the "individualization" of diagnosis and treatment, though hopefully our earlier discussion of how we evaluate medical therapies has shown why it is actually a deep problem with TCM herbalism and other varieties of alternative medicine.

The selection of remedies is equally subjective. Particular plants, and most often complex mixtures of plants as well as animal products (such as black bear bile, rhinoceros horn, dried seahorses, and many others), are determined appropriate for particular conditions based on a variety of sources. Traditional Chinese Medicine texts, some thousands of years old, are still often used to guide the selection of remedies. As I discussed earlier, this is simply trusting the individual observations and opinions of practitioners, including some who lived long before any modern scientific understanding of physiology or health.

The historical determination of the uses of plants in medicine often rely on superficial characteristics of plants interpreted through the general theories of TCM. This is a variety of the "sympathetic magic" I discussed in the section on homeopathy, and it is often called the "doctrine of signatures" in herbalism. For example, red plants are viewed as stimulating circulation or relieving the stagnation of fluids or energies based on the perception of red as a vigorous or active color. Roots of plants are thought more likely to support patients with deficiencies and flowers or bark to disperse infectious agents or parasites from the outer regions of the body, based on the locations of these structures in the overall anatomy of the plant.[3]

One of the most significant guides to the utility of plant remedies has been thought to be taste. Plants with pungent odors or spicy taste are thought to be stimulating or warming and to be good for relieving pain. Bitter-tasting plants, on the other hand, might be used for calming or slowing bodily functions, such as reducing fever or inflammation. Some TCM herbalist, and others, appear to believe strongly that this sort of personal experience of a plant's properties is even more useful than any scientific analysis of its constituents or effects. For example:

> Theoretical knowledge is sterile compared with traditional herbalists' approach of tasting each herb, experiencing its unique qualities, and discerning its properties.
>
> Observing herbs and tasting them directly…is of great benefit, as is taking the herbs for a course of therapy to experience the effects.

Placebos for Pets?

Herbalists who follow this path will know at a deep experiential level what it is they are prescribing.[3]

Unfortunately, there is no consistent scientific evidence to support this sort of intuitive, subjective kind of association between appearance or taste and medicinal effects. Certainly, the use of thousands of plants in TCM and other herbal traditions for nearly every imaginable problem has led to some chance associations that can be cited as evidence for this. Cinchona bark, for example, is bitter, and it does turn out to have a compound in it that can attack the parasite responsible for malaria, which might then reduce the fever that is a characteristic symptom of this disease. However, the vast majority of such associations have not been shown to be real, and it is easy to find many more counter-examples. For example, Cinchona bark, like artemisinin, would be of no use for fevers from most causes other than malaria, such as viral infection, bacterial infection, auto-immune disease, cancer, and so on.

And it would be easy for different individuals or cultures to assign entirely different significance to the same features of a given plant. A red plant could just as easily be claimed to reduce bleeding or inflammation based on its color as to stimulate circulation or movement of fluids. And instead of using Lungwort to treat breathing problems based on its vague similarity in shape to a human lung, it could be argued to be useful for skin disease because of its spots.

In fact, nearly all herbal remedies have been used for a great variety of unrelated medical problems based on the slippery and subjective nature of the doctrine of signatures. In addition to breathing problems, for example,

215

lungwort was used in the Western tradition to treat dysentery, excessive menstrual bleeding, wounds, and other ills.[3]

A currently popular herbal product originating in the TCM system is ginseng root. It has a vaguely humanoid shape, which has been the basis for much of the purported medical uses for it.

This shape has traditionally been interpreted as masculine, and this has been used as a basis for claiming the plant can function as a general tonic to "strengthen" health and combat weakness. This seems a bit sexist to me, since some ginseng roots seem rather feminine.

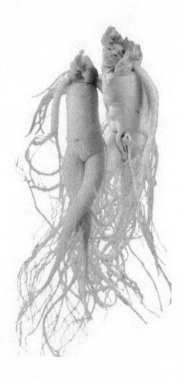

And some frankly don't look much like humans to me at all!

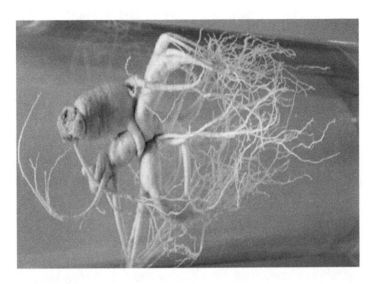

In any case, this general "strengthening" application has led to the use of ginseng in virtually any medical condition, from fatigue to infection, liver disease, cough, fever, vomiting, anxiety and even, somewhat counterintuitively, in pregnancy. So varied are its uses, the scientific name, Panax, actually comes from the Greek cognate of the Latin word "panacea," which means a cure-all.

Such varied use is sometimes claimed as an example of the superiority of herbal medicine over scientific medicine, since the concept of a cure-all has been largely abandoned in scientific medicine in the face of our failure to find any such remedy that survives scientific testing. However, it is more likely that the variety of uses to which ginseng has been put is actually an example of the vague, subjective nature of traditional herbal prescribing.

A great deal of scientific research has gone into trying to validate the many proposed benefits of ginseng. While this evidence is mixed and not entirely conclusive (which is nearly always the case for herbal medicine research, as I will discuss shortly), it does not support the claims that this magical root can support and strengthen nearly any patient with any problem, despite its "manly" appearance and all the anecdotal, trial-and-error use that has been made of it.[26]

There are many other examples of the unscientific system TCM uses to define medical problems and assign treatments, including herbal remedies. Even though the plants used in these remedies undoubtedly contain many chemical compounds with potential uses in medicine, this kind of mystical traditional system is unlikely to be effective in identifying the benefits, or the dangers, of these compounds. The dominance of such traditional folk systems in herbal medicine is one of the greatest barriers to unlocking the true potential of plant-based medicines. The systematic, scientific path taken by Dr. Tu is a much more productive and promising approach.

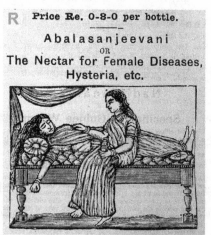

P. Gopalacharlu, Ayurvedic Medicines from the Welcome Collection Gallery under Creative Commons by SA 4.0

Ayurvedic Herbal Medicine

Ayurveda, a folk medicine tradition from India, is a metaphoric system with strong resemblances to both TCM and European humoral medicine.[3] The reason for the similarities in these geographically distinct systems is an interesting puzzle. Herbalists will often argue that they arise from some underlying truth about health and disease. Perhaps folk medicine traditions commonly identify disease as an imbalance in opposing forces, for example, because this is a true core principle in human biology, even if different systems may characterize the details of these forces and their manipulation quite differently.

Skeptics, on the other hand, are more likely to argue that the similarities result from consistent features in human reasoning that lie in our biology and largely transcend cultural context. We all have brains that see agency or purpose where there is only randomness and that look for patterns we can identify and manipulate, so we all find what we are predisposed to seek. This seems the most plausible explanation to me.

There is also a case to be made for historical communication between the cultures of Europe, India, and China that can explain some of the correspondences between different herbal medicine traditions. Perhaps the mystical energy forces associated with disease in Ayurveda (Purusha and Prakruti) are rough analogues of the forces discussed in TCM (Yin and Yang), and perhaps the vital energy called Prana in Ayurveda seems similar to the force known as Qi in TCM, because of a shared historical scaffolding of concepts behind both traditions.[27]

Whatever the origins, there are many general correspondences between Ayurveda and TCM that make them quite similar systems in the outline, though very different in the details of diagnostic and therapeutic practices. Metaphorical forces like cold and damp, wind and heat, and various proposed relationships between climate and time of day and temperament and others are also believed to characterize patients and their illnesses. Disease is viewed as an imbalance among the various forces and constituents of the spiritual and physical aspects of living things, and the goal of medical treatment is to identify the imbalance in metaphorical terms and then provide treatments, including herbal remedies, to restore balance.

As in TCM, herbs are categorized in terms of their inherent "energy" based on taste and other features. In both systems, combinations of herbs, often unique to individual practitioners who keep their recipes secret, are used more often than single plants. The prescription of herbs for medical problems traditionally takes no account of the scientific medical diagnosis or the chemical constituents of the plants. For convenience, however, Ayurvedic and TCM practitioners will sometimes list likely herbal remedies to employ for specific conditions named according to conventional medical practice. Such "integrative medicine" approaches claim the benefits of folk medicine tradition without adhering strictly to the diagnostic and therapeutic systems of those traditions while also claiming to be "scientific" despite the near total lack of scientific clinical research showing the practices to be safe and effective.

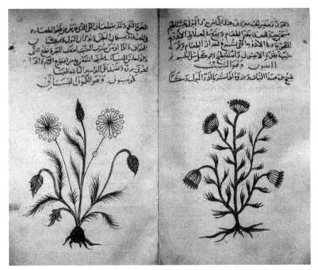

Arabic Herbal Medicine Guidebook

OTHER HERBAL TRADITIONS

European, Middle Eastern, and Native American cultures have a long history of using herbal remedies, but the herbal traditions of China and India are probably more commonly practiced today. With the rise of scientific medicine in the West, humoral medicine and other indigenous herbal traditions were largely abandoned. Some herbalists have revived the use of traditional Western plant remedies, even though they generally have not brought back the system of humorism. The use of particular herbal remedies for specific problems is more often based not on a general theoretical system, as in Ayurveda and TCM, but on historical sources recommending these practices, general herbalist principles like those discussed earlier (detoxification, tonics, doctrine of signatures, and so on), or on the basis of limited scientific research on the properties of particular plants and plant chemicals. Western herbalism tends to be more of an integrative medicine practice, borrowing

221

from science and folk medicine, and less purely traditionalist than TCM and Ayurveda.

There are also herbal remedies that appear to have been invented out of whole cloth by individuals. Essiac and Bach flower essences are two examples of this.

Essiac Tea is a concoction invented by a Canadian nurse in the 1920s.[28,29] She claimed it to be a traditional Native American herbal remedy, but there is no objective historical evidence for this. It contains a variety of plant ingredients, but the inventor and the company that subsequently bought the rights to the remedy have never disclosed a verified, consistent formula, and the particular herbs in the mixture appear to have changed over time.[30,31] This is a common and potentially dangerous characteristic of many herbal remedies, which I will return to in the section on the safety of herbal medicine.

Essiac has been primarily marketed for cancer treatment, though many other claims have been made for it, from detoxification to boosting immune function to breaking down mucus and lowering cholesterol.[31,32] The limited research done on this product hasn't supported any of these claims, in people or in animals. Some test tube and lab animal studies show effects that might potentially have benefits,[33,34,35] but other studies find no effect,[30,36,37] and there is even evidence Essiac could make some cancers grow faster.[38] There is no clinical trial evidence, in humans or in animals, to suggest real-world benefits.[30,39,40] This is an example of a remedy that has persisted in use without either a rationale from a specific folk tradition or any plausible scientific theory for why it should be safe or beneficial.

Placebos for Pets?

A similarly idiosyncratic example of the varieties of herbal medicine can be found in Bach flower essences. Dr. Edward Bach was a physician and homeopath in England in the late nineteenth and early twentieth centuries. He eventually gave up his medical practice to focus full-time on developing a system of treatment based on elements of homeopathy and his own ideas about health and disease.[41]

A classic vitalist, Bach believed that all disease was primarily spiritual in origin and due to negative emotions. These emotions are the manifestation of a conflict between the divine energy of the spirit and the limitations and weaknesses of the physical body and the mind. He became convinced that certain flowers possess unique energetic resonances that can help dispel negative feelings and re-establish balance between body and spirit.[41]

Dr. Bach identified the healing properties of specific flowers intuitively, by touching a flower or putting a petal on his tongue and then observing changes in his own feelings. He compiled an extensive list of specific flowers and combinations indicated for specific emotions and situations. The most popular Bach remedy currently is Rescue Remedy®, a mixture of five flower essences purported to be calming during sudden emotional crises.[41,42]

Dr. Bach initially treated people with dew from flowers, which he believed absorbed the signature energy of the plant, but because of the limited quantity of dew which could be produced he began instead to soak flowers in water and then collect this. The water was then mixed 1:1 with brandy and this stock solution dispensed to patients. The patient generally would take several drops of the stock solution directly or mixed into a beverage. The Dr. Edward Bach Centre continues to produce flower essences by these methods and holds the rights to the term Bach Flower Essence, though other manufacturers make products produced in a similar manner under other brand names.

Due to the extreme dilution of the remedies, flower essences contain only very small quantities of alcohol, and they are unlikely to contain much in the way of residual chemicals from the plants used in their preparation. In this way, they resemble homeopathic remedies, but they are produced and used according to a different system, and they do sometimes have actual chemical compounds in them, if only alcohol in many cases.

Despite the implausible ideas behind these products, several clinical studies of Bach flower remedies have been conducted in humans. They consistently show no effect, and it is pretty clear that Bach flower remedies are nothing more than a placebo.[42–46] Unfortunately, this information seems to do little to discourage their use.

Bach flower essences and Essiac are only two examples of many plant-based remedies in current use in the developed world which do not come from the dominant lineages of TCM or Ayurveda. The plausibility of claims made for such products is often difficult to evaluate since there is no coherent theory behind how they might work. Products like Rescue Remedy® and Essiac lack any controlled scientific research to support their use, relying on testimonial and anecdote as folk remedies always have. Now that we understand why this kind of evidence isn't reliable, let's take a look at what better evidence there might be for herbal remedies.

DOES IT WORK?

I have cheated a bit and discussed this question some already. A global answer to whether "herbal medicine" as a category is effective is impossible since the question is too vague to be meaningful. The theories behind much herbal prescribing, from TCM, Ayurveda, vitalism, and other approaches, are implausible from a scientific perspective. This doesn't mean they can't be true, only that much of established scientific knowledge and methodology would have to be wrong if they are true, and that's not a bet I would take.

In terms of scientific research on specific herbal remedies, there is actually quite a large literature to investigate. Herbalists often point to the existence of TCM and herbal medicine journals and the sheer number of research articles as proof that their field is "scientific" and their methods work. Sadly, this is not necessarily true. Homeopathy has dedicated journals and thousands of scientific articles published about it, and a careful, thorough reading of this material shows it is worthless. Acupuncture has an even larger and more impressive research literature, yet even so there is little compelling evidence to support specific claims made for acupuncture treatment in real patients. Are you tired of hearing that the devil is in the details yet?

In general, the research literature in herbal medicine supports a number of specific claims:

1. Plants contain a large number of chemical compounds with many interesting effects on the physiology of animals.

2. Some of these effects have the potential to be useful as medical treatments.

3. A small percentage of these compounds have been tested in animal models of disease or on a small scale in humans. This testing suggests some may be clinically useful, but such testing often fails to accurately predict the safety and efficacy of medicines once they are used widely in real patients.

4. There is reasonable clinical trial evidence in humans supporting some specific claims for a small number of herbal remedies.

5. There is virtually no high-quality clinical trial evidence for herbal remedies in companion animals.

6. Those herbal remedies which have shown some beneficial effects in clinical trials also have potential risks.

Because herbal medicine is such a huge and diverse subject that does not allow meaningful generalizations about whether it "works" or not, this is probably the best we can do in terms of an overall conclusion based on the evidence. The theories and methods of traditional herbal prescribe are implausible and haven't been proven correct, but some specific herbal products likely are beneficial for particular clinical problems in humans. Decisions about whether to use a particular remedy have to be made on a case-by-case basis.

A couple of representative examples may help to illustrate both the complexities of the evidence and decisions about using herbal medicines and how you can use our core three questions to evaluate claims about particular herbal treatments.

CANNABIS

What Is It?

Medical marijuana for humans has been a hot topic for many years. Much of the debate about it has focused on ethical and legal issues that aren't directly answerable through scientific research. Participants in these debates often gravitate towards ideological extremes. For some, any use of marijuana, medical or recreational, is immoral and dangerous. For those at the other extreme, marijuana is a perfect, risk-free cure for anything from depression to cancer.

In the last several years, these debates have migrated to veterinary medicine, with both extremes well represented. It has grown easier and more common for animal owners to provide their pets with cannabis-based remedies, both marijuana itself and products specifically produced for companion animals.

Cannabis sativa contains a bewildering variety of chemical compounds. Some have been shown to have significant effects on many different body systems, from the brain to the intestinal tract to the immune system. There is, therefore, good reason to believe cannabis-derived medicine could have real benefits, as well as real risks, in veterinary patients.

The chemical compound responsible for psychological effects associated with recreational cannabis is tetrahydrocannabinol (THC). While some studies have evaluated medical uses for this compound, its obvious side effects limit its use in people. And it turns out that dogs, at least, are even more sensitive to THC than humans, so it is unlikely to be a useful drug in veterinary patients.

The other main compound of interest is cannabidiol (CBD). This lacks most of the psychological effects of THC but seems to be responsible for some of the potential medical benefits of cannabis. There are also many, many other chemicals in the cannabis plant, as in all plants, and these may also turn out to be useful, individually or in combination. However, for now the best data involve CBD.

This, of course, is the scientific perspective. Traditional Chinese Medicine has been aware of the cannabis plant for centuries, and like most folk herbal traditions, beliefs about it and uses for the different parts of the plant have varied wildly. Contemporary TCM is mostly limited to using hemp seeds as a laxative, and there is not extensive use of other parts of the plant containing THC, CBD, and most of the chemical compounds of interest to scientific medicine. Historical sources, however, list a fascinating variety of apparently unrelated uses for the various parts of the plant[47]:

> Break accumulations, relieve impediments, and disperse pus, dispels wind, relieves pain, and settles tetany
> Treats headache, menstrual irregularities, itching, convulsions, anemia, and dry cough
> Indicated for "bone marrow wind toxin"
> Take one pill every morning facing the sun and after 100 days one will see ghosts [This appears to be both an intended effect and a potential risk since other sources say "excessive consumption causes one to see ghosts and run about frenetically"]
> Treats '120 types of malign wind' as well as itching, and expels all malign wind and blood; it was also indicated to treat lack of free flow following menstruation.
> Treats "agitation, hysteria, spasmodic cough, and nerve pain"[47]

The Ayurvedic perspective on cannabis is somewhat similar to the Chinese Medicine perspective. While some uses are identified in historic texts, it was not viewed as an important herbal remedy. According to one source, "cannabis is sharp, heating and light in its quality...increases humoral bile and removes humoral phlegm...stimulates delusions, slows speech, and raises the heat of the digestive fire." However, "it is only ever recommended in miniscule doses, and always in combination with other more sattvic herbs to balance the tamasic effects of cannabis."[48] More attention is devoted to the spiritual imbalances created by recreational use than to potential health benefits, and it is generally viewed negatively in traditional sources.

Such a hodgepodge of clinical symptoms and vague spiritual maladies that cannabis is purported to create or relieve is typical for the broad and fanciful way in which herbs are evaluated in traditional folk medicine. While it is always possible to find particular uses that correspond to those demonstrated for specific compounds derived from the plant, this is not evidence that traditional uses correspond to modern medical practice. When folk tradition casts a wide enough net, claiming numerous vague uses for many plant remedies, it will catch some legitimate use from time to time, just as a sufficiently vague horoscope will sometimes seem to predict actual events. As we have already seen with *Artemesia*, Traditional Chinese Medicine employed the cannabis plant for centuries without developing a consistent, effective, rational understanding of the real risks and benefits of the plant, as scientific medicine is now beginning to do.

Ayurveda, similarly, was aware of the plant and made use of it, but the spiritual perspective of the approach led to a focus on the negative impact of marijuana use on the progress towards enlightenment, rather than a rational empirical approach to discovering its medical risks and benefits. The haphazard nature of traditional trial-and-error and anecdote-based medicine is simply not an efficient, reliable method for evaluating herbs and making effective use of the potential in herbal medicines.

Does It Work?

There have been quite a few studies on cannabis-derived medicines in humans, though these have been limited by legal restrictions. A comprehensive review by the US National Academies of Science, Engineering, and Medicine identified strong evidence that cannabis can reduce nausea in patients getting cancer treatment and can help those suffering from chronic pain.[49] There is also compelling evidence that CBD can reduce seizures in children with a particular kind of epilepsy that is very difficult to control.[50]

There are very few published studies of cannabis in veterinary patients, though recent changes in relevant laws and in public attitudes have stimulated a great deal of interest, and several studies are now ongoing. At this point, we have some basic information about how CBD is absorbed and metabolized in dogs, which suggests that it may be useful as a drug if given in the right form.[51,52] We also have one small clinical trial in dogs with arthritis showing meaningful improvements in pain and lameness.

Though this was a pretty good clinical trial, one study of sixteen dogs is not even close to the level of evidence that would be expected before a drug could be used in people, so it still has to be viewed as tentative. It certainly does not justify all the claims made for cannabis products, from treating pain and nausea to relieving dementia and even stopping cancer. These claims go far beyond even the evidence in humans, much less the far weaker data for animals. At this time, there is reason for optimism about the potential of cannabis-based medicines in veterinary patients, but there is very little real evidence, and nearly all the claims made for cannabis products on the market are unsupported.

Is It Safe?

In humans, many of the risks associated with marijuana use are psychological and likely due to THC. Substance abuse, auto accidents, and exacerbation of some psychiatric disorders in people are serious concerns, but they don't likely apply to veterinary use of CBD and other cannabis compounds. In general, cannabis does not appear to have serious, short-term side effects that significantly limit its medical use in humans.[49]

However, it is clear that marijuana exposure can have toxic effects on dogs and cats.[53,54] Pets are typically exposed to marijuana through ingesting edible forms, and they experience symptoms that range from mild to severe, though such exposure is rarely fatal. The primary compound responsible for this toxicity is THC, though it is possible that other compounds could also have undesirable effects, and we don't yet have enough evidence in dogs and cats to know.

There is also evidence that the greater availability of marijuana associated with legalization for human medical or recreational use can increase the incidence of marijuana poisoning in pets.[55] Many products intended for humans contain chocolate or other substances that pose a greater risk to pets than cannabis itself. There is little information on the safety of cannabis-based medical products aimed at the veterinary market, and there are no studies at all on long-term use. A survey of owners using such products did report low rates of undesirable effects, but this is only anecdotal.[56]

There is also concern about the consistency and labeling accuracy of medical cannabis products. Some states in the US that allow medical marijuana use in humans have standards for labeling and quality control testing. However, there is evidence cannabis products are frequently inconsistent in composition and labeling despite these regulations.[57,58] Even if CBD or other chemicals in cannabis have beneficial effects, patients won't experience these if they are buying products that don't contain the level of CBD they claim or that have other undisclosed ingredients that might be harmful. Given the complete absence of regulation or testing for veterinary cannabis-derived remedies, it is impossible to evaluate the consistency or labeling of these products, but they are likely to be at least as unreliable as products intended for human use. This issue of quality control is a major problem with herbal medicine generally, which I will talk more about when we get to the question of safety.

Bottom Line

Cannabis is a great example of a plant with lots of potential medical benefits that were never identified by the trial-and-error practices of folk herbalism but which science has begun to uncover. So far, there is substantial evidence for only a couple of uses in humans. As far as veterinary research, there is limited clinical trial evidence only for the use of CBD to treat arthritis in dogs. Lots of other possible uses remain untested. There is also a tremendous problem with lack of regulation and quality assurance for veterinary canna-bis-based products, so while CBD itself seems to pose little direct health risk, it is unclear how risky using particular cannabis products might be.

Right now, CBD might be a reasonable thing to try for dogs with ar-thritis pain, once better-demonstrated treatments, such as weight loss and conventional pain medications, have been tried. However, there is a great deal of research going on, and as more evidence appears we will be better able to make reliable choices about what kind of cannabis-based remedies to use, how to use them, and what the likely risks and benefits are. This is how scientific herbal medicine can and should work, and if we stick to the slow but tried-and-true scientific methods, other plant-derived remedies may turn out to be safe and useful medicines as cannabis seems to be.

GINKGO BILOBA

What Is It?

Ginkgo serves as a different kind of example of herbal medicine than cannabis. Despite a long history of medical and recreational use, the true medicinal potential of cannabis has largely been missed by folk medicine tradition. This is partly due to the inherent haphazard nature of folk medicine generally, and also to the influence of the obvious recreational effects on attitudes towards the plant, which continues to impede appropriate scientific research into its risks and benefits. Science is beginning to overcome both the limitations of traditional methods for evaluating the potential of cannabis and the negative attitudes associated with it by illustrating the reality of the risks (less dire than portrayed by both TCM and Ayurvedic spiritualism and Western cultural moralism) and the benefits (potentially greater than understood by folk medical traditions though likely less than the extremes promoted by modern herbalists).

Ginkgo, on the other hand has been widely accepted as a treatment in both Chinese Medicine and modern Western Herbalism. There has also been a fair bit of scientific research on the plant, and there is widespread belief that it is a herbal medicine success story, an example of traditional herbal medicine eventually validated by science. That narrative, however, has some serious holes in it.

Chinese Medicine theory classifies ginkgo as sweet, astringent, bitter, and energetically neutral (neither warming nor cooling), except for the root, which is classified as warming. Historical sources vary on the meridians or channels it supposedly interacts with, most agreeing the lung channel and some suggesting heart, bladder, and kidney. All of these categorizations, of course, correspond to the unscientific folk beliefs underlying TCM, not the scientific conceptions of organ function. The effects of ginkgo to "astringe lung and kidney Qi deficiency" or to "tonify heart" are fanciful concepts employed before there was any real understanding of anatomy and physiology.[59] Whatever the true effects of chemicals in the ginkgo plant, employing such concepts to guide the use of this herb makes little sense.

Because of this reliance on folk concepts to determine the application of ginkgo, the traditional uses for this plant in Chinese medicine were varied and not rationally connected to any specific mechanism of action. Different parts of the plant have been recommended for conditions as varied as asthma and chest pain, vaginal discharge and problems with urination. Modern herbalism has dramatically expanded the list of purported uses for ginkgo to include circulatory problems, Alzheimer's disease and other forms of dementia, depression, memory enhancement, tinnitus, hemorrhoids and diseases of the retina.[59,60] Such a laundry list of unrelated diseases all supposedly treated by one remedy is always a warning sign of unscientific and unrealistic claims.

Like most plants, *Ginkgo biloba* contains an enormous variety of chemical compounds.[61,62] Obviously, these exist to perform functions of relevance to the plant, such as defense against being eaten, not as a pharmacy for humans. However, extensive laboratory research has identified and categorized many of these chemical compounds and found some intriguing effects on isolated tissues of lab animals, such as rats and mice. By itself, this doesn't tell us if we or our pets should take ginkgo, it simply opens up avenues of research that might or might not lead to safe and effective medicines. Many of these avenues have been explored by scientists in the last few decades, and the results can help us answer the second of our standard questions...

Does It Work?

As you know by this point, a confident answer to this question can only be found when we focus on multiple, high-quality clinical studies of specific products or preparations for particular diseases in the type of patient we want to treat. A study showing increased blood flow to the brain in healthy mice doesn't mean ginkgo is effective in treating humans with Alzheimer's disease. A small single study in humans looking at the use of ginkgo for memory loss doesn't tell us if dogs with canine cognitive dysfunction syndrome should be given ginkgo. The devil is in the details, and our conclusions always have to be proportional to the strength of evidence that is specific to the question we are asking.

This is tough with herbal remedies like ginkgo that are touted as treatments for multiple unrelated problems. Despite hundreds of clinical trials involving various ginkgo products for various medical conditions, the National Center for Complementary and Integrative Health in the US still admits "there is no conclusive evidence that ginkgo is helpful for any health condition."[63] It is possible to find specific studies, and even systematic reviews that conclude there is a benefit for particular conditions, but the limitations in the research and the contradictory nature of different studies still makes it impossible to confidently claim there are any scientifically proven benefits for ginkgo. The evidence is sufficiently weak and murky that different analyses come to different conclusions, which is not typically the case with clearly and unequivocally effective treatments.

This may be surprising to you, as it was to me, given how widely ginkgo is used and believed, even by mainstream, conventional medical doctors, that this is an example of a herbal remedy with proven benefits. Unfortunately, that confidence and use is based on a shaky foundation of evidence.

Studies of ginkgo for brain disease in humans have been mixed, with no clear benefits in treating Alzheimer's disease or dementia or in preventing or slowing cognitive decline in the elderly.[64–68] There is also no strong evidence for benefits in treating tinnitus,[69] circulatory problems, including high blood pressure[70] and stroke,[71] altitude sickness,[72] asthma,[73] premenstrual symptoms, or glaucoma.[74] Many other purported uses have been evaluated, but the evidence is too limited to draw firm conclusions. Overall, this adds up to a lot of people taking ginkgo without any conclusive evidence that they are getting any benefit from it.

What about use in veterinary patients? Not surprisingly, there are plenty of lab studies in mice and rats, and a few in dogs, but no reliable clinical trial evidence for naturally occurring disease in dogs and cats. The few studies that have been done have serious methodological limitations.[75,76] These are preliminary kinds of studies which help clarify our hypotheses, but they don't show that ginkgo has real benefits for any specific problem in our pets.

Veterinary herbalists often assume benefits seen in humans (whether proven scientifically or simply assumed from traditional use and personal experience) should also be found in animals, so ginkgo is recommended for problems in veterinary patients that resemble those it is used for in people. A number of products marketed for cognitive dysfunction syndrome (a behavioral disorder analogous to dementia in people) contain ginkgo. However, we've already seen that there is no convincing evidence ginkgo is beneficial for people with dementia, and you know that extrapolating from people to animal patients is a dodgy proposition. This use for ginkgo hasn't been validated in any meaningful way.

There has been one published report of ginkgo extract given to elderly dogs with behavioral problems, but it involved no placebo or blinding or other controls bias at all, so the fact that the authors report overwhelmingly positive effects says more about their existing beliefs and expectations than about whether or not ginkgo might be useful for dogs with cognitive dysfunction.[77] Such small, uncontrolled studies in humans also tended to have encouraging results, but these disappeared when proper controls were used in subsequent trials. This is yet another example of the importance of proper methods to make sure our research studies are reliable and not misleading or a waste of time and resources.

A combination product marketed for cognitive dysfunction in dogs contains ginkgo along with other ingredients, and there have been a couple of studies looking at this product.[76,77] These are small studies, often with little or no controls for bias or funded by the manufacturer, and they have other important limitations. They seem to show some beneficial effects, but whether these are real, and whether they are due to ginkgo or some other component of the product, is unclear. We can have little confidence in the conclusions of such research, especially given the much stronger study evidence in humans that has failed to find convincing benefits of ginkgo for dementia in people.

At this point, it really isn't clear if there are any meaningful benefits to various ginkgo-derived remedies. As the evidence grows, we may find some, or we may find that, as often happens, the encouraging early trials were misleading and bigger, better studies contradict them. Right now, the only honest answer to the question "Does it work?" is "Not so far as we can tell."

Is It Safe?

There have been some concerns about risks associated with ginkgo products. This, as I've said before, would be a good sign in some ways since any product with real benefits will inevitably have some risks. It is clear that the raw ginkgo seeds can be toxic to the brain, causing unconsciousness and seizures. The risk of such symptoms from cooked seeds or preparations of ginkgo leaves appears to be lower, but the exact concentration of toxic agents in the plant often aren't known in specific ginkgo products since these are not regulated or tested consistently.[78,79,80]

Minor side effects are commonly reported by people taking ginkgo, such as headache, dizziness, and constipation. Whether the remedy is truly the cause of these symptoms is difficult to determine in everyday use. Allergic reactions have also been seen to ginkgo preparations.[78,79]

One of the most significant concerns has been about the potential that ginkgo might cause bleeding. There are several cases in the medical literature of people experiencing abnormal blood clotting and bleeding while taking ginkgo preparations. However, formal reviews of this literature do not find a clear or consistent causal relationship in such cases, and the risk of bleeding for healthy people taking ginkgo is likely low.[81] Most experts do recommend avoiding use of ginkgo in combination with other medicines or herbal products that might increase bleeding risk or in people with a known blood clotting disorder.

There have been some worrying reports of an increased risk of certain cancers, specifically in the liver and thyroid gland, in lab animals given high doses of ginkgo over a prolonged period.[78,82] This is the kind of risk that is very difficult to identify in humans when there is widespread use of herbal products without any formal surveillance for long-term effects, so such lab studies are important in giving us an idea of what to look out for. However, such rodent studies often do not accurately predict risks or benefits in humans or other species, so it is not clear that this is a real risk for people or veterinary patients taking ginkgo.

Finally, there are many reports of negative interactions between ginkgo and other medicines.[83,84,85] This shouldn't be surprising to anyone who understands that both drugs and herbal remedies are chemicals that interact with the physiology of patients who take them and with each other in incredibly complex ways. I've already discussed why the belief that because herbal remedies are, in some ill-defined sense, "natural" they should be inherently safe is a dangerous misconception. Plant chemicals are inherently no more likely to do good or to cause harm than any other chemical, regardless of whether we call them "herbal remedies" or "drugs." The main difference between herbs and drugs is that herbal remedies typically have not been through a rigorous scientific process, such as that described above for arte-misinin, that allows us to understand the interactions and risks and benefits much better than we can with simple trial and error.

Ginkgo can enhance or interfere with the absorption, activity, and me-tabolism of prescription or over-the-counter medicines depending on the detailed pharmacology of these drugs. Some of the compounds in the plant alter the way the liver processes other drugs, which may lead to too much or too little of these medicines in the patient's system. As mentioned already, there is some concern ginkgo may affect blood clotting, so there are concerns about using it with other medicines that effect the clotting system. Such in-teractions are complicated and difficult to predict, but in some individuals they can lead to serious harm.

There is virtually no research looking at the safety of ginkgo in veteri-nary patients. No dramatic and obvious risks are apparent, but we haven't been looking very hard for them. All we can do is hope that the safety in dogs and cats approximates that in humans and lab animals and hope for the best, but this is not a very satisfying approach, especially given the lack of strong reason to expect real benefits.

Bottom Line

Ginkgo provides an example of a herbal remedy with a very different history from that of cannabis. Cannabis was somewhat neglected by herbal medicine tradition and restricted legally for many years, and now science has begun to discover several potential uses for it. Ginkgo has a long history of traditional use and widespread adoption beyond the confines of Chinese medicine or other herbal traditions, yet science has not consistently found good evidence to support the claims made for it. While the risks of ginkgo are probably low for healthy individuals not taking many other medicines or herbal products, the case for meaningful benefits is weak. Science is always evolving, of course, and the possible risks and benefits of this plant will likely become clearer with more research. So far, though, it seems like most of the time and money spent on ginkgo has not been spent well.

IS IT SAFE?

As I said at the outset, herbal medicines are among the most promising of alternative therapies because they contain active chemical compounds that can be identified and evaluated and that often interact with the physiology of animals in interesting, and potentially beneficial, ways. This, of course, also means herbal remedies are likely to pose some risk since not all these interactions are likely to be benign. Specific dangers from particular herbal products can be identified, but often there is minimal research directed at finding such effects, so safety is more often assumed than proven. This may be sufficient to protect us against dramatic, common short-term harm, but such a casual, haphazard approach is not likely to identify less common, less apparent, and long-term injury.

Even the extensive research required of pharmaceuticals sometimes fails to uncover important risks that only become apparent through post-marketing monitoring once these medicines have gone into widespread use. The relative lack of pre-market research and absence of any structured post-marketing monitoring system makes it likely that patients are being harmed by some of these products and we simply don't know about it.

Unfortunately, it is possible to find many examples of individuals harmed by herbal medications. In 1998, Sandra Stay was a 56-year-old mother of six working in the catering industry in England. She had suffered for many years from psoriasis, an uncomfortable skin condition that conventional medicine can help manage but cannot cure. Out of desperation, Sandra saw a Chinese Medicine doctor and was prescribed a herbal remedy. She took the remedy for three years and felt that it helped her skin condition. Then, in 2001, she began having headaches, nausea, and other symptoms. Eventually, it was discovered that she had severe and irreversible kidney damage from Aristolochia, one of the ingredients in the herbal remedy she had been taking. Sandra will have to have regular dialysis treatments for the rest of her life.[86] Many other people have experienced this same injury, and despite evidence showing that this herb is dangerous, and no evidence showing it has any benefits, it continues to be used in Chinese herbal remedies.[87,88,89]

An even more dramatic example of the dangers of herbal products is the case of bloodroot, sometimes known as black salve.[90–93] This plant-based product is often recommended for both topical and internal use as a cancer treatment. It is claimed that it kills only cancer cells and spares healthy tissue. However, there are numerous reports of cases like this.

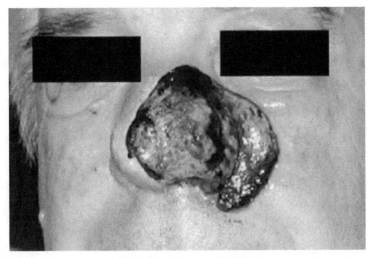

Image from Eastman (2011).[94]

This is a picture of a 63-year-old man who treated a suspected skin cancer with black salve and experienced severe burns, losing half of his nose. Despite this, he continued to treat not only skin lesions with this herbal product but elected to take an oral version when he was diagnosed with colon cancer, from which he eventually died.[94]

There is some evidence that bloodroot derivatives can kill cancer cells in lab experiments. However, they do not reliable spare healthy cells, and there are no clinical trials showing they work in real patients or that they are worth the risk.[90,92]

Other examples of specific harm caused to human patients by herbal remedies include liver cancer associated with herbs containing Aristolochia,[95,96,97] liver damage caused by kava, kratom, khat, pennyroyal, comfrey, and many other herbal products,[98,99,100] heart rhythm abnormalities from aconite,[101] electrolyte abnormalities and muscle damage caused by licorice,[102] low blood sugar and other negative effects associated with ginseng use,[103] heart attacks and strokes caused by ephedra,[104,105,106] and many others.

In veterinary patients, as always, there is less evidence, but serious harm has been seen with some herbal remedies, including severe chemical burns from bloodroot. A report in the Journal of the American Veterinary Medical Association in 2011 identified two golden retrievers who had benign tumors injected with a bloodroot product. Both experienced localized tissue damage, and one developed a huge area of dead tissue that had to be surgically removed. This dog required multiple treatments under anesthesia and physical therapy to regain full function due to the size and severity of this wound.[107]

Other direct injures from herbal preparations reported in pets include seizures and even death from tea tree oil and other essential oils,[108–111] anemia from garlic,[112] liver damage from pennyroyal, comfrey, and many of the herbs that cause this problem in humans,[113,114] seizures and heart problems due to ephedra,[115] and others.[116,117]

Unfortunately, reports received by veterinarians or pet poison control services of adverse reactions to herbal remedies are often not followed up with active research, so the details of what risks these products pose in which species at what dose, and so on, are often unknown. Even without aggressive monitoring, it is not difficult to find examples of direct harm from toxic components in herbal remedies. The real question is how many other examples of such harm could we find if we looked harder?

There are many dangers to herbal medicine that are less obvious than direct toxic effects. One that this field of alternative medicine has in common with most others is the harm that comes from delaying or avoiding effective science-based treatment in favor of using herbal remedies. Most herbal products haven't been effectively evaluated scientifically, and they cannot be relied upon as effective medicine solely based on traditional use or anecdotes. Sadly, people and pets suffer and die needlessly from distrust of science-based medicine and reliance on unproven "natural" alternatives.[118–124]

As I mentioned while discussing *Ginkgo biloba*, the chemicals in herbal remedies can also harm patients by interacting with prescription medications. Plant compounds can add to the effects of conventional medicines, they can block these effects, and they can either delay or hasten the normal metabolism and excretion of pharmaceuticals. All of these interactions can lead to harm, and often there is insufficient scientific research on herbal remedies to effectively predict when such interactions will occur.[117,125–129] It is also common for human patients and for pet owners not to tell their doctors about the use of herbal remedies. This makes it difficult to identify any harmful interactions between such remedies and other medications.

I always ask my clients if they are giving any medicine to their pets. If they say "No," I always follow up by asking specifically about vitamins, supplements, and herbal remedies. Very often clients will then admit to using some of these products. Unfortunately, the inaccurate characterization of alternative remedies as "natural" and inherently different from conventional medicines misleads people into thinking that they aren't medicines and that they don't have any potential risks. It is crucial that you tell your veterinarian about *anything* you give your pet so they can help evaluate the usefulness and safety of such products both in light of your pet's medical condition and in combination with any prescription medications your vet may want to recommend.

One risk of herbal remedies that I alluded to when discussing cannabis is the risk associated with limited regulation and quality control of herbal products. Testing of such products has frequently found potentially dangerous plant chemicals, heavy metals and other toxins, and even pharmaceuticals as contaminates of herbal remedies, all of which can be harmful.[130–147] A popular category of herbal products are so-called "herbal Viagra," plant mixtures supposed to treat erectile dysfunction in men as effectively as the drug Viagra (sildenafil) without the risks. Quite a few such products have been pulled from the market after being found to contain actual Viagra, or related pharmaceuticals.[148–151] Apart from the fact that there is no reason to believe any herbal remedies can treat this condition, or that those which should be any safer than a thoroughly tested prescription medicine, the fact that people who believe this are being sold a drug they don't even know they are taking is dishonest and dangerous. Without appropriate regulatory oversight, such problems are common in the herbal medicine market.

There is no question that there are significant risks to herbal remedies. Direct harm is sometimes caused by the plant chemicals themselves, which are rarely sufficiently tested scientifically to ensure they are safe and effective to use in people or pets. Historical tradition and personal experience are simply not adequate to identify the risks these compounds pose. Unfortunately, the misguided belief that herbal remedies can be assumed safe has led to inadequate regulation, testing, and monitoring. This potentially allows real harm to go undetected and leads to poor quality control for herbal products, including adulteration with toxins and pharmaceuticals. Finally, inadequate testing leaves us guessing about the effects of herbal remedies, and this undoubtedly harms patients with serious illness who are misled into taking these untested remedies and delaying appropriate diagnosis and scientific medical treatment.

BOTTOM LINE

As well as being among the most promising of alternative therapies, herbal medicine is one of the most dangerous. With few exceptions, giving your pet homeopathy is likely to do nothing at all for them. Giving them a herbal product, however, could potentially help or harm them, and most of the time we don't know which outcome we'll get. Rolling the dice may be fun in Vegas, but it's not a wise way to make medical choices for our beloved animal companions.

Herbal remedies should absolutely be analyzed and tested rigorously, as has been done for artemisinin and is being done with cannabis. Pharmacognosy, the scientific process of evaluating plants for medicinal use, is the best way to mine this rich resource of potential medicines. Many truly effective medicines have been found this way, and undoubtedly many more wait to be discovered among the millions of chemical compounds in traditional herbal remedies and other plants.

However, developing this resource means leaving behind the unscientific theories and unreliable methods of traditional herbalism. Traditional folk medicine can provide interesting observations that stimulate hypotheses for scientific testing. It cannot reliably show us which herbal remedies are safe and effective for specific conditions and which aren't. For that we need good, strong science.

Proponents of herbal medicine sometimes claim it is unfair to expect rigorous scientific testing of herbal remedies for animals since this is expensive and time-consuming. This would not be a compelling argument even if true because without such testing we're just playing a game of chance with our pets' health. Whether or not scientific testing is feasible, it is the only way to know what works and what is safe in herbal medicine, and folk theories, tradition, and anecdotes simply aren't a reliable substitute.

However, the claim that applying the same standards of evidence to herbs as we apply to pharmaceutical medicines is impossible is frankly untrue and disingenuous. The herbal medicine industry is worth billions of dollars annually worldwide. Companies in this industry make plenty of profit, but they spend a much lower share of this on research than pharmaceutical companies. Is this because Big Pharma is simply a more altruistic group of companies? Of course not! The difference is that the law requires proper scientific testing of conventional medicines because it is understood such testing is necessary to protect patients. There is no valid reason to apply a lesser standard or do less to protect patients from herbal remedies. We can and should treat all claims about all kinds of medicine equally, evaluating the plausibility of underlying theories and performing all the basic research and clinical studies necessary to find what works and discard what doesn't.

A truly science-based herbalism is a real and exciting potential field of medicine. Proper evaluation of herbal remedies for safety and effectiveness, accompanied by appropriate regulation to ensure quality of herbal products, would likely be of great use to veterinarians and pet owners looking for more and better ways to protect health and treat disease. Unfortunately, efforts at achieving this kind of scientific approach to herbal medicine are currently very few, and they are impeded by the reliance of most herbalists on folk tradition and personal clinical experience. The general philosophical perspective of alternative medicine, which I discussed in Chapter 1, gets in the way of a more reliable and productive scientific approach to herbal remedies.

Hopefully, the more veterinarians and pet owners understand about why traditional approaches to herbalism, such as TCM and Ayurveda, are not very useful and how science can more effectively find the real risks and benefits hidden in plants, the more the discipline of herbal medicine will move away from unreliable folk beliefs and towards a rigorously scientific herbalism that will reap real benefits for our pets and ourselves.

"Herbal medicine's been around for thousands of years!" Indeed it has...and the stuff that worked became 'medicine'. And the rest of it is just a nice bowl of soup and some potpourri.

- Dara O Briain

[1] Faurant C. From bark to weed: the history of artemisinin. *Parasite.* 2011;18(3):215-218. doi:10.1051/parasite/2011183215

[2] Su X-Z, Miller LH. The discovery of artemisinin and the Nobel Prize in Physiology or Medicine. *Sci China Life Sci.* 2015;58(11):1175-1179. doi:10.1007/s11427-015-4948-7

[3] Wynn S. *Veterinary Herbal Medicine.* St. Louis Mo.: Mosby Elsevier; 2007.

[4] Schoen AM, Wynn SG. *Complementary and Alternative Veterinary Medicine : Principles and Practice.* 1 ed. St.Louis (Misuri): Mosby; 1998.

[5] Allen J, Montalto M, Lovejoy J, Weber W. Detoxification in naturopathic medicine: a survey. *J Altern Complement Med.* 2011;17(12):1175-1180. doi:10.1089/acm.2010.0572

[6] Farrell DJ, Bower L. Fatal water intoxication. *J Clin Pathol.* 2003;56(10):803-804..

[7] Chawla A, Lavania AK. OXYGEN TOXICITY. *Med journal, Armed Forces India.* 2001;57(2):131-133. doi:10.1016/S0377-1237(01)80133-7

[8] Ernst E. Alternative detox. *Br Med Bull.* 2012;101(1):33-38. doi:10.1093/bmb/lds002

[9] Lee SWS, Tang H, Wan J, Mai X, Liu C. A cultural look at moral purity: wiping the face clean. *Front Psychol.* 2015;6:577. doi:10.3389/fpsyg.2015.00577

[10] Curtis VA. Dirt, disgust and disease: a natural history of hygiene. *J Epidemiol Community Health.* 2007;61(8):660-664. doi:10.1136/jech.2007.062380

[11] Huang JY, Ackerman JM, Newman GE. Catching (up with) magical contagion: A review of contagion effects in consumer cntexts. *J Assoc Consum Res.* 2017;2(4):430-443. doi:10.1086/693533

[12] Davey GCL. Disgust: the disease-avoidance emotion and its dysfunctions. *Philos Trans R Soc Lond B Biol Sci.* 2011;366(1583):3453-3465. doi:10.1098/rstb.2011.0039

[13] Rozin P, Nemeroff C, Wane M, Sherrod A. Operation of the sympathetic magical law of contagion in interpersonal attitudes among Americans. *Bull Psychon Soc.* 1989;27(4):367-370. doi:10.3758/BF03334630

[14] Fazil M, Nikhat S. Qai (emesis): from ancient to modern era and its therapeutic efficacy in various disorders. *J Drug Deliv Ther.* 2016;6(4):63-68. doi:10.22270/jddt.v6i4.1292

[15] Lamphere L. Symbolic elements in Navajo ritual. *Southwest J Anthropol.* 25:279-305. doi:10.2307/3629279

[16] Abenavoli L, Capasso R, Milic N, Capasso F. Milk thistle in liver diseases: past, present, future. *Phyther Res.* 2010;24(10):1423-1432. doi:10.1002/ptr.3207

[17] Sarker SD. Pharmacognosy in modern pharmacy curricula. *Pharmacogn Mag.* 2012;8(30):91-92. doi:10.4103/0973-1296.96545

[18] Singer MS, Mace KC, Bernays EA. Self-Medication as adaptive plasticity: Increased ingestion of plant toxins by parasitized caterpillars. May RC, ed. *PLoS One.* 2009;4(3):e4796. doi:10.1371/journal.pone.0004796

[19] Ansari MA, Khandelwal N, Kabra M. A Review on zoopharmacognosy. *Int J Pharm Chem Sci*. 2013;2(1):246-253.

[20] Hoppe-Dominik B. Grass-eating leopards: Wolves turned into sheep? *Naturwissenschaften*. 1988;75(1):49-50. doi:10.1007/BF00367444

[21] Hart B. Why do dogs and cats eat grass? *Vet Med*. 2008;103(12):648-649.

[22] Bjone SJ, Brown WY, Price IR. *Grass Eating Patterns in the Domestic Dog, Canis Familiaris*. Rec Adv Anim Nutr Austr. 2007;16:45-49.

[23] Sueda KLC, Hart BL, Cliff KD. Characterisation of plant eating in dogs. *Appl Anim Behav Sci*. 2008;111(1-2):120-132. doi:10.1016/J.APPLANIM.2007.05.018

[24] McKenzie SJ, Brown WY, Price IR. Reduction in grass eating behaviours in the domestic dog, Canis familiaris, in response to a mild gastrointestinal disturbance. *Appl Anim Behav Sci*. 2010;123(1-2):51-55. doi:10.1016/J.APPLANIM.2009.12.003

[25] Xie H. *Traditional Chinese Veterinary Medicine : Fundamental Principles*. Reddick Fla.: Chi Institute; 2007.

[26] Shergis JL, Zhang AL, Zhou W, Xue CC. *Panax ginseng* in randomised controlled rtrials: A Systematic review. *Phyther Res*. 2013;27(7):949-965. doi:10.1002/ptr.4832

[27] Buell PD, May T, Ramey D. Greek and Chinese horse medicine: déjà vu all over again. *Sudhoffs Arch*. 2010;94(1):31-56.

[28] LeMoine L. Essiac: an historical perspective. *Can Oncol Nurs J*. 1997;7(4):216-221..

[29] Kaegi E. Unconventional therapies for cancer: 1. Essiac. The Task Force on Alternative Therapies of the Canadian Breast Cancer Research Initiative. *CMAJ*. 1998;158(7):897-902..

[30] Ulbricht C, Weissner W, Hashmi S, et al. Essiac: systematic review by the natural standard research collaboration. *J Soc Integr Oncol*. 2009;7(2):73-80.

[31] Essiac Facts. Essiac Tea Benefits for Health. http://essiacfacts.com/essiac-tea-benefits-for-health/. Accessed December 2, 2018.

[32] Essiac Facts. Essiac Tea for Dogs and Other Pets. http://essiacfacts.com/essiac-tea-for-dogs-and-other-pets/. Accessed December 2, 2018.

[33] Seely D, Kennedy DA, Myers SP, et al. In vitro analysis of the herbal compound Essiac. *Anticancer Res*. 27(6B):3875-3882..

[34] Tai J, Cheung S, Wong S, Lowe C. In vitro comparison of Essiac and Flor-Essence on human tumor cell lines. *Oncol Rep*. 2004;11(2):471-476..

[35] Ottenweller J, Putt K, Blumenthal EJ, Dhawale S, Dhawale SW. Inhibition of prostate cancer-cell proliferation by Essiac®. *J Altern Complement Med*. 2004;10(4):687-691. doi:10.1089/acm.2004.10.687

[36] Leonard BJN, Kennedy DA, Cheng F-C, Chang K-K, Seely D, Mills E. An in vivo analysis of the herbal compound essiac. *Anticancer Res*. 26(4B):3057-3063.

[37] Eberding A, Madera C, Xie S, Wood CA, Brown PN, Guns ES. Evaluation of the antiproliferative effects of Essiac™ on *in vitro* and *in vivo* models of prostate cancer compared to paclitaxel. *Nutr Cancer*. 2007;58(2):188-196. doi:10.1080/01635580701328396

[38] Kulp KS, Montgomery JL, Nelson DO, et al. Essiac® and Flor-Essence® herbal tonics stimulate the in vitro growth of human breast cancer cells. *Breast Cancer Res Treat*. 2006;98(3):249-259. doi:10.1007/s10549-005-9156-x

[39] Zick SM, Sen A, Feng Y, Green J, Olatunde S, Boon H. Trial of Essiac to ascertain its effect in women with breast cancer (TEA-BC). *J Altern Complement Med*. 2006;12(10):971-980. doi:10.1089/acm.2006.12.971

[40] Cassileth BR. Essiac. *Oncology*. 2011;11(25).

[41] Bach, E. Wheeler, FJ. *The Bach Flower Remedies*. New York, NY.: McGraw-Hill; 1997.

[42] Armstrong NC, Ernst E. A randomized, double-blind, placebo-controlled trial of a Bach Flower Remedy. *Complement Ther Nurs Midwifery*. 2001;7(4):215-221. doi:10.1054/CTNM.2001.0525

[43] Walach H, Rilling C, Engelke U. Efficacy of Bach-flower remedies in test anxiety: a double-blind, placebo-controlled, randomized trial with partial crossover. *J Anxiety Disord*. 15(4):359-366.

[44] Pintov S, Hochman M, Livne A, Heyman E, Lahat E. Bach flower remedies used for attention deficit hyperactivity disorder in children—A prospective double blind controlled study. *Eur J Paediatr Neurol*. 2005;9(6):395-398. doi:10.1016/j.ejpn.2005.08.001

[45] Thaler K, Kaminski A, Chapman A, Langley T, Gartlehner G. Bach Flower Remedies for psychological problems and pain: a systematic review. *BMC Complement Altern Med*. 2009;9(1):16. doi:10.1186/1472-6882-9-16

[46] Ernst E. Bach flower remedies: a systematic review of randomised clinical trials. *Swiss Med Wkly*. 2010;140:w13079. doi:10.4414/smw.2010.13079

[47] Brand EJ, Zhao Z. Cannabis in Chinese Medicine: Are some traditional indications referenced in ancient literature related to cannabinoids? *Front Pharmacol*. 2017;8:108. doi:10.3389/fphar.2017.00108

[48] McConaghay D. The Ayurvedic Approach to Marijuana. *Gaia*. April 2014.

[49] National Academies of Sciences *The Health Effects of Cannabis and Cannabinoids*. National Academies Press (US); 2017. doi:10.17226/24625

[50] Thiele EA, Marsh ED, French JA, et al. Cannabidiol in patients with seizures associated with Lennox-Gastaut syndrome (GWPCARE4): a randomised, double-blind, placebo-controlled phase 3 trial. *Lancet (London, England)*. 2018;391(10125):1085-1096. doi:10.1016/S0140-6736(18)30136-3

[51] Bartner L. Assessment of safety, toxicity, and pharmacokinetics of cannabidiol in healthy dogs. In: *Proceedings of the 2017 ACVIM Forum*. National Harbor, MD; 2017.

[52] Gamble L-J, Boesch JM, Frye CW, et al. Pharmacokinetics, safety, and clinical efficacy of cannabidiol treatment in osteoarthritic dogs. *Front Vet Sci*. 2018;5:165. doi:10.3389/fvets.2018.00165

[53] Donaldson C. Marijuana exposure in animals. *Vet Med*. 2002;97(6):437-439.

[54] Janczyk P, Donaldson CW, Gwaltney S. Two hundred and thirteen cases of marijuana toxicoses in dogs. *Vet Hum Toxicol*. 2004;46(1):19-21.

[55] Meola SD, Tearney CC, Haas SA, Hackett TB, Mazzaferro EM. Evaluation of trends in marijuana toxicosis in dogs living in a state with legalized medical marijuana: 125 dogs (2005-2010). *J Vet Emerg Crit Care*. 2012;22(6):690-696. doi:10.1111/j.1476-4431.2012.00818.x

[56] Kogan LR, Hellyer PW, Robinson NG. Consumers' perceptions of hemp products for animals. *Scientific Report*. Vol 42.; 2016..

[57] Vandrey R, Raber JC, Raber ME, Douglass B, Miller C, Bonn-Miller MO. Cannabinoid dose and label accuracy in edible medical cannabis products. *JAMA*. 2015;313(24):2491. doi:10.1001/jama.2015.6613

[58] Thomas BF, Pollard GT. Preparation and distribution of cannabis and cannabis-derived dosage formulations for investigational and therapeutic use in the United States. *Front Pharmacol*. 2016;7:285. doi:10.3389/fphar.2016.00285

[59] Dharmandanda S, Fruehauf H. Ginkgo: Cultural background and medicinal usage in China. *J Chinese Med*. 1998;56(40).

[60] TCM Chinese Herbs, Health Benefits of GingKo. Available at: https://www.tkithealth.com/tag/active-components-of-ginkgo/ Accessed June 23, 2019.

[61] van Beek TA. Chemical analysis of Ginkgo biloba leaves and extracts. *J Chromatogr A*. 2002;967(1):21-55. doi:10.1016/S0021-9673(02)00172-3

[62] Ude C, Schubert-Zsilavecz M, Wurglics M. Ginkgo biloba extracts: A review of the pharmacokinetics of the active ingredients. *Clin Pharmacokinet*. 2013;52(9):727-749. doi:10.1007/s40262-013-0074-5

[63] National Center for Complementary and Integrative Medicine. Ginkgo. Available at: https://nccih.nih.gov/health/ginkgo/ataglance.htm. Accessed June 23, 2019.

[64] Birks J, Grimley Evans J. Ginkgo biloba for cognitive impairment and dementia. *Cochrane Database Syst Rev*. January 2009. doi:10.1002/14651858.CD003120.pub3

[65] Weinmann S, Roll S, Schwarzbach C, Vauth C, Willich SN. Effects of Ginkgo biloba in dementia: systematic review and meta-analysis. *BMC Geriatr*. 2010;10(1):14. doi:10.1186/1471-2318-10-14

[66] Yang G, Wang Y, Sun J, Zhang K, Liu J. Ginkgo biloba for mild cognitive impairment and alzheimer's disease: A systematic review and meta-analysis of randomized controlled trials. *Curr Top Med Chem*. 2016;16(5):520-528.

[67] Charemboon T, Jaisin K. Ginkgo biloba for prevention of dementia: a systematic review and meta-analysis. *J Med Assoc Thai.* 2015;98(5):508-513.

[68] Yuan Q, Wang C, Shi J, Lin Z. Effects of Ginkgo biloba on dementia: An overview of systematic reviews. *J Ethnopharmacol.* 2017;195:1-9. doi:10.1016/j.jep.2016.12.005

[69] Hilton MP, Zimmermann EF, Hunt WT. Ginkgo biloba for tinnitus. *Cochrane Database Syst Rev.* March 2013. doi:10.1002/14651858.CD003852.pub3

[70] Xiong XJ, Liu W, Yang XC, et al. Ginkgo biloba extract for essential hypertension: A systemic review. *Phytomedicine.* 2014;21(10):1131-1136. doi:10.1016/j.phymed.2014.04.024

[71] Zeng X, Liu M, Yang Y, Li Y, Asplund K. Ginkgo biloba for acute ischaemic stroke. *Cochrane Database Syst Rev.* October 2005. doi:10.1002/14651858.CD003691.pub2

[72] Murdoch D. Altitude sickness. *BMJ Clin Evid.* 2010;2010:1209.

[73] Huntley A, Ernst E. Herbal medicines for asthma: a systematic review. *Thorax.* 2000;55(11):925-929. doi:10.1136/THORAX.55.11.925

[74] Kang JM, Lin S. Ginkgo biloba and its potential role in glaucoma. *Curr Opin Ophthalmol.* 2018;29(2):116-120. doi:10.1097/ICU.0000000000000459

[75] Reichling J, Frater-Schröder M, Herzog K, Bucher S, Saller R. Reduction of behavioural disturbances in elderly dogs supplemented with a standardised Ginkgo leaf extract. *Schweiz Arch Tierheilkd.* 2006;148(5):257-263. doi:10.1024/0036-7281.148.5.257

[76] Araujo JA, Landsberg GM, Milgram NW, Miolo A. Improvement of short-term memory performance in aged beagles by a nutraceutical supplement containing phosphatidylserine, Ginkgo biloba, vitamin E, and pyridoxine. *Can Vet J = La Rev Vet Can.* 2008;49(4):379-385..

[77] Osella MC, Re G, Odore R, et al. Canine cognitive dysfunction syndrome: Prevalence, clinical signs and treatment with a neuroprotective nutraceutical. *Appl Anim Behav Sci.* 2006;105(4):297-310. doi:10.1016/j.applanim.2006.11.007

[78] Mei N, Guo X, Ren Z, Kobayashi D, Wada K, Guo L. Review of *Ginkgo biloba* -induced toxicity, from experimental studies to human case reports. *J Environ Sci Heal Part C.* 2017;35(1):1-28. doi:10.1080/10590501.2016.1278298

[79] Roland P-D, Nergård C. Ginkgo biloba - effekt, bivirkninger og interaksjoner. *Tidsskr Den Nor legeforening.* 2012;132(8):956-959. doi:10.4045/tidsskr.11.0780

[80] National Library of Medicine. Ginkgo. *Drugs and Lactation Database.* 2018. Available at: http://www.ncbi.nlm.nih.gov/pubmed/30000868. Accessed December 3, 2018.

[81] Kellermann AJ, Kloft C. Is there a risk of bleeding associated with standardized *Ginkgo biloba* extract therapy? A systematic review and meta-analysis. *Pharmacotherapy.* 2011;31(5):490-502. doi:10.1592/phco.31.5.490

[82] Rider C V, Nyska A, Cora MC, et al. Toxicity and carcinogenicity studies of Ginkgo biloba extract in rat and mouse: liver, thyroid, and nose are targets. *Toxicol Pathol.* 2014;42(5):830-843. doi:10.1177/0192623313501235

[83] Bressler R. Herb-drug interactions: interactions between Ginkgo biloba and prescription medications. *Geriatrics*. 2005;60(4):30-33.

[84] Abad MJ, Bedoya LM, Bermejo P. An update on drug interactions with the herbal medicine Ginkgo biloba. *Curr Drug Metab*. 2010;11(2):171-181.

[85] Unger M. Pharmacokinetic drug interactions involving *Ginkgo biloba*. *Drug Metab Rev*.2013;45(3):353-385. doi:10.3109/03602532.2013.815200

[86] Chinese medicine has caused kidney failure and even cancer. So how safe are these popular "cures." *Daily Mail*. Published March 2, 2010. Available at: https://www.dailymail.co.uk/health/article-1254746/Chinese-medicine-caused-kidney-failure-cancer-So-safe-popular-cures.html. Accessed June 23, 2019.

[87] Jadot I, Declèves A-E, Nortier J, Caron N. An integrated view of aristolochic acid nephropathy: Update of the literature. *Int J Mol Sci*. 2017;18(2):297. doi:10.3390/ijms18020297

[88] Cosyns J-P. Aristolochic acid and "Chinese herbs nephropathy." *Drug Saf*. 2003;26(1):33-48. doi:10.2165/00002018-200326010-00004

[89] Debelle FD, Vanherweghem J-L, Nortier JL. Aristolochic acid nephropathy: A worldwide problem. *Kidney Int*. 2008;74(2):158-169. doi:10.1038/ki.2008.129

[90] Eastman KL, McFarland L V., Raugi GJ. A review of topical corrosive Black Salve. *J Altern Complement Med*. 2014;20(4):284-289. doi:10.1089/acm.2012.0377

[91] Lim A. Black salve treatment of skin cancer: a review. *J Dermatolog Treat*. 2018;29(4):388-392. doi:10.1080/09546634.2017.1395795

[92] Croaker A, King GJ, Pyne JH, Anoopkumar-Dukie S, Liu L. A review of Black Salve: Cancer specificity, cure, and cosmesis. *Evidence-Based Complement Altern Med*. 2017;2017:1-11. doi:10.1155/2017/9184034

[93] Croaker A, King GJ, Pyne JH, Anoopkumar-Dukie S, Simanek V, Liu L. Carcinogenic potential of sanguinarine, a phytochemical used in 'therapeutic' black salve and mouthwash. *Mutat Res Mutat Res*. 2017;774:46-56. doi:10.1016/j.mrrev.2017.09.001

[94] Eastman KL, McFarland L V., Raugi GJ. Buyer beware: A black salve caution. *J Am Acad Dermatol*. 2011;65(5):e154-e155. doi:10.1016/j.jaad.2011.07.031

[95] Shaw D. Toxicological risks of Chinese herbs. *Planta Med*. 2010;76(17):2012-2018. doi:10.1055/s-0030-1250533

[96] Grollman AP, Marcus DM. Global hazards of herbal remedies: lessons from Aristolochia: The lesson from the health hazards of Aristolochia should lead to more research into the safety and efficacy of medicinal plants. *EMBO Rep*. 2016;17(5):619-625. doi:10.15252/embr.201642375

[97] Ng AWT, Poon SL, Huang MN, et al. Aristolochic acids and their derivatives are widely implicated in liver cancers in Taiwan and throughout Asia. *Sci Transl Med*. 2017;9(412):eaan6446. doi:10.1126/scitranslmed.aan6446

[98] Gordon P, Khojasteh SC. A decades-long investigation of acute metabolism-based hepatotoxicity by herbal constituents: a case study of pennyroyal oil. *Drug Metab Rev.* 2015;47(1):12-20. doi:10.3109/03602532.2014.990032

[99] Bunchorntavakul C, Reddy KR. Review article: herbal and dietary supplement hepatotoxicity. *Aliment Pharmacol Ther.* 2013;37(1):3-17. doi:10.1111/apt.12109

[100] Mei N, Guo L, Fu PP, Fuscoe JC, Luan Y, Chen T. Metabolism, genotoxicity, annd carcinogenicity of comfrey. *J Toxicol Environ Heal Part B.* 2010;13(7-8):509-526. doi:10.1080/10937404.2010.509013

[101] Chan TYK. *Aconitum* alkaloid poisoning because of contamination of herbs by aconite roots. *Phyther Res.* 2016;30(1):3-8. doi:10.1002/ptr.5495

[102] Nazari S, Rameshrad M, Hosseinzadeh H. Toxicological effects of *Glycyrrhiza glabra* (licorice): A review. *Phyther Res.* 2017;31(11):1635-1650. doi:10.1002/ptr.5893

[103] Paik DJ, Lee CH. Review of cases of patient risk associated with ginseng abuse and misuse. *J Ginseng Res.* 2015;39(2):89-93. doi:10.1016/j.jgr.2014.11.005

[104] Kim EJY, Chen Y, Huang JQ, et al. Evidence-based toxicity evaluation and scheduling of Chinese herbal medicines. *J Ethnopharmacol.* 2013;146(1):40-61. doi:10.1016/j.jep.2012.12.027

[105] Fleming RM. Safety of ephedra and related anorexic medications. *Expert Opin Drug Saf.* 2008;7(6):749-759. doi:10.1517/14740330802510915

[106] Food and Drug Administration, HHS. Final rule declaring dietary supplements containing ephedrine alkaloids adulterated because they present an unreasonable risk. Final rule. *Fed Regist.* 2004;69(28):6787-6854. http://www.ncbi.nlm.nih.gov/pubmed/14968803. Accessed December 7, 2018.

[107] Childress MO, Burgess RCF, Holland CH, Gelb HR. Consequences of intratumoral injection of an herbal preparation containing blood root (*Sanguinaria canadensis*) extract in two dogs. *J Am Vet Med Assoc.* 2011;239(3):374-379. doi:10.2460/javma.239.3.374

[108] Genovese AG, McLean MK, Khan SA. Adverse reactions from essential oil-containing natural flea products exempted from Environmental Protection Agency regulations in dogs and cats. *J Vet Emerg Crit Care.* 2012;22(4):470-475. doi:10.1111/j.1476-4431.2012.00780.x

[109] Benson K. Essential Oils and Cats. Pet Poison Helpline. Available at: https://www.petpoisonhelpline.com/blog/essential-oils-cats/. Accessed June 23,2019

[110] Marshall J. Essential Oils and Dogs. Pet Poison Helpline. Available at: https://www.petpoisonhelpline.com/pet-safety-tips/essential-oils-dogs/. Accessed June 23, 2019.

[111] Khan SA, McLean MK, Slater MR. Concentrated tea tree oil toxicosis in dogs and cats: 443 cases (2002–2012). *J Am Vet Med Assoc.* 2014;244(1):95-99. doi:10.2460/javma.244.1.95

[112] Gugler K, Piscitelli CM, Dennis J. Hidden dangers in the kitchen: Common foods toxic to dogs and cats. *Compend Contin Educ Pract Vet.* 2013;35(7).

[113] Means C. Selected herbal toxicities in dogs and cats. In: *Poisonous Plants: Global Research and Solutions.* Wallingford: CABI; :554-559. doi:10.1079/9781845932732.0554

[114] Sudekum M, Poppenga RH, Raju N, Braselton WE. Pennyroyal oil toxicosis in a dog. *J Am Vet Med Assoc.* 1992;200(6):817-818.

[115] Ooms TG, Khan SA, Means C. Suspected caffeine and ephedrine toxicosis resulting from ingestion of an herbal supplement containing guarana and ma huang in dogs: 47 cases (1997-1999). *J Am Vet Med Assoc.* 2001;218(2):225-229..

[116] Poppenga RH. Risks associated with the use of herbs and other dietary supplements. *Vet Clin North Am Equine Pract.* 2001;17(3):455-77, vi-vii..

[117] Poppenga RH. Herbal medicine: Potential for intoxication and interactions with conventional drugs. *Clin Tech Small Anim Pract.* 2002;17(1):6-18. doi:10.1053/svms.2002.27785

[118] Boivin J, Schmidt L. Use of complementary and alternative medicines associated with a 30% lower ongoing pregnancy/live birth rate during 12 months of fertility treatment. *Hum Reprod.* 2009;24(7):1626-1631. doi:10.1093/humrep/dep077

[119] Boström H, Rössner S. Quality of alternative medicine--complications and avoidable deaths. *Qual Assur Heal care Off J Int Soc Qual Assur Heal Care.* 1990;2(2):111-117.

[120] Roy A, Lurslurchachai L, Halm EA, Li X-M, Leventhal H, Wisnivesky JP. Use of herbal remedies and adherence to inhaled corticosteroids among inner-city asthmatic patients. *Ann Allergy, Asthma Immunol.* 2010;104(2):132-138. doi:10.1016/j.anai.2009.11.024

[121] Yun YH, Lee MK, Park SM, et al. Effect of complementary and alternative medicine on the survival and health-related quality of life among terminally ill cancer patients: a prospective cohort study. *Ann Oncol.* 2013;24(2):489-494. doi:10.1093/annonc/mds469

[122] Johnson SB, Park HS, Gross CP, Yu JB. Use of Alternative Medicine for Cancer and Its Impact on Survival. *JNCI J Natl Cancer Inst.* 2018;110(1):121-124. doi:10.1093/jnci/djx145

[123] Johnson SB, Park HS, Gross CP, Yu JB. Complementary medicine, refusal of conventional cancer therapy, and survival among patients with curable cancers. *JAMA Oncol.* 2018;4(10):1375. doi:10.1001/jamaoncol.2018.2487

[124] Ma H, Carpenter CL, Sullivan-Halley J, Bernstein L. The roles of herbal remedies in survival and quality of life among long-term breast cancer survivors--results of a prospective study. *BMC Cancer.* 2011;11:222. doi:10.1186/1471-2407-11-222

[125] Ulbricht C, Chao W, Costa D, Rusie-Seamon E, Weissner W, Woods J. Clinical evidence of herb-drug interactions: a systematic review by the natural standard research collaboration. *Curr Drug Metab.* 2008;9(10):1063-1120.

[126] Zuo Z, Huang M, Kanfer I, Chow MSS, Cho WCS. Herb-drug interactions: Systematic review, mechanisms, and therapies. *Evidence-Based Complement Altern Med*. 2015;2015:1-1. doi:10.1155/2015/239150

[127] Asher GN, Corbett AH, Hawke RL. Common herbal dietary supplement-drug interactions. *Am Fam Physician*. 2017;96(2):101-107.

[128] Izzo AA, Hoon-Kim S, Radhakrishnan R, Williamson EM. A critical approach to evaluating clinical efficacy, adverse events and drug interactions of herbal remedies. *Phyther Res*. 2016;30(5):691-700. doi:10.1002/ptr.5591

[129] Alissa EM. Medicinal herbs and therapeutic drugs interactions. *Ther Drug Monit*. 2014;36(4):413-422. doi:10.1097/FTD.0000000000000035

[130] Kim H, Hughes PJ, Hawes EM. Adverse events associated with metal contamination of traditional chinese medicines in korea: A clinical review. *Yonsei Med J*. 2014;55(5):1177. doi:10.3349/ymj.2014.55.5.1177

[131] Posadzki P, Watson L, Ernst E. Contamination and adulteration of herbal medicinal products (HMPs): an overview of systematic reviews. *Eur J Clin Pharmacol*. 2013;69(3):295-307. doi:10.1007/s00228-012-1353-z

[132] Kosalec I, Cvek J, Tomić S. Contaminants of medicinal herbs and herbal products. *Arch Ind Hyg Toxicol*. 2009;60(4):485-501. doi:10.2478/10004-1254-60-2009-2005

[133] Efferth T, Kaina B. Toxicities by herbal medicines with emphasis to traditional Chinese medicine. *Curr Drug Metab*. 2011;12(10):989-996.

[134] Tang G, Tu X, Feng P. Lead Poisoning caused by traditional chinese medicine: A case report and literature review. *Tohoku J Exp Med*. 2017;243(2):127-131. doi:10.1620/tjem.243.127

[135] Ernst E. Toxic heavy metals and undeclared drugs in Asian herbal medicines. *Trends Pharmacol Sci*. 2002;23(3):136-139. doi:10.1016/S0165-6147(00)01972-6

[136] Lynch E, Braithwaite R. A review of the clinical and toxicological aspects of 'traditional' (herbal) medicines adulterated with heavy metals. *Expert Opin Drug Saf*. 2005;4(4):769-778. doi:10.1517/14740338.4.4.769

[137] Byard RW, Musgrave I, Maker G, Bunce M. What risks do herbal products pose to the Australian community? *Med J Aust*. 2017;206(2):86-90.

[138] Ernst E. Adulteration of Chinese herbal medicines with synthetic drugs: a systematic review. *J Intern Med*. 2002;252(2):107-113.

[139] de Carvalho LM, Moreira AP, Martini M, Falcão T. The illegal use of synthetic pharmaceuticals in herbal formulations: an overview of adulteration practices and analytical investigations. *Forensic Sci Rev*. 2011;23(2):73-89.

[140] Zovko Končić M. Getting more than you paid for: Unauthorized "natural" substances in herbal food supplements on EU market. *Planta Med*. 2018;84(06/07):394-406. doi:10.1055/s-0044-100042

[141] Calahan J, Howard D, Almalki A, Gupta M, Calderón A. Chemical adulterants in herbal medicinal products: A review. Planta Med. 2016;82(06):505-515. doi:10.1055/s-0042-103495

[142] Srirama R, Santhosh Kumar JU, Seethapathy GS, et al. Species adulteration in the herbal trade: Causes, consequences and mitigation. Drug Saf. 2017;40(8):651-661. doi:10.1007/s40264-017-0527-0

[143] Huang WF, Wen KC, Hsiao ML. Adulteration by synthetic therapeutic substances of traditional Chinese medicines in Taiwan. J Clin Pharmacol. 1997;37(4):344-350.

[144] Burkhard PR, Burkhardt K, Haenggeli CA, Landis T. Plant-induced seizures: reappearance of an old problem. J Neurol. 1999;246(8):667-670.

[145] Blacksell L, Byard RW, Musgrave IF. Forensic problems with the composition and content of herbal medicines. J Forensic Leg Med. 2014;23:19-21. doi:10.1016/J.JFLM.2014.01.008

[146] Ahmad B, Ashiq S, Hussain A, Bashir S, Hussain M. Evaluation of mycotoxins, mycobiota, and toxigenic fungi in selected medicinal plants of Khyber Pakhtunkhwa, Pakistan. Fungal Biol. 2014;118(9-10):776-784. doi:10.1016/J.FUNBIO.2014.06.002

[147] Coghlan ML, Haile J, Houston J, et al. Deep sequencing of plant and animal dna contained within traditional chinese medicines reveals legality issues and health safety concerns. DeSalle R, ed. PLoS Genet. 2012;8(4):e1002657. doi:10.1371/journal.pgen.1002657

[148] Kee C-L, Ge X, Gilard V, Malet-Martino M, Low M-Y. A review of synthetic phosphodiesterase type 5 inhibitors (PDE-5i) found as adulterants in dietary supplements. J Pharm Biomed Anal. 2018;147:250-277. doi:10.1016/j.jpba.2017.07.031

[149] Patel DN, Li L, Kee C-L, Ge X, Low M-Y, Koh H-L. Screening of synthetic PDE-5 inhibitors and their analogues as adulterants: Analytical techniques and challenges. J Pharm Biomed Anal. 2014;87:176-190. doi:10.1016/j.jpba.2013.04.037

[150] Nissan R, Poperno A, Stein GY, et al. A case of hepatotoxicity induced by adulterated "Tiger King", a Chinese herbal medicine containing sildenafil. Curr Drug Saf. 2016;11(2):184-188..

[151] Skalicka-Woźniak K, Georgiev MI, Orhan IE. Adulteration of herbal sexual enhancers and slimmers: The wish for better sexual well-being and perfect body can be risky. Food Chem Toxicol. 2017;108(Pt B):355-364. doi:10.1016/j.fct.2016.06.018

7|
DIETARY SUPPLEMENTS

The difficulty lies not so much in developing new ideas as in escaping from old ones.

- John Maynard Keynes

INTRODUCTION

Dietary supplements are, by far, the most popular and widely used of the treatments I will talk about. Surveys find that dietary supplement use varies from country to country, but in many developed nations 50-70% of adults report using some kind of supplement, and many children are given supplement products as well.[1-9] Pet owners also commonly give supplements to their animals, though at somewhat lower rates. About 30% of dog owners and 20% of cat owners in one survey reported using dietary supplements for their pets.[10]

The popularity of supplements makes them a very profitable product. The dietary supplement industry is worth hundreds of billions of dollars worldwide, and while the majority of this is the market for humans, veterinary supplements are still a billion-dollar a year business.[11,12]

People report taking supplements for various reasons, but most commonly they use them to improve their overall health and energy level, to lose weight, or to treat specific medical problems.[8,9] Pet owners mostly report giving supplements to prevent or treat specific health problems in their pets.[10] They willingly spend a portion of their limited resources for pet healthcare on supplements hoping that this investment will pay off in terms of better health for their pets and possible less expense and risk from conventional medical treatments. Let's take a look at whether this is a sound investment or not.

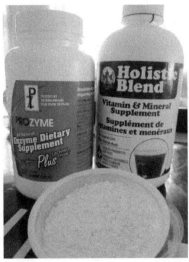

Veterinary Supplements 2010 by Rhona-Mae Arca under Creative Commons by SA 2.0

WHAT IS IT?

Defining a dietary supplement can be tricky, and there is no single, universally accepted definition. Legal definitions for the term vary from country to country, and these may not always correspond to what ordinary people think of as a dietary supplement. In general, a dietary supplement is some substance, often but not always found in foods, that is taken in concentrated form and is intended to have some beneficial effect on health. Pretty vague, eh? Sometimes dietary supplements are legally classified as foods, sometimes they are considered drugs, and sometimes the same substance can be in both categories depending on how it is labeled and used. Herbal remedies are sometimes considered dietary supplements, but they are also given their own regulatory category in some places.

Ultimately, there is no hard and fast rule for what a dietary supplement really is. If we are isolating chemicals and concentrating them in pills or liquids and then taking them to affect our health, how are these not drugs? If these supplements are foods, not drugs, then why are we taking them at high doses in pills rather than just eating more of the foods they come from? A lot of the claims made for supplements try to confuse us by suggesting they can have the same effects as drugs but that they are safer because they are foods rather than drugs. This makes little sense from the perspective of biology, or even basic logic!

The best we can probably do for now is to consider a dietary supplement to be a nutrient or other chemical typically found in food that is taken in concentrated form to prevent or treat some specific health condition. This should allow us to look at the evidence for the effectiveness and safety of dietary supplements and make some judgements about how much confidence to have in health claims made for them. As pet owners, our goal is to protect and improve the health of our pets and to minimize the risk of anything we give them, so looking critically at supplements as medical treatments and evaluating them scientifically is the best way to achieve this goal.

Because supplements are so widely accepted and used, you may be wondering if they belong in a book that is mostly about alternative medicine. Just as it is difficult to clearly define dietary supplements, it is also difficult to classify them as either science-based or alternative medical treatments. They can be either depending on how we evaluate and use them. Unlike herbal remedies, most dietary supplements do not have a theoretical rationale based in historical folk medicine traditions or philosophical views that are incompatible with a scientific perspective. Most supplements are used based on at least some plausible rationale drawn from established scientific evidence in the fields of nutrition and physiology, and most have at least had some testing in preclinical laboratory settings. This is a much more promising starting point than folk wisdom or spiritual beliefs.

If a dietary supplement is backed by a scientifically plausible theory for how it could work, if it is rigorously tested in the lab and in animal models to identify any risks and benefits it might have, and if it is then run through the clinical trial process and accumulates solid evidence of safety and efficacy, then it is simply another tool in the toolbox of science-based medicine, and there is nothing alternative about it. There are some supplements that have been developed and used in this way.

Unfortunately, however, many supplements are promoted and used without enduring this scientific testing process. Many show some promise in early, preclinical studies, and they become popular and profitable treatments without finishing the process and going through the critical and necessary step of clinical studies in real patients. Just like *Gingko biloba*, which I discussed in the last chapter, supplements that are used without proper testing often turn out to be less useful, or less safe, than hoped once this testing is ultimately done.

Skipping steps in the scientific process wastes time and resources, and it ultimately hurts patients. Those who may choose an insufficiently tested supplement over a proven therapy because they believe it to be safer or more effective based on low-quality evidence can be harmed by the supplement or by delaying truly effective treatment. And in veterinary medicine, where resources for research and treatment are scarce and where euthanasia is an option when these resources run out, money and time wasted on ineffective treatments can be very dangerous for our animal patients.

Of course, going beyond the available evidence and skipping steps in the scientific process may just be sloppy medicine, not necessarily alternative medicine. However, supplements are often used on the basis of many of the philosophical principles I discussed in Chapter 1 that inform and characterize alternative medicine. They may be assumed to be safer and more effective than conventional treatments because they are "natural," which is our old nemesis the Appeal to Nature Fallacy rearing its head again. And supplements may be recommended confidently on the basis of personal experience and anecdote even when scientific research shows they don't work, which is typical of the preference given to anecdote over data in the alternative medicine community. In many cases, the approach to the use of these products is typical of alternative medicine approaches in general.

Dietary supplements are popular in both conventional and alternative medicine, but they tend to be used and promoted more aggressively by those skeptical of the value and safety of conventional treatments, often in place of these treatments. Just as dietary supplements occupy something of a grey area between food and medicine, so they occupy a shifting and ill-defined space between science-based and alternative medicine. For this reason, I think they are worth talking about here since they fit some of the patterns that characterize the other therapies I have discussed.

GENERAL CONCEPTS IN DIETARY SUPPLEMENT USE

Surveys indicate that there are many reasons why people choose supplements for themselves and for their pets, but there are a number of recurring themes and beliefs people have about supplements in general that influence when and how they use them. Looking at some of these concepts may help you take a more critical and scientific perspective when making decisions about using supplements in your own pets.

If Some is Good; More is Better

The most popular dietary supplements for humans are vitamins and minerals.[8,9] These are nutrients which are essential for life and normal health, though they are only needed in very small quantities. Too little of these micronutrients can lead to illness. Some of the most terrible and intractable diseases in human history were the result of vitamin and mineral deficiencies. Children with rickets suffered from soft, deformed bones due to insufficient Vitamin D. Sailors and other travelers would lose hair and teeth, bleed from the gums, and suffer from severe infections caused by scurvy, a lack of Vitamin C. Blindness, nerve and brain disease, heart problems, and many other terrible symptoms were once common due to a lack of essential vitamins, minerals, and other nutrients in the diet.

Identifying and curing nutritional deficiency diseases has been one of the great successes in scientific medicine. Vitamin and mineral supplements, in food and taken directly in pills or other forms, can have miraculous effects at preventing and reversing these conditions. Most of us are at least vaguely familiar with this history, and even today we can see the impact of nutritional supplements on health in developing nations. Blindness in children due to Vitamin A deficiency is still widespread in Africa and Asia, and interventions such as encouraging breastfeeding, supplementing foods, and growing new crop varieties with more of this vitamin have a dramatic impact on the health and well-being of these children.

My mother was a nurse, and for most of my childhood and adolescence, I accompanied her once a month to volunteer at a medical clinic for children in Mexico. As I grew and learned to speak Spanish, I got to know a lot of the mothers who brought their children to the clinic. Many had seen the power of vitamin supplements directly, and even when they and their children had adequate nutrition and did not suffer from nutrient deficiency diseases, they often asked for vitamins and other supplements for their children. They saw these as nearly magical substances which could ward of and cure disease. And for some diseases, this is certainly true. But much of the time, the problems these women and their children faced were not due to nutrient deficiencies, and the money and time spent using them could have been more effective if spent on finding and treating the real causes of their health issues.

Because of personal or cultural familiarity with the dramatic success of nutritional supplements in preventing and treating so many awful diseases, there is a tendency to mythologize these products and to imagine that if we can gain such great health benefits by taking enough to prevent a deficiency, we might get even more benefit by taking even more of these supplements.

Placebos for Pets?

Unfortunately, the idea that if some is good more is better is danger-ously mistaken in biology and medicine. Many dietary supplements contain chemicals which we need in very specific amounts. Too little is bad for us, but so is too much. Vitamins in particular, and supplements more generally, are often assumed to be benign since they are found naturally in the food we eat. As you will see when we talk about the risks of supplements, this is quite clearly not true.

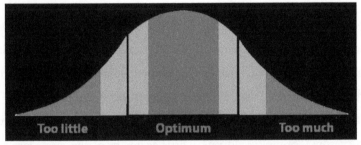

Image from Zwart, S. Ironing out nutrition's bell-shaped curve.[13] ©J. Robinson

This diagram illustrates how most nutrients work in terms of health. There is an optimum or ideal range for how much of a nutrient we need. This varies with species, the particular nutrient, age, sex, genetics, and many other factors. We typically can't know exactly what the level of a given nu-trient might be for a particular individual, but we know that for a specific population (for example, human males from 15 to 65 years old), there is a "green zone" in which the level of a nutrient will have the best possible effect on those aspects of health it influences. In the "yellow zone" we may not have the best possible levels of the nutrient, but we usually don't have sig-nificant diseases associated with it. At the extreme levels, both too little and too much of most nutrients, we can see health problems.

This is only a rough approximation of the story and, of course, the devil is in the details (where have I heard that before?). But looking at the levels of most nutrients, such as vitamins and minerals, in this way will help you to make better choices about supplements. As I will discuss in more detail later, there is very little evidence to suggest that taking more of these nutrients beyond the amount needed to avoid deficiency is beneficial to health, and there are clear cases in which it is actively harmful.

Boosting the Immune System

One of my favorite experiments when I was teaching undergraduate biology was giving the students a Petri dish, a culture medium for growing bacteria, and fungal organisms. I would tell the students they could put anything they wanted on the nutrient material in the dish (except body fluids, for obvious safety reasons). Some would put a little water from the classroom water fountain in the dish; others would touch the medium with their favorite pen, the sandwich they had brought for lunch, or other personal items; some would simply set the open Petri dish on their desk for a little while. Invariable, all the dishes grew a variety of colorful bacteria and fungi, and invariably the students were horrified by the presence of so many invisible microorganisms all around them. We swim in a sea of living organisms of which we are mostly unaware.

So why aren't we sick all the time? Well, not all the microorganisms around us are harmful, and some are even beneficial for our health, which I will talk more about shortly. But the main reason we can live happily and healthily awash in microorganisms is that we have an immune system. This is a set of defenses, from physical barriers like our skin to specialized blood cells that attack and eat potentially harmful germs. Our immune system is always on and always protecting us, and most of the time we aren't even aware of it.

Since many of us have heard about the immune system and its ability to fight off not only infectious invaders but the growth of abnormal and cancerous cells within our own bodies, we know how important it is for our immune systems to function well. And most of us also know that some things can weaken our immune system and make us vulnerable to diseases we might otherwise resist. Malnutrition,[14] poor sleep,[15] stress (though that's a slippery concept as well),[16,17] many diseases, some drugs, even natural aspects of our life cycle such as being young or old[18,19] can make us more vulnerable to infectious disease.

In the quest for good health, for ourselves and our pets, we sometimes look for ways to strengthen or "boost" our immune systems. This seems like a sensible idea, but it is not as straightforward as it sounds. We can certainly support optimal function of our immune system by avoiding things that weaken it. Not drinking and smoking,[20,21] sleeping enough, eating a balanced and nutritionally appropriate diet, and exercising all support normal immune system function (though some of these, such as exercise, are examples of things with an optimum level, and too much can weaken the immune system even though the right amount will strengthen it).[22]

One rationale for taking dietary supplements is that they can boost the immune system. Though this is taking things a bit out of order, I can tell you now that there is virtually no evidence this is true. While enough of many nutrients is essential for normal immune function, it has not been convincingly demonstrated that more than enough of any nutrient makes a normal, already healthy immune system any stronger. It is also not clear that supplements can compensate for other factors that may weaken the immune system. Taking vitamins, for example, when you are older and have a naturally weaker immune system than you once did does not appear to be very useful in preventing infections.[23,24] And certainly, supplements aren't going to get you off the hook for smoking or drinking too much or many of the other behaviors that weaken the immune system. More to the point for our pets, who don't typically engage in such self-destructive behavior, there is no compelling evidence that supplements will compensate for age, pregnancy, illness, or other things that weaken the immune system in pets.

The other question people often forget to ask is, "Even if we can boost our immune system, should we?" When your immune system is activated to fight off an infection, for example, you often feel pretty lousy. Boosting your immune system might mean having a fever, a runny nose, and feeling achy and tired all the time, since those are all natural effects of heightened immune system function. Overactive immune systems also cause more serious problems. Allergies are essentially an excessive and improperly targeted activation of our immune systems. When your pet with environmental allergies is chewing on her paws and scratching at her inflamed skin, she doesn't need her immune system boosted, she needs it turned down! Finally, autoimmune diseases are serious, often deadly examples of excessive and inappropriate immune system function. Activating or ramping up the function of our pets' immune system, even if we could do so, isn't necessarily a good idea for improving their health.

Placebos for Pets?

If supplements are to be useful in terms of immune function, we have to ensure that they are providing an optimum amount of an essential nutrient or that they have some specific, proven effect that reduces the risk of illness in our pets and doesn't create unpleasant or dangerous symptoms of excessive immune system function. We cannot blithely assume that supplements are necessary or are safe and effective in supporting immune system function without appropriate evidence, despite the dramatic, often illogical claims of the folks selling us supplements.

Antioxidants

I'll be honest here, I didn't really enjoy basic chemistry much in school. Even though I took courses in chemistry repeatedly, in high school, college, and graduate school, I never felt especially excited by oxidation and reduction and other chemical reactions. I'm going to guess that many of you reading this book aren't chemists and may not feel entirely in command of the details of basic chemistry. If I say that ascorbic acid participates in redox reactions with molecules that have an unpaired valence electron, you might just put the book down and go have a cup of tea. But if I say that Vitamin C is a natural antioxidant, that might sound a little more comprehensible and appealing.

My point is that "antioxidants" are widely viewed as good for our health and "free radicals" are seen as bad, even though most of us don't really understand much about what that means. The antioxidant craze is an example of a legitimate and interesting scientific hypothesis that has been sloppily popularized and turned into a lucrative marketing tool for supplements well before there was good evidence that the hypothesis was true or could lead to effective health interventions.

Here I will try to explain the hypothesis simply and then look at why calling something an antioxidant doesn't necessarily mean it is useful and you should give it to your pet.

A natural product of chemical reactions happening in our bodies, and those of our pets, are substances called free radicals or reactive oxygen species (ROS). These ROS are very quick to react with other chemicals, and that can lead to damage to important molecules in cells, and ultimately to dysfunction the cells and tissues. The reason we don't all melt away immediately in an oxidative conflagration is, of course, that our bodies have natural antioxidant systems in place to neutralize ROS and both prevent and repair the damage they can do. Some nutrients, such as Vitamin C and Vitamin E, are utilized as part of these natural antioxidant mechanisms.

These systems aren't perfect, of course, so damage from ROS does sometimes accumulate, and it has been shown to be one factor in the process of ageing and the development of some diseases. Despite the enthusiasm of some early researchers, oxidative damage is not the sole cause of illness or ageing, and reducing or eliminating it would not keep us from getting old or developing cancer. However, oxidative damage is a proven risk factor for some diseases and does play a role in the changes that come with age, and there is reason to believe that some manipulations of this process might be beneficial in some cases.[23]

As you may have come to expect by now, however, there are few perfect heroes or absolute villains in biology. It turns out that ROS aren't just a cause of damage in our bodies, they also perform a variety of vital, beneficial functions. The immune system uses ROS, for example, to kill harmful bacteria and to destroy cancer cells before they can get established and make us sick.[25,26] Some laboratory research even suggests reducing the production of ROS may accelerate rather than retard ageing.[27] This should make us think twice about trying to wipe out these molecules.

The research on antioxidant supplements has been extensive and expensive and has gone on for decades. There is no "final word" on the subject, as is typical for science in general, but there is a growing consensus that: oxidative damage is only one of many factors involved in ageing and illness; natural antioxidant systems work pretty well by themselves; and while some antioxidants such as vitamins are necessary at normal levels in the diet to help control ROS, excessive consumption of these as supplements not only doesn't seem to have health benefits, it can actually do harm. Multiple studies in people have shown that high doses of antioxidant vitamins do not effectively prevent illness, and they can sometimes increase the risk of cancer and other diseases.[28–33]

There is little direct research on antioxidant supplementation, in food or as nutritional supplements, for producing health benefits in dogs and cats. A handful of studies show some potentially promising effects on markers of oxidative damage, and a couple seem to show some clinical benefits, but the evidence is scant and weak.[34–48] The harmful effects of antioxidant supplementation in humans has only emerged with studies of large numbers of individuals over periods of time far longer than typical veterinary trials, so while few specific safety risks are known for common antioxidants, the assumption of safety is not justified for most.

Brennen McKenzie

The bottom line is that most of the claims concerning the benefits of antioxidants are based on theory or indirect and limited evidence. The specific antioxidant given, the form in which it is given, the other components of the diet, the species, health status, and individual makeup of each animal, and many other factors all influence the effects of antioxidants. Whether such effects are strong enough to be clinically significant, and whether they are beneficial or harmful if they do have a real effect, is a complicated question, and simplistic, strong claims are not justified. Using antioxidant supplements in your pets is a roll of the dice. You might protect them, you might put them at risk, and you probably won't ever be able to tell which you are doing because the complexity of biology makes individual cases unreliable predictors of the true benefits and risks of such products.

DOES IT WORK?

As I'm sure you will expect at this point, there is no way to talk about whether dietary supplements in general work or don't work. Every individual supplement, ideally every particular product, should be tested at each level, from theory, to preclinical lab studies, to clinical trials, in the specific species and for the specific problem it is meant to treat or prevent. As you have probably also come to realize, this kind of comprehensive scientific evidence is rare in veterinary medicine, so most of the time we have to make decisions about what to give our pets based on lower quality evidence and extrapolating from studies in humans. This is less than ideal, and since it can easily lead us to the wrong decision, we should also be careful not to have too much confidence in our judgements and to be open to changing our minds when there is new and better evidence, even if this contradicts our own experiences.

For the most part, veterinary supplements are loosely regulated, with even less control than for supplements marketed for humans, and these in turn are less tightly monitored than conventional medicines.[49-52] Governments tend to focus on monitoring what companies say about their supplements more than on the effects of the products themselves. In the human market, most companies can't say a supplement prevents, treats, or cures a particular disease unless they have scientific evidence for this, as is required for drugs. Most get around this with vague claims that their products "support" or "enhance" or "boost" some normal function.

Veterinary supplements are sometimes expected to follow similar rules, and in some jurisdictions are effectively not regulated much at all. In general, the supplement industry is a classic "buyer beware" market in which you can't trust that claims of safety or effectiveness have been proven scientifically or are endorsed by government health authorities.

Because a high level of evidence is not required before marketing for supplements, it doesn't exist for most. Lab animal and test tube research predominates, and when clinical trials are done they are often funded and conducted by manufacturers, meaning a significant risk of bias in the results. I will discuss a couple of examples of the most popular supplements to illustrate the challenges in evaluating their effects scientifically. Our usual approach and standards for assessing a treatment apply to dietary supplements, so these examples are intended mostly as a roadmap for the process you might want to apply to any other products you are considering, along with the evaluation of possible risks, which I will address a bit later. A few other popular supplements will also be evaluated in Chapter 9.

EXAMPLES OF DIETARY SUPPLEMENTS

GLUCOSAMINE

What Is It

Glucosamine has remained among the most popular supplements for decades, in both humans and animals. Global glucosamine sales are expected to be worth over US$1 billion by 2020, and glucosamine was the single largest product in the nearly US$600 million veterinary supplement market in 2014.[53,54]

Glucosamine is rarely the only constituent in supplement products, and it is most often combined with chondroitin sulfate and other chemicals in supplements used primarily to treat and prevent arthritis. Both glucosamine and chondroitin are produced naturally in mammals, and they are normal components of the fluid that lubricates joints.[55] These compounds are also produced in shellfish and some fungi, and supplement products on the market contain a variety of different chemical forms of these compounds from various sources. This contributes to some confusion about the results of research studies and the evaluation of particular products.

Oral supplementation of glucosamine has been hypothesized to help prevent or treat arthritis and the pain associated with it by various mechanisms, from mechanical lubrication of joints to reducing inflammation and other chemical reactions in arthritic joints that contribute to the symptoms and progression of the disease.[55]

276

Does It Work?

Because arthritis is very common, and joint supplements containing glucosamine are consequently very popular, there has been more research than usual done on this substance. As a result, it is a good example of how a scientific evaluation of a supplement should look.

The basic theories behind the use of glucosamine, involving the chemistry of joints and the effects glucosamine has in test tubes on other chemicals and cells found in joints, are plausible and well-studied. There is certainly good reason to think glucosamine might be useful based on this kind of basic scientific knowledge. There are also many lab animal studies looking at various forms of glucosamine, alone and in combination with lots of other substances. These are mixed, and not all show a clear benefit, though some do. At the level of preclinical evidence, then, glucosamine might work, but the results are not completely clear or consistent.

In dogs, there have been four clinical trials of various glucosamine-containing products, with multiple systematic reviews and narrative reviews published critically evaluating this literature (sorry, cat owners, no clinical trials published for glucosamine as a supplement yet, only one for a diet which contained glucosamine and other joint supplement ingredients).[56–59] These studies involved a total of about 170 dogs treated for 1-5 months. By veterinary standards, this is a lot of evidence! And the winner is...

Unfortunately, the evidence isn't entirely conclusive. Some of the studies showed some improvement in subjective measures of pain and in function compared with a placebo, others didn't. A couple of studies also looked at objective measures of effect (using a device to measure the amount of weight a dog will put on an arthritic limb).[60,61] Neither of these studies showed any effect of glucosamine on these objective measures, which suggests that even with the intent of blinding investigators to which treatment the dogs were getting, some kind of bias or placebo effect may have been at work in these trials. Some of the studies also compared glucosamine to a non-steroidal anti-inflammatory drug (NSAID), which is the standard treatment for arthritis pain in dogs. The NSAIDs clearly had greater benefits than the glucosamine in these studies.[60,62]

These studies used different products, different doses, different populations of dogs, and different ways of measuring the effect of the supplement, so it is hard to compare them. Proponents of glucosamine, and other supplement or alternative treatments that don't perform well in multiple clinical trials often cite such differences to claim that the negative results don't mean the treatments don't work, only that the studies didn't use the right form, dose, or variety of the treatment. This is a legitimate point, but it raises a tricky problem.

With the hundreds of different glucosamine-containing supplements on the market, and all the differences we will inevitably see between arthritis patients and researchers in different studies, we could easily conduct many hundreds of clinical trial, find all negative results, and still not completely rule out the possibility that the treatment would work if used in some form or manner we haven't yet tested. As a practical matter, we have to make decisions based on the best evidence currently available. We can always change our minds later if there is new or better evidence, but we shouldn't get so carried away by our understanding of the limitations in research studies that we start ignoring their findings and go back to relying on our theories or anecdotes. So while the evidence is limited and imperfect, so far it doesn't look good for glucosamine, at least in dogs.

As proud as we can be of the amount of clinical trial evidence we have in dogs for glucosamine, which is more than we often have to base our decisions on, it is still worth taking a look at the evidence in humans. While extrapolation from research in people is perilous, the amount and quality of the evidence in human medicine is often far greater than in veterinary medicine, and we can't afford to ignore it entirely. In the case of glucosamine, our four clinical trials and three systematic reviews look pretty paltry compared with the human literature. There are over 150 systematic reviews of glucosamine arthritis studies listed in the US National Library of Medicine's PubMed database, and hundreds of clinical trials. These involve thousands of patients, some studied for several years.[55,63–77]

Even with so much greater an evidence base, the conclusions of the reviews are not all in agreement. Most conclude that there is little reason to think glucosamine has significant benefits for humans with arthritis. Some studies do show positive effects, but the better the controls for bias and error, and the less involvement supplement manufacturers have in funding and conducting the studies, the less likely we are to see any benefit. Recommendations from organizations of specialists in arthritis treatment vary, some suggesting glucosamine might be worth taking and others recommending against it.[78,79]

At most, there might be a very small effect for some subgroups of people with particular kinds of arthritis, but overall, the human literature is no more convincing than the studies in dogs about the benefits of glucosamine in arthritis patients. The lack of clear and definitive evidence that glucosamine works in people despite decades of research and hundreds of studies is, itself, pretty good reason to conclude there is no dramatic benefit to be found.

So if the evidence suggests glucosamine probably doesn't do much, if anything, to treat pain or slow the progression of arthritis, why is it still so popular? In this regard, glucosamine is a great example of how the supplement market works. As patients, and pet owners, dealing with chronic and incurable diseases, we want something active to do to combat these conditions. Our psychological need to do something can easily overcome our intellectual understanding that what we are doing may not really work. And all the biases and errors I talked about in Chapter 1 come into play so that it almost always seems to us, at least at first, like the supplement we are using helps, even if there is more reliable objective evidence to suggest it probably doesn't.

Supplement makers are also free to cater to our desire to act, and they are typically allowed to at least imply, if not state outright, that their products are effective even when the evidence doesn't show that. The rules are set by politicians, not scientists. They tend to favor our desire to have options, even if they are not truly helpful, and to favor the interests of business who profit from selling supplements and who are often involved and influential in the political domain.

The supplement industry is also free to encourage our fear of science-based therapies such as NSAIDs. Because we have more and better evidence for such treatments, since it is required by regulators, we also have a better understanding of the risks. No truly effective therapy is completely without risks, so once we've understood the benefits of a treatment, we will also be aware of at least some of the potential harm it can do. In the case of

NSAIDs, the risks are real, though they are pretty small compared to the benefits for most pets. Promoters of glucosamine and other supplements are free to encourage our fears of these risks and to exaggerate them while claiming better and safer results from their products, which don't have to undergo anything like the level of scrutiny traditional medicines are subjected to.

Proponents of glucosamine, and other supplements and alternative therapies, will often say, "If so many people swear by it, it must work!" This is another classic logic error, known as the *ad populum* fallacy. As we've seen with bloodletting, acupuncture, and other treatments I've discussed, it is easy and common for many people to swear by a therapy that doesn't actually work. In the case of supplements like glucosamine, the economic environment, the legal and regulatory context, and basic human psychology all favor the continued use of ineffective treatments, not only when there is little evidence for them but even when the bulk of the evidence suggests they don't work. Apart from products with dramatic and direct harm, our current methods of evaluating and regulating dietary supplements does a poor job of helping us distinguish the useful from the useless. And as we will see later, often the system doesn't even help us avoid products which are clearly harmful.

Is It Safe?

Fortunately, in the case of glucosamine the answer is probably "Yes." While the evidence for benefit is poor, very little evidence of serious harm has turned up in the human or veterinary research. Mild complaints, such as nausea and diarrhea, show up in some patients, but they are not very common or severe. More serious concerns have been raised about possible effects on blood clotting or the maintenance of proper blood sugar levels, but these don't seem to be truly significant problems given the enormous numbers of people and pets who are taking glucosamine products without any obvious harm.[80,81]

Bottom Line

We have more and better-quality evidence concerning glucosamine than for most dietary supplements used in pets, largely because it is a wildly popular and profitable product. The bulk of the evidence, in humans and in dogs, suggests it probably doesn't do much to help patients with arthritis. We cannot absolutely rule out some benefit from some types of glucosamine in some cases, but given the volume of research over several decades, if it were a powerful therapy for most patients, we would know this by know. Claims to the contrary are based on anecdote and wishful thinking, not science.

Many supplements are marketed and used by consumers with the idea that they might or might not be helpful but at least using them can't hurt. As we shall see when we talk about supplement safety in general, this is frequently not true. However, in the case of glucosamine, this is a pretty fair assessment. It might help some patients, it probably won't help most, and it is unlikely to do any direct harm.

The main disadvantages to using glucosamine are the cost and the risks of delaying more effective treatment. Most pet owners don't have unlimited resources, and it is frustrating to see people spend these on something that probably isn't doing much, only to have difficulty affording appropriate testing and treatment when it is needed. And because the evidence suggests glucosamine isn't likely to be very effective, it should not be seen as a substitute for treatments that do work. The risks of NSAIDs are well understood and generally small, and they clearly do relieve pain in our pets. I find it hard to see animals suffering unnecessarily with arthritis because their owners have excessive fear of NSAIDS and other proven medicines or are mistakenly convinced that glucosamine or other alternatives are effective.

While I appreciate these owners care for their pets and are trying to do the best for them, it is still hard to watch my patients suffer when they shouldn't have to. One of my hopes for this book is that you will learn the best approaches for evaluating the treatment options available to you, and this will help you to make the best, most evidence-based choices you can for your pets.

PROBIOTICS

What Is It?

It has been said that there are ten times as many bacterial cells as human cells in the average human body.[82] It has been said, but it's probably not true.[83] Still, there is undoubtedly a large and complex ecology of microorganisms living in and on every individual mammal, and this ecology has multifaceted and important health effects.[84] Microorganisms produce important nutrients, influence immune function and digestion, and have other beneficial effects on health.[84] Disruption of this ecosystem can have negative health effects, as anyone who has suffered from antibiotic-associated diarrhea can attest!

Our growing understanding of the importance of commensal microorganisms has led to the hope that we may be able to deliberately alter the microbial flora of healthy animals and veterinary patients to achieve targeted health benefits. Microorganisms, usually bacteria or yeast, that are administered to prevent or treat disease are known as probiotics, and a lucrative industry has emerged to produce and sell such organisms.[53,85] They are consistently in the top ten supplements sold for both human and animal use.

There are certain characteristics an organism has to have to make a potential probiotic. Obviously, it can't be something that is going to make the patient taking it ill. It also needs to be able to survive passing through the stomach, a bag full of acid designed as much for killing off potentially infectious organisms as for digesting our food. After making it through the stomach, the organism then needs to establish itself in the gut of the patient and be able reproduce and interact with other organisms and with the patient. It is generally thought that the beneficial effects of probiotics require these organisms to survive transit through the stomach and to colonize the intestines, though there are some studies suggesting that even dead probiotic organisms, in sufficient quantities, can have effects on the health of the patient taking them.[86,87]

If ever there was a perfect example of my now too familiar principle that the devil is in the details, it is the field of probiotics. There are hundreds, perhaps thousands of different organisms living throughout the guts of humans and their pets, many of which haven't even been identified yet. This complex ecology is constantly changing, and it is influenced by our genes, the other people and animals we live with, the foods we eat, the medicines we take, and many other factors we don't fully understand.

For probiotics administered as a supplement to have health effects, they have to enter and function in this ecology in a reliable and predictable way.

Simply dropping a few *Lactobacillus* in a cup of yoghurt into this environment is unlikely to have a large impact on health. One infectious disease specialist and humorist, Dr. Mark Crislip, has likened taking probiotics to planting a putting green in the middle of the Amazon rainforest. It's hard to imagine this remaking the entire ecological system.

How exactly probiotics influence health isn't clear, and there are probably multiple mechanisms.[88,89,90] They may crowd out other organisms that do us harm, they may influence the activity of our own immune systems, they may change the ecological balance of the gut in ways that promote beneficial activity by other organism, and there may be other mechanisms we know nothing about. Simplistic explanations, such as the common claim that probiotics "balance" the gut, are not accurate or helpful.

Deciding whether a probiotic is going to be useful for our pets requires thinking about what the problem is we are trying to solve, what the state of their microbial ecosystem is and how it got that way, what particular organisms have been shown to meet the criteria for a useful probiotic and what kind of evidence there is that these actually solve the problem we are dealing with. We then also have to think about which products to use, since even the same organism can be more or less helpful depending on how it is produced, packaged, and administered. Whew, I'm tired already!

Does It Work?

By now you know I'm not going to give you a simple answer. There is good preclinical evidence that probiotics might work. Some organisms have potentially useful effects in lab animal studies, so there is reason to believe they could be useful in actual patients. And in humans, there is an overwhelming body of clinical research on a huge variety of different types of probiotic bacteria and yeast. A search of the Pubmed database shows over 1,000 systematic reviews evaluating over 2,500 clinical trials!

This extensive literature involves studies of many different kinds of probiotics in various populations and with many different medical conditions. For most specific diseases or probiotic products, the evidence is mixed and inconclusive. There is, however, pretty good evidence in humans that probiotics can help with several types of diarrhea (traveler's diarrhea, antibiotic-associated diarrhea, and some cases caused by viral infections).[91–100] They also appear useful in preventing some types of allergic skin disease in children,[101,102] and they may help some people with chronic inflammatory bowel disease.[103,104] There are many, many other possible uses for which the evidence is limited or conflicting.

And what about our pets? Probiotics have been recommended for a variety of problems in dogs and cats. Many of these are the same as the conditions probiotics are used for in humans, including diarrhea and inflammatory bowel disease, as well as viral upper respiratory infection and kidney disease. A handful of studies have been done looking at these and other uses.[105,106] Some proponents have also suggested everyone should take probiotics because they can improve or protect health even in individuals without any apparent disease, but there is no reliable human or veterinary research evidence to support this.[105] Below are some common uses for which probiotics have been recommended and brief summaries of the available evidence.

1. Acute Diarrhea

There are several studies showing beneficial effects on probiotics on prevention and treatment of acute diarrhea in dogs and cats.[105–110]

These studies are small, employ a variety of different probiotic products, and have some significant methodological limitations. There are also studies that have failed to find significant effects of probiotics for diarrhea.[105,111]

Overall, the existing evidence for the value of probiotics in preventing and treating acute diarrhea is encouraging, though still not robust.

2. Chronic Intestinal Disease

There are also encouraging studies showing effects of probiotics on the intestinal ecology in dogs with food sensitivities and inflammatory bowel disease.[105,112] However, there are no definitive studies showing significant and sustained improvement in long-term symptoms for dogs or cats with chronic intestinal disease.

3. Skin Allergies

Because probiotics have various effects on the immune system, several studies have looked at the potential value of probiotic treatment in the management of allergic skin disease.[105,113,114] Once again, there are some encouraging results, but predictable, durable, and meaningful improvement in real-world use has not yet been shown.

4. Upper Respiratory Infections

A single pilot study has been reported evaluating probiotic use in cats with an upper respiratory viral infection.[115] The study was small, and results were mixed and did not show a convincing beneficial effect. As with allergic skin disease, additional research is warranted, but there isn't much basis for clinical use at this point.

5. Chronic Kidney Disease

   Some preliminary studies in dogs, rats and pigs have suggested probiotics might reduce the buildup of metabolic toxins or otherwise
   benefit patients with chronic kidney disease.[116, 117] Uncontrolled observations in cats and dogs have also suggested some such effects,
   but of course you know that the risk of bias is very high for such
   anecdotal evidence.[116] At least one commercial probiotic has been
   marketed for this purpose and has been the subject of several studies.[116,118,119] Though small and with significant limitations, these
   controlled studies have not found any convincing evidence of a
   meaningful impact of this probiotic on kidney disease in dogs or
   cats.

So the short answer (or is it too late for that?) to the question "Does It
Work?" is "Sometimes." Specific probiotics have proven useful for specific
health problems. There is pretty good evidence for several products in diarrhea in humans, cats, and dogs. There is less evidence, but still encouraging
data on the treatment of chronic intestinal disease. I expect more uses for
probiotics will be found, and in the future we will have a large and well-
documented selection of living organisms that we can reliably use to control
different health problems. Right now, though, we are just at the very beginning of discovering what probiotics can and can't do, and most of the claims
you are likely to hear about them are not based on solid scientific evidence.

Is It Safe?

Whenever there is limited research evidence, it is impossible to be certain of
not only the efficacy but the safety of medical therapies. Both actual and

theoretical risks from probiotics have been discussed in the human medical literature. Generally, probiotics are considered safe in people with healthy, functional immune systems, though not all the potential risks are well characterized.[120,121] There have been rare cases of serious infection and even death associated with probiotic organisms in people with abnormal immune function, such as those with an immunosuppressive disease or on chemotherapy or other medications that can impede the immune system.

Some evidence of negative effects has been reported in veterinary species as well.[122] One study in foals found that a probiotic actually made diarrhea symptoms worse rather than better. Another study found that use of a probiotic increased the chances that dogs would harbor potentially dangerous *Salmonella* bacteria.[123]

There are also concerns about indirect risks, such as the transmission of antibiotic resistance genes from probiotic species to potentially infectious organism. This led to the refusal of one regulatory agency, the European Food Safety Authority, to approve the use of a commercial veterinary probiotic when the constituent organism was found to be resistant to the antibiotic clindamycin.[124] Despite such concerns and the uncertainty of limited evidence, probiotics have been widely available and frequently used, in research and clinical settings, without many reports of obvious harm to veterinary patients, so the risks are likely quite low.

Is It Safe?

Just as the effectiveness of supplements has to be evaluated on a case-by-case basis, so we have to look closely at the potential risks of each specific supplement individually. However, there are some general concerns with dietary supplements that apply broadly throughout the industry.

Because there is inconsistent and often minimal regulation, the ingredients in supplements are frequently misrepresented by manufacturers. This can lead to poor efficacy even when a supplement should be helpful if the active ingredient is of poor quality or perhaps not even present at all in a specific product you buy for your pets. Probiotics are a stark example of this. Studies of both human and veterinary probiotic products have found that a large percentage of them are incorrectly or misleadingly labeled.[125,126,127] Some have minor deficiencies, such as misspelled or incorrect species names for the organisms they are supposed to contain. Many have more serious problems, such as contamination with unintended organisms, lower levels of the intended organisms than promised or, in some cases, no live organisms at all! Even if there is good evidence that some probiotics can help your dog recover faster from a case of diarrhea, you aren't going to get these benefits from a product with little or no probiotic in it. There are similar serious problems with labeling and quality control for many other types of dietary supplements as well.

It is often assumed that the risk of dietary supplements is negligible. This is usually an expression of the Appeal to Nature Fallacy, since any substance which has a meaningful effect on the body for good is likely to have some unintended or undesirable effects as well. It is important to remember, also, that safety is frequently related to dose, and that even supplements which are safe when used as intended can be dangerous when taken at higher doses, intentionally or accidentally. While joint supplements for dogs, for example, seem to be pretty safe in clinical studies, there have been a number of cases of severe injury and even death from overdoses of these supplements.[128,129] Many veterinary dietary supplements are designed to be tasty and appealing to our pets to make it easier to administer them, and this can lead to our animals, especially dogs, eating far too much of such supplements if they get the chance.

More worrisome than accidental overdose is the presence of poisonous ingredients in supplements that aren't supposed to be there. A large and growing number of humans have ended up in the hospital, often with life-threatening disease such as kidney failure or liver failure, due to undisclosed or illicit ingredients in dietary supplements. Supplement manufacturers have been known to put unidentified herbal ingredients or even illegal prescription drugs into supplement products. Products intended for weight loss, for muscle building, for increasing energy, and for treating sexual dysfunction have turned out to contain amphetamines, anabolic steroids, and prescription medications like Viagra which are intended to create the effects the manufacturer claims, often without real evidence, that consumers will get from the dietary supplement itself. This has led to serious illness and death in people taking such supplements, and the evidence suggests the rates of harm from supplement products is growing.[130-144]

Finally, there is sometimes real risk even from the intended ingredients in supplements taken at the recommended dose. The fact that we often have very little, if any, clinical trial research on most supplement products means we cannot be confident about their effectiveness or their safety.

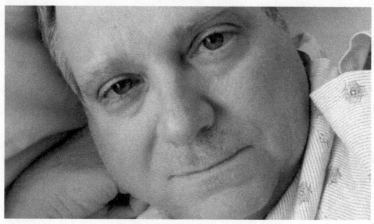

© Jim McCants, from[145]

Jim McCants was fifty years old and determined to take good care of himself. He increased his exercise, started improving his diet and trying to lose weight, and he started taking an antioxidant supplement made from green tea. Unfortunately, Jim became one of a growing number of people taking such supplements who developed liver failure as an unintended result.[145]

We don't know exactly why the chemical compounds in such supplements sometimes damage the liver because there is no requirement for the necessary research to be done before marketing these products. It may be the dose, the way the products are made, or individual genetic factors. What we do know is that people like Jim, who are already healthy, can suffer severe harm from these supplements, and that the risk is unpredictable.

Plenty of other supplements have turned out to have unexpected risks, even those we might assume to be the most benign. Vitamin E has been associated with an increased risk of cancer, heart attacks and strokes in several studies.[31,32,33,146–150] Men taking high doses of B vitamins have a higher risk of lung cancer than those not taking this supplement.[151] Some studies have even shown a higher overall risk of death in people taking vitamin supplements compared with people not taking them.[152,153]

Non-vitamin supplements have also been associated with a variety of risks, from minor uncomfortable symptoms to severe injury. Tens of thousands of people are admitted to hospital emergency rooms every year for symptoms related to dietary supplement use, and this is for a class of products that we often don't know for sure even have any real benefits.[142]

In the veterinary world, there is much less research and monitoring of supplement use and adverse effects. There is no particular reason to think supplements marketed to our pets are any safer than those marketed for human use, but we don't look very hard to monitor the safety of such products, so it is difficult to say how much harm they may be doing. Without real evidence, pet owners are in the uncomfortable position of simply having to hope for the best if they choose to use most of the available products.

That may be reasonable if your pet has a serious illness and there are no proven treatments that are likely to help, but it seems a needless risk in healthy pets. Our desire to have control over the fate of our animal friends and to protect them from harm is laudable, but we must also be rational and careful in the choices we make for our pets. Balancing risks and benefits is always necessary in making decisions about any treatment or preventative we use, and this is true of dietary supplements as well. This is made more difficult by the lack of reliable research evidence for most veterinary supplements, but a cautious and skeptical approach can still help us make good decisions for our pets.

Brennen McKenzie

If fifty million people say a foolish thing, it is still a foolish thing.

- Anatole France

[1] Kobayashi E, Nishijima C, Sato Y, Umegaki K, Chiba T. The prevalence of dietary supplement use among elementary, junior high, and high school students: A nationwide survey in Japan. *Nutrients*. 2018;10(9):1176. doi:10.3390/nu10091176

[2] Kobayashi E, Sato Y, Umegaki K, Chiba T. The prevalence of dietary supplement use among college students: a nationwide survey in Japan. *Nutrients*. 2017;9(11):1250. doi:10.3390/nu9111250

[3] Lentjes MAH, Welch AA, Luben RN, Khaw K-T. Differences in dietary supplement use and secular and seasonal trends assessed using three different instruments in the EPIC-Norfolk population study. *J Diet Suppl*. 2013;10(2):142-151. doi:10.3109/19390211.2013.790336

[4] Hutchinson J, Burley VJ, Greenwood DC, Cade JE. General supplement use, subsequent use and cancer risk in the UK Women's Cohort Study. *Eur J Clin Nutr*. 2014;68(10):1095-1100. doi:10.1038/ejcn.2014.85

[5] Rovira M-A, Grau M, Castañer O, Covas M-I, Schröder H. Dietary supplement use and health-related behaviors in a Mediterranean population. *J Nutr Educ Behav*. 2013;45(5):386-391. doi:10.1016/j.jneb.2012.03.007

[6] Kofoed CLF, Christensen J, Dragsted LO, Tjønneland A, Roswall N. Determinants of dietary supplement use – healthy individuals use dietary supplements. *Br J Nutr*. 2015;113(12):1993-2000. doi:10.1017/S0007114515001440

[7] Lieberman HR, Marriott BP, Williams C, et al. Patterns of dietary supplement use among college students. *Clin Nutr*. 2015;34(5):976-985. doi:10.1016/j.clnu.2014.10.010

[8] Kantor ED, Rehm CD, Du M, White E, Giovannucci EL. Trends in dietary supplement use among US adults from 1999-2012. *JAMA*. 2016;316(14):1464. doi:10.1001/jama.2016.14403

[9] Dickinson A, Blatman J, El-Dash N, Franco JC. Consumer usage and reasons for using dietary supplements: report of a series of surveys. *J Am Coll Nutr*. 2014;33(2):176-182. doi:10.1080/07315724.2013.875423

[10] Burns K. Assessing pet supplements. *JAVMA News*. January, 2017. Available at: https://www.avma.org/News/JAVMANews/Pages/170115a.aspx. Accessed June 23, 2019.

[11] Reed C. The Growing Pet Supplements Market. *Nutritional Outlook*. March, 2017. Available at: http://www.nutritionaloutlook.com/trends-business/growing-pet-supplements-market. Accessed June 23, 2019.

[12] Grand View Research. *Dietary Supplements Market Size, Share & Trend Analysis Report By Ingredient (Botanicals, Vitamins, Minerals, Amino Acids, Enzymes), By Product, By Application, By End-Use, And Segment Forecasts, 2019 - 2025*. 2019. Available at: https://www.grandviewresearch.com/industry-analysis/dietary-supplements-market. Accessed June 23, 2019.

[13] Zwart S. Ironing out nutrition's bell-shaped curve. A Lab Aloft (International Space Station Research). 2015. Available at: https://blogs.nasa.gov/ISS_Science_Blog/2015/02/24/ironing-out-nutritions-bell-shaped-curve/ Accessed September 12, 2018.

[14] Schaible UE, Kaufmann SHE. Malnutrition and infection: complex mechanisms and global impacts. *PLoS Med*. 2007;4(5):e115. doi:10.1371/journal.pmed.0040115

[15] Irwin MR. Why sleep is important for health: a psychoneuroimmunology perspective. *Annu Rev Psychol*. 2015;66(1):143-172. doi:10.1146/annurev-psych-010213-115205

[16] Segerstrom SC, Miller GE. Psychological stress and the human immune system: a meta-analytic study of 30 years of inquiry. Psychol Bull. 2004;130(4):601-630. doi:10.1037/0033-2909.130.4.601

[17] Dhabhar FS. Effects of stress on immune function: the good, the bad, and the beautiful. *Immunol Res*. 2014;58(2-3):193-210. doi:10.1007/s12026-014-8517-0

[18] Simon AK, Hollander GA, McMichael A. Evolution of the immune system in humans from infancy to old age. *Proceedings Biol Sci*. 2015;282(1821):20143085. doi:10.1098/rspb.2014.3085

[19] Weyand CM, Goronzy JJ. Aging of the immune system. mechanisms and therapeutic targets. *Ann Am Thorac Soc*. 2016;13(Supplement_5):S422-S428. doi:10.1513/AnnalsATS.201602-095AW

[20] Szabo G, Saha B. Alcohol's effect on host defense. *Alcohol Res*. 2015;37(2):159-170.

[21] Qiu F, Liang C-L, Liu H, et al. Impacts of cigarette smoking on immune responsiveness: Up and down or upside down? *Oncotarget*. 2017;8(1):268-284. doi:10.18632/oncotarget.13613

[22] Krüger K, Mooren F-C, Pilat C. The Immunomodulatory effects of physical activity. *Curr Pharm Des*. 2016;22(24):3730-3748..

[23] El-Kadiki A, Sutton AJ. Role of multivitamins and mineral supplements in preventing infections in elderly people: systematic review and meta-analysis of randomised controlled trials. *BMJ*. 2005;330(7496):871. doi:10.1136/bmj.38399.495648.8F

[24] Gariballa S. Vitamin and mineral supplements for preventing infections in older people. *BMJ*. 2005;331(7512):304-305. doi:10.1136/bmj.331.7512.304

[25] Pizzino G, Irrera N, Cucinotta M, et al. Oxidative stress: Harms and benefits for human health. *Oxid Med Cell Longev*. 2017;2017:8416763. doi:10.1155/2017/8416763

[26] Pham-Huy LA, He H, Pham-Huy C. Free radicals, antioxidants in disease and health. *Int J Biomed Sci*. 2008;4(2):89-96.

[27] Yee C, Yang W, Hekimi S. The intrinsic apoptosis pathway mediates the pro-longevity response to mitochondrial ROS in C. elegans. *Cell*. 2014;157(4):897-909. doi:10.1016/j.cell.2014.02.055

[28] Bjelakovic G, Nikolova D, Gluud LL, Simonetti RG, Gluud C. Mortality in randomized trials of antioxidant supplements for primary and secondary prevention. *JAMA.* 2007;297(8):842. doi:10.1001/jama.297.8.842

[29] Bjelakovic G, Nikolova D, Gluud LL, Simonetti RG, Gluud C. Antioxidant supplements for prevention of mortality in healthy participants and patients with various diseases. *Cochrane Database Syst Rev.* 2012;(3):CD007176. doi:10.1002/14651858.CD007176.pub2

[30] Bjelakovic G, Nikolova D, Gluud C. Antioxidant supplements and mortality. *Curr Opin Clin Nutr Metab Care.* 2013;17(1):1. doi:10.1097/MCO.0000000000000009

[31] Sesso HD, Buring JE, Christen WG, et al. Vitamins E and C in the prevention of cardiovascular disease in men. *JAMA.* 2008;300(18):2123. doi:10.1001/jama.2008.600

[32] Paulsen G, Cumming KT, Holden G, et al. Vitamin C and E supplementation hampers cellular adaptation to endurance training in humans: a double-blind, randomised, controlled trial. *J Physiol.* 2014;592(8):1887-1901. doi:10.1113/jphysiol.2013.267419

[33] Schürks M, Glynn RJ, Rist PM, Tzourio C, Kurth T. Effects of vitamin E on stroke subtypes: meta-analysis of randomised controlled trials. *BMJ.* 2010;341:c5702. doi:10.1136/BMJ.C5702

[34] Piercy RJ, Hinchcliff KW, DiSilvestro RA, et al. Effect of dietary supplements containing antioxidants on attenuation of muscle damage in exercising sled dogs. *Am J Vet Res.* 2000;61(11):1438-1445.

[35] Freeman LM. Focus on nutrition: antioxidants in cancer treatment: helpful or harmful? *Compend Contin Educ Vet.* 2009;31(4):154-158.

[36] Hall JA, Chinn RM, Vorachek WR, et al. Influence of dietary antioxidants and fatty acids on neutrophil mediated bacterial killing and gene expression in healthy Beagles. *Vet Immunol Immunopathol.* 2011;139(2-4):217-228. doi:10.1016/j.vetimm.2010.10.020

[37] Milgram NW, Head E, Zicker SC, et al. Learning ability in aged beagle dogs is preserved by behavioral enrichment and dietary fortification: a two-year longitudinal study. *Neurobiol Aging.* 2005;26(1):77-90. doi:10.1016/j.neurobiolaging.2004.02.014

[38] Siwak CT, Tapp PD, Head E, et al. Chronic antioxidant and mitochondrial cofactor administration improves discrimination learning in aged but not young dogs. *Prog Neuro-Psychopharmacology Biol Psychiatry.* 2005;29(3):461-469. doi:10.1016/j.pnpbp.2004.12.011

[39] Milgram NW, Araujo JA, Hagen TM, Treadwell B V., Ames BN. Acetyl- l -carnitine and α-lipoic acid supplementation of aged beagle dogs improves learning in two landmark discrimination tests. *FASEB J.* 2007;21(13):3756-3762. doi:10.1096/fj.07-8531com

[40] Zicker SC, Wedekind KJ, Jewell DE. Antioxidants in veterinary nutrition. *Vet Clin North Am Small Anim Pract.* 2006;36(6):1183-1198. doi:10.1016/j.cvsm.2006.08.002

[41] Di Cerbo A, Centenaro S, Beribè F, et al. Clinical evaluation of an antiinflammatory and antioxidant diet effect in 30 dogs affected by chronic otitis externa: preliminary results. *Vet Res Commun*. 2016;40(1):29-38. doi:10.1007/s11259-015-9651-4

[42] Plevnik Kapun A, Salobir J, Levart A, Tav ar Kalcher G, Nemec Svete A, Kotnik T. Vitamin E supplementation in canine atopic dermatitis: improvement of clinical signs and effects on oxidative stress markers. *Vet Rec*. 2014;175(22):560-560. doi:10.1136/vr.102547

[43] Barrouin-Melo SM, Anturaniemi J, Sankari S, et al. Evaluating oxidative stress, serological- and haematological status of dogs suffering from osteoarthritis, after supplementing their diet with fish or corn oil. *Lipids Health Dis*. 2016;15(1):139. doi:10.1186/s12944-016-0304-6

[44] Snigdha S, de Rivera C, Milgram NW, Cotman CW. Effect of mitochondrial cofactors and antioxidants supplementation on cognition in the aged canine. *Neurobiol Aging*. 2016;37:171-178. doi:10.1016/j.neurobiolaging.2015.09.015

[45] Sechi S, Fiore F, Chiavolelli F, Dimauro C, Nudda A, Cocco R. Oxidative stress and food supplementation with antioxidants in therapy dogs. *Can J Vet Res*. 2017;81(3):206-216.

[46] Marshall RJ, Scott KC, Hill RC, et al. Supplemental Vitamin C appears to slow racing greyhounds. *J Nutr*. 2002;132(6):1616S-1621S. doi:10.1093/jn/132.6.1616S

[47] Head E, Murphey HL, Dowling ALS, et al. A combination cocktail improves spatial attention in a canine model of human aging and alzheimer's disease. *J Alzheimer's Dis*. 2012;32(4):1029-1042. doi:10.3233/JAD-2012-120937

[48] Hesta M, Ottermans C, Krammer-Lukas S, et al. The effect of vitamin C supplementation in healthy dogs on antioxidative capacity and immune parameters. *J Anim Physiol Anim Nutr (Berl)*. 2009;93(1):26-34. doi:10.1111/j.1439-0396.2007.00774.x

[49] Center for Veterinary Medicine USF and DA. *CPG Sec. 690.100 Nutritional Supplements for Companion Animals*. Office of Regulatory Affairs; 1995. Available at: https://www.fda.gov/ICECI/ComplianceManuals/CompliancePolicyGuidanceManual/ucm074708.htm. Accessed December 11, 2018.

[50] Coppens P, da Silva MF, Pettman S. European regulations on nutraceuticals, dietary supplements and functional foods: A framework based on safety. *Toxicology*. 2006;221(1):59-74. doi:10.1016/j.tox.2005.12.022

[51] Larsen LL, Berry JA. The regulation of dietary supplements. *J Am Acad Nurse Pract*. 2003;15(9):410-414..

[52] Dwyer JT, Coates PM, Smith MJ. Dietary supplements: Regulatory challenges and research resources. *Nutrients*. 2018;10(1). doi:10.3390/nu10010041

[53] Packaged Facts. *Pet Supplements in the U.S., 5th Edition*. Rockville, MD; 2015. Available aty: https://www.packagedfacts.com/Pet-Supplements-8773200/. Accessed December 11, 2018.

[54] Grand View Research. *Glucosamine Market Analysis By Application (Nutritional Supplements, Food & Beverages, Dairy Products) And Segment Forecasts To 2022.* 2016. Available at: https://www.grandviewresearch.com/industry-analysis/glucosamine-market. Accessed December 11, 2018.

[55] Vasiliadis HS, Tsikopoulos K. Glucosamine and chondroitin for the treatment of osteoarthritis. *World J Orthop.* 2017;8(1):1-11. doi:10.5312/wjo.v8.i1.1

[56] Aragon CL, Hofmeister EH, Budsberg SC. Systematic review of clinical trials of treatments for osteoarthritis in dogs. *J Am Vet Med Assoc.* 2007;230(4):514-521. doi:10.2460/javma.230.4.514

[57] Sanderson RO, Beata C, Flipo R-M, et al. Systematic review of the management of canine osteoarthritis. *Vet Rec.* 2009;164:418-424. doi:10.1136/vr.164.14.418

[58] Vandeweerd JM, Coisnon C, Clegg P, et al. Systematic review of efficacy of nutraceuticals to alleviate clinical signs of osteoarthritis. *J Vet Intern Med.* 2012;26(3):448-456. doi:10.1111/j.1939-1676.2012.00901.x

[59] Bhathal A, Spryszak M, Louizos C, Frankel G. Glucosamine and chondroitin use in canines for osteoarthritis: A review. *Open Vet J.* 2017;7(1):36-49. doi:10.4314/ovj.v7i1.6

[60] Moreau M, Dupuis J, Bonneau NH, Desnoyers M. Clinical evaluation of a nutraceutical, carprofen and meloxicam for the treatment of dogs with osteoarthritis. *Vet Rec.* 2003;152(11):323-329..

[61] Gupta RC, Canerdy TD, Lindley J, et al. Comparative therapeutic efficacy and safety of type-II collagen (uc-II), glucosamine and chondroitin in arthritic dogs: pain evaluation by ground force plate. *J Anim Physiol Anim Nutr (Berl).* 2012;96(5):770-777. doi:10.1111/j.1439-0396.2011.01166.x

[62] McCarthy G, O'Donovan J, Jones B, McAllister H, Seed M, Mooney C. Randomised double-blind, positive-controlled trial to assess the efficacy of glucosamine/chondroitin sulfate for the treatment of dogs with osteoarthritis. *Vet J.* 2007;174(1):54-61. doi:10.1016/j.tvjl.2006.02.015

[63] Eriksen P, Bartels EM, Altman RD, Bliddal H, Juhl C, Christensen R. Risk of bias and brand explain the observed inconsistency in trials on glucosamine for symptomatic relief of osteoarthritis: A meta-analysis of placebo-controlled trials. *Arthritis Care Res (Hoboken).* 2014;66(12):1844-1855. doi:10.1002/acr.22376

[64] Harrison-Muñoz S, Rojas-Briones V, Irarrázaval S. Is glucosamine effective for osteoarthritis? *Medwave.* 2017;17(Suppl1):e6867-e6867. doi:10.5867/medwave.2017.6867

[65] Runhaar J, Rozendaal RM, van Middelkoop M, et al. Subgroup analyses of the effectiveness of oral glucosamine for knee and hip osteoarthritis: a systematic review and individual patient data meta-analysis from the OA trial bank. *Ann Rheum Dis.* 2017;76(11):1862-1869. doi:10.1136/annrheumdis-2017-211149

[66] Black C, Clar C, Henderson R, et al. The clinical effectiveness of glucosamine and chondroitin supplements in slowing or arresting progression of osteoarthritis of the knee: a systematic review and economic evaluation. *Health Technol Assess (Rockv)*. 2009;13(52):1-148. doi:10.3310/hta13520

[67] Dostrovsky NR, Towheed TE, Hudson RW, Anastassiades TP. The effect of glucosamine on glucose metabolism in humans: a systematic review of the literature. *Osteoarthr Cartil*. 2011;19(4):375-380. doi:10.1016/j.joca.2011.01.007

[68] Gallagher B, Tjoumakaris FP, Harwood MI, Good RP, Ciccotti MG, Freedman KB. Chondroprotection and the Prevention of Osteoarthritis Progression of the Knee. *Am J Sports Med*. 2015;43(3):734-744. doi:10.1177/0363546514533777

[69] Chan KOW, Ng GYF. A review on the effects of glucosamine for knee osteoarthritis based on human and animal studies. *Hong Kong Physiother J*. 2011;29(2):42-52. doi:10.1016/J.HKPJ.2011.06.004

[70] Liu X, Machado GC, Eyles JP, Ravi V, Hunter DJ. Dietary supplements for treating osteoarthritis: a systematic review and meta-analysis. *Br J Sports Med*. 2018;52(3):167-175. doi:10.1136/bjsports-2016-097333

[71] Ogata T, Ideno Y, Akai M, et al. Effects of glucosamine in patients with osteoarthritis of the knee: a systematic review and meta-analysis. *Clin Rheumatol*. 2018;37(9):2479-2487. doi:10.1007/s10067-018-4106-2

[72] Simental-Mendía M, Sánchez-García A, Vilchez-Cavazos F, Acosta-Olivo CA, Peña-Martínez VM, Simental-Mendía LE. Effect of glucosamine and chondroitin sulfate in symptomatic knee osteoarthritis: a systematic review and meta-analysis of randomized placebo-controlled trials. *Rheumatol Int*. 2018;38(8):1413-1428. doi:10.1007/s00296-018-4077-2

[73] Towheed T, Maxwell L, Anastassiades TP, et al. Glucosamine therapy for treating osteoarthritis. *Cochrane Database Syst Rev*. 2005;(2):CD002946. doi:10.1002/14651858.CD002946.pub2

[74] Kongtharvonskul J, Anothaisintawee T, McEvoy M, Attia J, Woratanarat P, Thakkinstian A. Efficacy and safety of glucosamine, diacerein, and NSAIDs in osteoarthritis knee: a systematic review and network meta-analysis. *Eur J Med Res*. 2015;20(1):24. doi:10.1186/s40001-015-0115-7

[75] Zeng C, Wei J, Li H, et al. Effectiveness and safety of glucosamine, chondroitin, the two in combination, or celecoxib in the treatment of osteoarthritis of the knee. *Sci Rep*. 2015;5(1):16827. doi:10.1038/srep16827

[76] Bhathal A, Spryszak M, Louizos C, Frankel G. Glucosamine and chondroitin use in canines for osteoarthritis: A review. *Open Vet J*. 2017;7(1):36. doi:10.4314/ovj.v7i1.6

[77] Bruyère O, Altman RD, Reginster J-Y. Efficacy and safety of glucosamine sulfate in the management of osteoarthritis: Evidence from real-life setting trials and surveys. *Semin Arthritis Rheum*. 2016;45(4):S12-S17. doi:10.1016/j.semarthrit.2015.11.011

[78] McAlindon TE, Bannuru RR, Sullivan MC, et al. OARSI guidelines for the non-surgical management of knee osteoarthritis. *Osteoarthr Cartil.* 2014;22(3):363-388. doi:10.1016/j.joca.2014.01.003

[79] Nelson AE, Allen KD, Golightly YM, Goode AP, Jordan JM. A systematic review of recommendations and guidelines for the management of osteoarthritis: The Chronic Osteoarthritis Management Initiative of the U.S. Bone and Joint Initiative. *Semin Arthritis Rheum.* 2014;43(6):701-712. doi:10.1016/j.semarthrit.2013.11.012

[80] Anderson JW, Nicolosi RJ, Borzelleca JF. Glucosamine effects in humans: a review of effects on glucose metabolism, side effects, safety considerations and efficacy. *Food Chem Toxicol.* 2005;43(2):187-201. doi:10.1016/J.FCT.2004.11.006

[81] Simon RR, Marks V, Leeds AR, Anderson JW. A comprehensive review of oral glucosamine use and effects on glucose metabolism in normal and diabetic individuals. *Diabetes Metab Res Rev.* 2011;27(1):14-27. doi:10.1002/dmrr.1150

[82] Sender R, Fuchs S, Milo R. Are we really vastly outnumbered? revisiting the ratio of bacterial to host cells in humans. *Cell.* 2016;164(3):337-340. doi:10.1016/j.cell.2016.01.013

[83] Sender R, Fuchs S, Milo R. Revised estimates for the number of human and bacteria cells in the body. *PLOS Biol.* 2016;14(8):e1002533. doi:10.1371/journal.pbio.1002533

[84] Zhang Y-J, Li S, Gan R-Y, Zhou T, Xu D-P, Li H-B. Impacts of gut bacteria on human health and diseases. *Int J Mol Sci.* 2015;16(4):7493-7519. doi:10.3390/ijms16047493

[85] Grand View Research. *Probiotics Dietary Supplements Market Analysis By Application (Food Supplements, Nutritional Supplements, Specialty Nutrients, Infant Formula), By Regions (North America, Europe, Asia Pacific, Middle East & Africa, CSA), And Segment Forecasts, 2018 - 2025.* San Francisco, CA; 2017.

[86] Behnsen J, Deriu E, Sassone-Corsi M, Raffatellu M. Probiotics: properties, examples, and specific applications. *Cold Spring Harb Perspect Med.* 2013;3(3):a010074. doi:10.1101/cshperspect.a010074

[87] Lahtinen SJ. Probiotic viability - does it matter? *Microb Ecol Health Dis.* 2012;23. doi:10.3402/mehd.v23i0.18567

[88] Singh VP, Sharma J, Babu S, Rizwanulla, Singla A. Role of probiotics in health and disease: a review. *J Pak Med Assoc.* 2013;63(2):253-257.

[89] Fong FLY, Shah NP, Kirjavainen P, El-Nezami H. Mechanism of action of probiotic bacteria on intestinal and systemic immunities and antigen-presenting cells. *Int Rev Immunol.* 2016;35(3):179-188. doi:10.3109/08830185.2015.1096937

[90] Bermudez-Brito M, Plaza-Díaz J, Muñoz-Quezada S, Gómez-Llorente C, Gil A. Probiotic mechanisms of action. *Ann Nutr Metab.* 2012;61(2):160-174. doi:10.1159/000342079

[91] Bae J-M. Prophylactic efficacy of probiotics on travelers' diarrhea: an adaptive meta-analysis of randomized controlled trials. *Epidemiol Health.* 2018;40:e2018043. doi:10.4178/epih.e2018043

[92] Mcfarland L V. Meta-analysis of probiotics for the prevention of traveler's diarrhea. *Travel Med Infect Dis.* 2007;5(2):97-105. doi:10.1016/j.tmaid.2005.10.003

[93] Goldenberg JZ, Ma SS, Saxton JD, et al. Probiotics for the prevention of Clostridium difficile-associated diarrhea in adults and children. *Cochrane Database Syst Rev.* 2013;(5):CD006095. doi:10.1002/14651858.CD006095.pub3

[94] Pinos Y, Castro-Gutiérrez V, Rada G. Are probiotics effective to prevent traveler's diarrhea? *Medwave.* 2016;16(Suppl5):e6807-e6807. doi:10.5867/medwave.2016.6807

[95] Blaabjerg S, Artzi D, Aabenhus R. Probiotics for the prevention of antibiotic-associated diarrhea in outpatients—A systematic review and meta-analysis. *Antibiotics.* 2017;6(4):21. doi:10.3390/antibiotics6040021

[96] Rondanelli M, Faliva MA, Perna S, Giacosa A, Peroni G, Castellazzi AM. Using probiotics in clinical practice: Where are we now? A review of existing meta-analyses. *Gut Microbes.* 2017;8(6):521-543. doi:10.1080/19490976.2017.1345414

[97] Salari P, Nikfar S, Abdollahi M. A meta-analysis and systematic review on the effect of probiotics in acute diarrhea. *Inflamm Allergy Drug Targets.* 2012;11(1):3-14.

[98] Allen SJ, Martinez EG, Gregorio G V, Dans LF. Probiotics for treating acute infectious diarrhoea. *Cochrane Database Syst Rev.* 2010;(11):CD003048. doi:10.1002/14651858.CD003048.pub3

[99] Applegate JA, Fischer Walker CL, Ambikapathi R, Black RE. Systematic review of probiotics for the treatment of community-acquired acute diarrhea in children. *BMC Public Health.* 2013;13 Suppl 3:S16. doi:10.1186/1471-2458-13-S3-S16

[100] Ahmadi E, Alizadeh-Navaei R, Rezai MS. Efficacy of probiotic use in acute rotavirus diarrhea in children: A systematic review and meta-analysis. *Casp J Intern Med.* 2015;6(4):187-195..

[101] Zuccotti G, Meneghin F, Aceti A, et al. Probiotics for prevention of atopic diseases in infants: systematic review and meta-analysis. *Allergy.* 2015;70(11):1356-1371. doi:10.1111/all.12700

[102] Cuello-Garcia CA, Brożek JL, Fiocchi A, et al. Probiotics for the prevention of allergy: A systematic review and meta-analysis of randomized controlled trials. *J Allergy Clin Immunol.* 2015;136(4):952-961. doi:10.1016/j.jaci.2015.04.031

[103] Saez-Lara MJ, Gomez-Llorente C, Plaza-Diaz J, Gil A. The role of probiotic lactic acid bacteria and bifidobacteria in the prevention and treatment of inflammatory bowel disease and other related diseases: A systematic review of randomized human clinical trials. *Biomed Res Int.* 2015;2015:1-15. doi:10.1155/2015/505878

[104] Derwa Y, Gracie DJ, Hamlin PJ, Ford AC. Systematic review with meta-analysis: the efficacy of probiotics in inflammatory bowel disease. *Aliment Pharmacol Ther.* 2017;46(4):389-400. doi:10.1111/apt.14203

[105] Jugan MC, Rudinsky AJ, Parker VJ, Gilor C. *Use of Probiotics in Small Animal Veterinary Medicine.* Vol 250.; 2017. Available at: https://avmajournals.avma.org/doi/pdf/10.2460/javma.250.5.519. Accessed October 29, 2018.

[106] Wynn SG. Probiotics in veterinary practice. *J Am Vet Med Assoc.* 2009;234(5):606-613. doi:10.2460/javma.234.5.606

[107] Herstad HK, Nesheim BB, L'Abée-Lund T, Larsen S, Skancke E. Effects of a probiotic intervention in acute canine gastroenteritis - a controlled clinical trial. *J Small Anim Pract.* 2010;51(1):34-38. doi:10.1111/j.1748-5827.2009.00853.x

[108] Kelley RL, Minikhiem D, Kiely B, et al. Clinical benefits of probiotic canine-derived Bifidobacterium animalis strain AHC7 in dogs with acute idiopathic diarrhea. *Vet Ther.* 2009;10(3):121-130..

[109] Rose L, Rose J, Gosling S, Holmes M. Efficacy of a probiotic-prebiotic supplement on incidence of diarrhea in a dog shelter: A randomized, double-blind, placebo-controlled trial. *J Vet Intern Med.* 2017;31(2):377-382. doi:10.1111/jvim.14666

[110] Gómez-Gallego C, Junnila J, Männikkö S, et al. A canine-specific probiotic product in treating acute or intermittent diarrhea in dogs: A double-blind placebo-controlled efficacy study. *Vet Microbiol.* 2016;197:122-128. doi:10.1016/J.VETMIC.2016.11.015

[111] Bybee SN, Scorza AV, Lappin MR. Effect of the probiotic enterococcus faecium sf68 on presence of diarrhea in cats and dogs housed in an animal shelter. *J Vet Intern Med.* 2011;25(4):856-860. doi:10.1111/j.1939-1676.2011.0738.x

[112] D'Angelo S, Fracassi F, Bresciani F, et al. Effect of *Saccharomyces boulardii* in dogs with chronic enteropathies: double-blinded, placebo-controlled study. *Vet Rec.* 2018;182(9):258-258. doi:10.1136/vr.104241

[113] Kim H, Rather IA, Kim H, et al. A double-blind, placebo controlled-trial of a probiotic strain *Lactobacillus sakei* probio-65 for the prevention of canine atopic dermatitis. *J Microbiol Biotechnol.* 2015;25(11):1966-1969. doi:10.4014/jmb.1506.06065

[114] Ohshima-Terada Y, Higuchi Y, Kumagai T, Hagihara A, Nagata M. Complementary effect of oral administration of *Lactobacillus paracasei* K71 on canine atopic dermatitis. *Vet Dermatol.* 2015;26(5):350-e75. doi:10.1111/vde.12224

[115] Lappin MR, Veir JK, Satyaraj E, Czarnecki-Maulden G. Pilot Study to Evaluate the Effect of Oral Supplementation of *Enterococcus Faecium* SF68 on Cats with Latent Feline Herpesvirus 1. *J Feline Med Surg.* 2009;11(8):650-654. doi:10.1016/j.jfms.2008.12.006

[116] Polzin DJ. Probiotic therapy of chronic kidney disease. In: *Proceedings of the 2011 ACVIM Forum.* Denver, CO; 2011.

[117] Lippi I, Perondi F, Ceccherini G, Marchetti V, Guidi G. Effects of probiotic VSL#3 on glomerular filtration rate in dogs affected by chronic kidney disease: A pilot study. *Can Vet J = La Rev Vet Can.* 2017;58(12):1301-1305.

[118] Kanakubo S, Ross H, Finke J. influence of azodyl on urea and water metabolism in uremic dogs. In: *Proceedings of the 2013 ACVIM Forum*. Seattle, WA; 2013.

[119] Rishniw M, Wynn SG. Azodyl, a synbiotic, fails to alter azotemia in cats with chronic kidney disease when sprinkled onto food. *J Feline Med Surg*. 2011;13(6):405-409. doi:10.1016/j.jfms.2010.12.015

[120] Didari T, Solki S, Mozaffari S, Nikfar S, Abdollahi M. A systematic review of the safety of probiotics. *Expert Opin Drug Saf*. 2014;13(2):227-239. doi:10.1517/14740338.2014.872627

[121] Hempel S, Newberry S, Ruelaz A, et al. Safety of probiotics used to reduce risk and prevent or treat disease. *Evid Rep Technol Assess (Full Rep)*. 2011;(200):1-645..

[122] Weese JS, Rousseau J. Evaluation of Lactobacillus pentosus WE7 for prevention of diarrhea in neonatal foals. *J Am Vet Med Assoc*. 2005;226(12):2031-2034..

[123] Vahjen W, Männer K. The effect of a probiotic Enterococcus faecium product in diets of healthy dogs on bacteriological counts of Salmonella spp., Campylobacter spp. and Clostridium spp. in faeces. *Arch Tierernahr*. 2003;57(3):229-233..

[124] EFSA Panel on Additives and Products or Substances used in Animal Feed. Scientific opinion on the safety and efficacy of Prostora Max (Bifidobacterium animalis) as a feed additive for dogs. *EFSA J*. 2012;10(12):2964.

[125] Weese JS, Martin H. Assessment of commercial probiotic bacterial contents and label accuracy. *Can Vet J = La Rev Vet Can*. 2011;52(1):43-46..

[126] Weese JS. Microbiologic evaluation of commercial probiotics. *J Am Vet Med Assoc*. 2002;220(6):794-797..

[127] Kolaček S, Hojsak I, Berni Canani R, et al. Commercial Probiotic Products. *J Pediatr Gastroenterol Nutr*. 2017;65(1):117-124. doi:10.1097/MPG.0000000000001603

[128] Nobles IJ, Khan S. Multiorgan dysfunction syndrome secondary to joint supplement overdosage in a dog. *Can Vet J = La Rev Vet Can*. 2015;56(4):361-364.

[129] Khan SA, McLean MK, Gwaltney-Brant S. Accidental overdosage of joint supplements in dogs. *J Am Vet Med Assoc*. 2010;236(5):509-510.

[130] Maughan R. Contamination of dietary supplements and positive drug tests in sport. *J Sports Sci*. 2005;23(9):883-889. doi:10.1080/02640410400023258

[131] ElAmrawy F, ElAgouri G, Elnoweam O, Aboelazayem S, Farouk E, Nounou MI. Adulterated and counterfeit male enhancement nutraceuticals and dietary supplements pose a real threat to the management of erectile dysfunction: A global perspective. *J Diet Suppl*. 2016;13(6):660-693. doi:10.3109/19390211.2016.1144231

[132] Brown AC. Heart toxicity related to herbs and dietary supplements: Online table of case reports. Part 4 of 5. *J Diet Suppl*. 2018;15(4):516-555. doi:10.1080/19390211.2017.1356418

[133] Brown AC. An overview of herb and dietary supplement efficacy, safety and government regulations in the United States with suggested improvements. Part 1 of 5 series. *Food Chem Toxicol.* 2017;107(Pt A):449-471. doi:10.1016/j.fct.2016.11.001

[134] Pawar RS, Grundel E. Overview of regulation of dietary supplements in the USA and issues of adulteration with phenethylamines (PEAs). *Drug Test Anal.* 2017;9(3):500-517. doi:10.1002/dta.1980

[135] Grisa A, Florio S, Bellia E, Cho S-C, Froum SJ. The role of dietary supplements in postsurgical bleeding: an update for the practitioner. *Compend Contin Educ Dent.* 37(10):690-695; quiz 696..

[136] Mathews NM. Prohibited contaminants in dietary supplements. *Sport Heal A Multidiscip Approach.* 2018;10(1):19-30. doi:10.1177/1941738117727736

[137] Navarro V. Herbal and dietary supplement hepatotoxicity. *Semin Liver Dis.* 2009;29(04):373-382. doi:10.1055/s-0029-1240006

[138] Cohen PA, Travis JC, Venhuis BJ. A methamphetamine analog (N,α -diethyl-phenylethylamine) identified in a mainstream dietary supplement. *Drug Test Anal.* 2014;6(7-8):805-807. doi:10.1002/dta.1578

[139] Marcus DM. Dietary supplements: What's in a name? What's in the bottle? *Drug Test Anal.* 2016;8(3-4):410-412. doi:10.1002/dta.1855

[140] Huang Y-C, Lee H-C, Lin Y-L, Tsai C-F, Cheng H-F. Identification of a new tadalafil analogue, dipropylaminopretadalafil, in a dietary supplement. *Food Addit Contam Part A.* 2016;33(6):953-958. doi:10.1080/19440049.2016.1184530

[141] Cohen PA, Maller G, DeSouza R, Neal-Kababick J. Presence of banned drugs in dietary supplements following FDA recalls. *JAMA.* 2014;312(16):1691. doi:10.1001/jama.2014.10308

[142] Geller AI, Shehab N, Weidle NJ, et al. Emergency department visits for adverse events related to dietary supplements. *N Engl J Med.* 2015;373(16):1531-1540. doi:10.1056/NEJMsa1504267

[143] Brown AC. Liver toxicity related to herbs and dietary supplements: Online table of case reports. Part 2 of 5 series. *Food Chem Toxicol.* 2017;107(Pt A):472-501. doi:10.1016/j.fct.2016.07.001

[144] Brown AC. Kidney toxicity related to herbs and dietary supplements: Online table of case reports. Part 3 of 5 series. *Food Chem Toxicol.* 2017;107(Pt A):502-519. doi:10.1016/j.fct.2016.07.024

[145] Quinn T. The food supplement that ruined my liver. BBC News. 2018. Available at: https://www.bbc.com/news/stories-45971416 Accessed June 23, 2019.

[146] Klein EA, Thompson IM, Tangen CM, et al. Vitamin E and the risk of prostate cancer. *JAMA.* 2011;306(14):1549. doi:10.1001/jama.2011.1437

[147] Lippman SM, Klein EA, Goodman PJ, et al. Effect of selenium and Vitamin E on risk of prostate cancer and other cancers. *JAMA.* 2009;301(1):39. doi:10.1001/jama.2008.864

[148] Byers T. Nutrition and lung cancer. *Am J Respir Crit Care Med*. 2008;177(5):470-471. doi:10.1164/rccm.200711-1681ED

[149] Wu Q-J, Xiang Y-B, Yang G, et al. Vitamin E intake and the lung cancer risk among female nonsmokers: a report from the Shanghai Women's Health Study. *Int J cancer*. 2015;136(3):610-617. doi:10.1002/ijc.29016

[150] Klein EA, Thompson IM, Tangen CM, et al. Vitamin E and the risk of prostate cancer: the Selenium and Vitamin E Cancer Prevention Trial (SELECT). *JAMA*. 2011;306(14):1549-1556. doi:10.1001/jama.2011.1437

[151] Ebbing M, Bønaa KH, Nygård O, et al. Cancer incidence and mortality after treatment with folic acid and Vitamin B. *JAMA*. 2009;302(19):2119. doi:10.1001/jama.2009.1622

[152] Mursu J, Robien K, Harnack LJ, Park K, Jacobs DR. dietary supplements and mortality rate in older women. *Arch Intern Med*. 2011;171(18):1625. doi:10.1001/archinternmed.2011.445

[153] Watkins ML, Erickson JD, Thun MJ, Mulinare J, Heath CW. Multivitamin use and mortality in a large prospective study. *Am J Epidemiol*. 2000;152(2):149-162. doi:10.1093/aje/152.2.149

8|
ALTERNATIVE NUTRITION

The hard but just rule is that if the ideas don't work, you must throw them away. Don't waste any neurons on what doesn't work. Devote those neurons to new ideas that better explain the data. Valid criticism is doing you a favor.

- Carl Sagan

FOOD IS LOVE

As a child, I was a big fan of the Peanuts cartoons. One of my favorite characters was Snoopy, a suave, bipedal beagle who wrote novels and engaged in breathtaking aerial combat with his nemesis, the Red Baron. Though Snoopy was unlike most other beagles I have known, he had one characteristic common to others of his breed, and indeed most dogs. When suppertime arrived, all other activities were forgotten, and he often launched into an exuberant, joyful suppertime dance. Every feeding was a celebration for Snoopy, a celebration not only of food but of the bond between dog and owner.

Few subjects generate the same intensity of emotion in pet owners as the question of what to feed our animal companions. Feeding our pets is the quintessential act of caring and love. And based on how most dogs and cats

307

act at feeding time, it certainly seems like a highlight of the relationship for them! There is also a deep sense in most pet owners that choosing a pet food has tremendous significance for the health and well-being of their pets. We all want to give our pets the best food, the food that will keep them active and happy and prevent illness for as long as possible. We have all been told most of our lives that what we eat affects our health, so we want to make good, healthy nutritional choices for our pets as well.

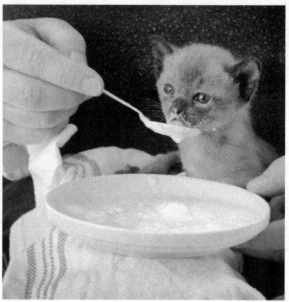

Food is Love 2002 by Mikael Moiner under Creative Commons by SA 2.0

The significance and emotion attached to feeding our pets can be good if it motivates us to think carefully about the food we choose to provide for them. However, the importance we place on this choice can also make us vulnerable to irrational decisions, and to exaggerated or unproven claims about nutrition and health. Like most medical subjects, nutrition is complicated and full of uncertainty and nuance, and our desire to find the perfect food to guarantee our pets' good health is all too easy to exploit by those selling pet food or promoting particular feeding ideologies. Even smart, rational people can get swept away by enthusiasm or diet fads that may not be based on reliable scientific principles or evidence.

As well as being an important part of the bond between us and our pets, their food is something we have control over. We naturally want to do everything we can to ensure our pets stay healthy, but many factors that influence the risk of disease are beyond our control. Food, at least, is something tangible and under our control that we know has an influence on health.

However, while the food we give our pets is important, it is not a magical elixir that will ward off illness. If we treat our pets' diet as one of many factors that each influence the risk of various diseases in small and complex ways, not as a quest for the one perfect food that will ensure a long and completely healthy life, then we are well on the way to avoiding magical thinking and poor decisions.

My goal in this chapter is not to provide specific advice on what to feed your pets. For one thing, this decision requires consideration of individual characteristics, such as breed, sex, age, lifestyle, and so on, and should be made by you in consultation with a vet who knows you and your animals. Instead, I want to focus on some of the more common and troublesome misconceptions and false claims about pet nutrition that you may encounter and help you distinguish reasonable, evidence-based nutritional advice from unscientific and unreasonable claims.

Brennen McKenzie

THE BASICS OF NUTRITION

Nutrition is a complex science, and the relationships between food and health are often indirect. The nutritional needs of our pets are influenced by individual characteristics and circumstances, and predicting the optimal diet to maximize health and minimize disease in any one pet is probably impossible, at least with our current level of understanding. However, there are basic principles about nutrition that don't change much with all of these factors and that are often misunderstood, or misrepresented, by those pushing one diet fad or another.

Calories

The first aspect of any diet to consider is how much energy it provides. In nutrition science, "energy" is not some vague or mystical force, but a measurable component of food that determines how much fuel the food provides for the activities and physiologic processes of your pet's body. If your pet is going to breathe, move, grow, or heal from illness, he or she needs energy, and this energy comes from food. The energy content of food is measured in calories (which is actually a shorthand for kilocalories, but this level of detail is more than we need here). Too few calories in their food and our pets lose weight and fail to thrive. Too many calories and, like us, they get overweight.

While the principle that the amount of energy taken in through food should match the amount of energy used in living is simple, as always real biology is more complicated than the theoretical biology. We have formulae for calculating the calorie needs of an individual pet, and they provide a good rough guideline. However, because there is tremendous individual variation in energy needs, such guidelines will still lead to overfeeding or underfeeding of many pets.

The only truly reliable measure of how many calories each pet needs to eat is how their body is responding to what they are fed. Body conditions scoring guidelines, like those of the World Small Animal Veterinary Association, are readily available to help determine if your pet is an appropriate weight. A dog or cat who is a healthy weight, who has a good-quality coat, is producing appropriate amounts of good-quality stool, and is happy and active is probably a pet who is getting an appropriate amount of energy in food. A pet who is overweight or underweight or in some other way is not thriving may not be getting the right number of calories for that pet, regardless of how much food our mathematical formulae, or your pet food package, says we should be feeding.

Finding the "right" calorie intake for a given pet is not an exact science but a science-informed process that also requires individual adjustment and some trial and error. This is also true for nearly every other aspect of choosing what to feed our pets. Theoretical considerations, and even good quality scientific research, can only take us so far. There is great variation between individuals and many other factors that influence the relationship between food and health, so all guidelines are only approximations.

Of course, our observations and anecdotes are just as unreliable when applied to nutrition as to any other medical subject, but they are also a necessary part of making choices about feeding, just as they are in every other medical question. Until we have perfect information, if such a thing is even possible, we have to make decisions based on the best information we have. Scientific research takes us much farther than personal observation alone, but it can't make our decisions for us. For better or worse (and I think it's for the better), we imperfect humans still have a vital role to play in choosing how we care for our pets, including what we feed them.

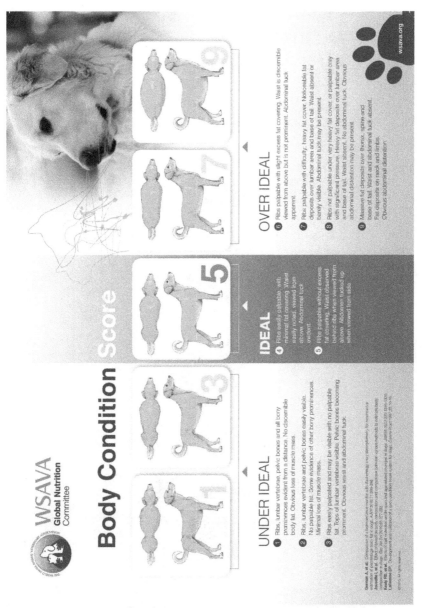

Image courtesy of World Small Animal Veterinary Association (WSAVA)

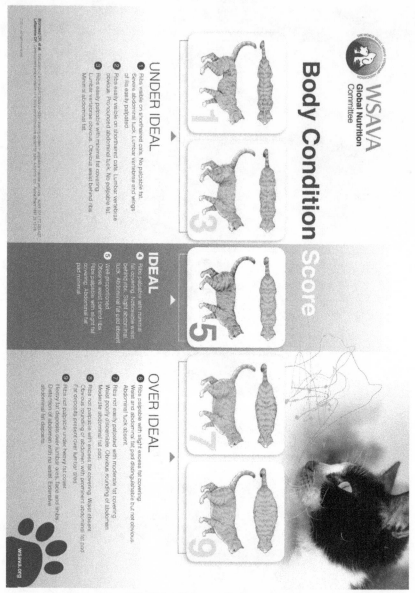

Image courtesy of World Small Animal Veterinary Association (WSAVA)

Macronutrients

After energy content, the main components of foods to know about are the macronutrients. These are the components of food eaten in the largest quantities and which provide most of the energy and nutrition in the food we eat. The main categories of macronutrients are carbohydrates, proteins, and fats. Some other vital substances which we need in fairly large amounts, such as water and certain minerals, are sometimes categorized as macronutrients, though they do not provide energy, as fats, proteins, and carbohydrates do, so for our purposes these are the three basic macronutrients.

We have a tendency to assign positive or negative value to the macronutrients, based largely on misunderstandings about what they are and their role in our bodies. For example, most people would think of proteins as "good" and associate them with strong muscles and other positive aspects of health. Fats, on the other hand, are usually viewed negatively and are associated with obesity, heart disease, and other health problems. More recently, carbohydrates have become a popular nutritional villain, and they are often blamed for various health problems. These oversimplifications, unfortunately, encourage sloppy thinking about nutrition and bad food choices.

Carbohydrates, proteins, and fats are all vital nutrients without which we cannot survive. Each category includes many different specific types. You have probably heard of simple and complex carbohydrates, of "good fats" and "bad fats," of essential and non-essential amino acids. None of these are inherently good or bad for our pets, and the health effects of macronutrients depends on the specific carbohydrates, fats, and proteins we eat as well as the proportion and relationships between them and all the many other individual factors that make nutrition such a complex science. A completely "fat

315

free" diet will probably kill you faster than one with too much "bad fat" in it, but both are less than ideal in the long run.

I will talk about specific macronutrients, and misconceptions about them, later in the chapter. For now, it is most important to understand that macronutrients come in a variety of types with different potential implications for health. If we reduce one macronutrient in a diet, say producing a low-carbohydrate food, we are automatically increasing the proportion of the other macronutrients. A low-carb diet is necessarily either a high-fat or a high-protein diet, while with a low-fat diet we automatically have more protein or more carbohydrate in it than a moderate-fat diet. Whether these changes are good or bad for our pets' health will depend on the nutritional needs of the individual and on the details of how we change the macronutrient content of the diet.

All of this means we cannot safely make simplistic generalizations about macronutrients and health. Carbohydrates and fats are neither inherently "bad" nor "good" for our pets' health. The devil is… (you know the rest). The health effects of specific macronutrients and relative amounts of them in a diet has to be evaluated by careful, rigorous scientific research and sensible observation of the condition of our pets, not assumed based on general theories about nutrition.

Micronutrients

As you might guess from the name, micronutrients are substances we require in our food in only very small quantities compared to the macronutrients, but they are still necessary to maintain normal health. The most familiar micronutrients are the vitamins and minerals we often hear touted as present in our breakfast cereal or other fortified foods. The discovery of micronutri-ents, and the elimination of once widespread deficiency diseases, such as scurvy and rickets, are part of the history of nutritional science that most people are familiar with. This represents one of the greatest achievements of science, and tremendous human and animal suffering has been prevented by understanding micronutrient requirements and providing the necessary nu-trients to prevent and cure such deficiency diseases.

Because we need micronutrients in such small amounts, the health ef-fects of deficiencies aren't always immediately apparent. And because the specific micronutrients, and the amount of each needed varies with species and, to a lesser extent, between individuals, it can be difficult to detect some health problems related to vitamin or mineral deficiencies, especially if the effects are subtle and develop over a long period of time. Ongoing research is continually improving our understanding of which nutrients are required and in what quantity to prevent micronutrient deficiencies.

However, there has been one negative effect of our dramatic successes in identifying and curing severe nutritional deficiency diseases. Many people have a tendency to believe because too little of some vitamins and minerals is bad, more of these in our diet must always be better for our health. This is a very dangerous misconception. Our bodies, and those of our animal companions, function best with an amount of each micronutrient in the diet that falls within an optimal range, and too much can be just as dangerous as too little. I discussed this concept in more detail in Chapter 7.

Studies in humans have identified serious health problems, from organ damage to increased cancer risk from both short-term and long-term intake of excessive amounts of even essential micronutrients.[1–12] While there is less evidence for pets, as always, toxic effects of excessive vitamins and minerals have been seen in dogs and cats. Often, this is due to pets accidentally eating vitamins intended for humans or overzealous supplementation by owners who are trying to improve their pets' health but who don't have an accurate understanding of nutrition and the role of micronutrients in health.[13,14,15] The key is that both too little and too much of a good thing can be a bad thing, and we should rely on scientific research to guide us in deciding how much of each micronutrient is best for our furry friends.

Science-based Pet Nutrition

As I have said already, it is crucial to remember that nutrition is one of many important factors that influences the health of our pets. We can certainly harm our pets with wildly inappropriate feeding choices. We may be able to improve or protect their health to some extent with specific manipulations of their diet, but often the evidence for this is a lot less clear. The perfect diet for any particular pet quite likely doesn't exist, and if it does we don't understand enough about the innumerable variables in nutrition and health to be able to identify it. On the whole, our pets are quite resilient and are able to live happy, healthy lives on a wide range of different diets. Broad categorizations of different diets as magical or terrible are rarely appropriate, but more nuanced evaluation based on scientific evidence can be helpful.

There is, perhaps surprisingly, quite a bit of evidence regarding dog and cat nutrition. Certainly, the claims of each individual brand of pet food to be better than every other brand are not supported by any kind of objective, reliable research data. Long-term trials in which groups of pets eat different foods for years and the impact on their health is assessed are impractical and not likely to be done. However, we have a strong understanding of the basic nutritional needs of cats and dogs, and we can certainly avoid serious deficiency diseases if we pay attention to this data.

We know less about the effect of excessive micronutrients over time, but there are some specific problems of this sort we can identify and prevent. Many reputable pet food companies conduct research on their products to identify potential health benefits, and research independent of the pet food industry is sometimes available as well.

There are some dramatic success stories in veterinary nutrition. Diets formulated for pets with kidney disease, for example, have been shown convincingly to improve the quality and length of life for pets with this condition. Diets formulated to dissolve certain kinds of bladder stones allow dogs and cats with this condition to avoid painful and expensive surgery. And the discovery that insufficient levels of the amino acid taurine caused one type of heart disease in cats led to the near elimination of this type of disease through changes in cat food formulation.[16]

Most of the positive impact of nutritional research in dogs and cats has been more subtle than these examples, but decades of study and refinement of pet foods has led to a situation in which most of our pets have good-quality nutrition that minimizes the risks of nutrition-associated disease. Undoubtedly, there is more to be learned, and we will likely continue to make both dramatic discoveries and small, incremental improvements in pet nutrition that lead to better health for our companions.

There is sometimes concern about the fact that most veterinary nutrition research is conducted and funded by companies selling pet foods. This is a legitimate issue since there is good evidence in human medicine that industry-funded research, particularly in the absence of strong regulatory oversight, does incorporate some bias that can affect the results and favor the interests of the funder. Good scientific methods for controlling bias, such as the blinding, randomization, placebo control groups and other methods I mentioned in Chapter 2, can go a long way towards reducing this potential source of bias in nutrition research studies. And findings that are consistent across multiple studies conducted by groups with different biases and interests are pretty likely to be true. We should always bear in mind the issue of funding bias when critically evaluating nutrition research, but it is not a reason to ignore the evidence we have or substitute much less reliable anecdotes or personal experiences.

MYTHS AND MISCONCEPTIONS ABOUT PET NUTRITION

This is a subject which could easily fill a book by itself. Because pet owners place such tremendous importance on deciding what to feed their companions, and because we tend to believe this choice has dramatic impact on our pets' health, we are ripe for manipulation by companies and individuals trying to sell us food or advice. Sorting through the maelstrom of claims on the Internet and in the pet section of the local bookstore, not to mention at our favorite dog park, daycare, groomer, breeder, or breed club, can be overwhelming. My hope is not to address every single claim you are likely to hear, but to use the general principles we have been applying throughout this book to a few of the most common examples of misinformation you may run across. Your own understanding of how to think critically about medical claims should help you deal sensibly with the many claims I don't have the space to cover.

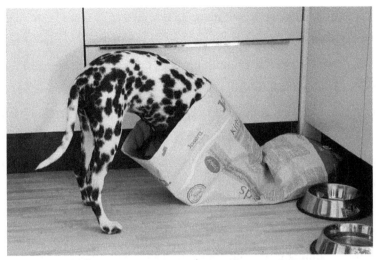

By Maja Dumat 2011 under Creative Commons by SA 2.0

Commercial Diets are Poison

Proponents of unconventional feeding practices often begin making their case with frightening claims about the ingredients and health effects of commercial dry and canned pet foods. You may have heard that these diets are full of sugar or nutritionally empty "by-products" and "fillers," or that they contain toxins, genetically modified ingredients (GMOs), or even the bodies of dead pets! Some of the more extreme advocates of alternative medicine and nutrition will tell you that commercial pet foods are "junk food" that cause cancer and other serious disease and that the pet food industry and veterinarians know this but don't do anything about it because they make money off of perpetuating illness in our pets. Such claims are truly horrifying, but fortunately they are also just scare tactics based on ignorance and a desire to frighten you into accepting alternative nutritional theories.

321

Of course, commercial pet diets are not perfect. Science is an ongoing process of refining and improving our understanding, and we never expect to reach a point where there is nothing more to learn. In retrospect, it is easy to see the flaws in the knowledge and reasoning of previous generations precisely because we have continued to build on and improve that knowledge. We are not yet in a position to say what is the optimal diet for every individual pet, and undoubtedly we will discover aspects of current diets that can be improved.

However, there is ample evidence to support the nutritional value of properly formulated commercial diets.[17] Decades of research has given us a solid understanding of the nutritional needs of dogs and cats, and modern pet foods do a very effective job of meeting these needs. We have even reached a point where we can prevent, cure, and reduce symptoms associated with specific health conditions using specially designed therapeutic diets.[18] Millions of dogs and cats around the world live long and healthy lives on commercial pet foods, so while they are not perfect or risk free, there is little reason to believe they are a major risk factor for disease in most animals, and there is certainly no good scientific evidence to support this idea.

Here are a few of the most pernicious myths about commercial pet foods.

Carbohydrates and Grains

These are popular villains in alternative narratives about nutrition these days. The ratio of the three macronutrients—carbohydrates, fat, and protein—are a key element in the formulation of pet diets. None of these are inherently "good" or "bad," and while the precise balance among them does have health

implications, especially in pets with specific medical conditions such as diabetes or kidney disease, the idea that commercial diets generally contain "too
much sugar" or other carbohydrates and that this causes disease is simply not
consistent with the evidence.[19]

Unlike humans, dogs and cats don't have to have carbohydrates in their
diet to survive. However, they can use this class of macronutrient perfectly
well as a source of calories.[20-25] Some non-digestible carbohydrates (often
known as "fiber") can have beneficial effects on the microbes that live in our
pets' guts, which can influence health, weight, stool consistency, and other
aspects of health.[26] Demonizing an entire class of nutrient is not rational or
justified.

This type of tactic has led to the predominance of "grain-free" diets, pet
foods in which carbohydrates from grains such as corn and wheat have been
replaced with other carbohydrate sources, such as potatoes, taro, legumes,
and others. There is absolutely no evidence to suggest such diets have health
benefits for our dogs. In fact, there is a new and growing concern that these
diets may actually increase the risk of some health problems. A small cluster
of dogs eating these diets have been found with a heart disease called dilated
cardiomyopathy that can be caused by a combination of genetic and dietary
risk factors. While it is too early to be sure that the grain-free diets are a
cause of this disease in these dogs, it illustrates the potential unanticipated
risks of a dietary fad not backed by research evaluating its potential benefits
and risks.[27,28,29]

As far as the claims that dietary carbohydrates of grains lead to cancer
or other disease in pets, these are pure speculation.[30] There are only a few
studies looking at diet and cancer risk in dogs and cats, and most of these

rely on owner recollections for data about diet, which has proven a very un-reliable approach in people. There are no studies at all showing restricting dietary carbohydrates reduces the risk of developing cancer in dogs and cats.

There are lab animal studies and epidemiologic research in humans which suggest *possible* relationships between carbohydrates in the diet and cancer. There are interesting features of the metabolism of cancer cells that suggest diet *might* have some influence on cancer progression and response to treatment. But there is no real-world, clinical trial evidence that supports the claim that dietary carbohydrates cause cancer in pets or that lower carbs will prevent or help treat cancer.

Carbohydrates are often seen as particularly dangerous to cats, who are truly obligate carnivores and so would naturally eat a high-fat/high-protein diet with few carbohydrates or grains in it, other than those found in the digestive system of herbivorous prey animals. However, research has demon-strated that cats can make use of carbohydrates in food as an energy source, and that these are not a significant risk factor for diabetes or other diseases often blamed on too much carbohydrate in commercial cat food.[19,20,25]

Perhaps the pet food ingredients most reviled in criticism of commercial pet foods are corn and wheat. The obsession in popular human nutrition lore about gluten has certainly contributed to this. However, many of the fears about gluten, in human and animal health, are unfounded. People with ce-liac disease can have negative health effects associated with eating gluten, and there are documented genetic cases of gluten sensitivity in a couple of dog breeds.[31,32] However, just as most people are not harmed by eating glu-ten, there is no evidence that this is a risk factor for disease in dogs and cats.[19] Abandoning wheat as a macronutrient source because of such fears simply leads to the substitution of other sources, and there is no guarantee these are safer or healthier. There is even some evidence that avoiding gluten can cause problems in people who do not have celiac disease.[33,34,35]

I have also heard advocates of alternative diets talk about "the menacing power of corn" as if it were inherently poisonous. This is simply silly, and it ignores decades of nutrition research showing the contrary.[19] Like every other food ingredient, corn is not inherently good or bad. It can contribute calories, protein, and essential fats to the diet, and it can be a safe ingredient in a balanced diet for both dogs and cats. It is obviously not appropriate as the sole food source for our pets, but no one is suggesting we use it that way, and claims that pet foods are "mostly corn" are demonstrably untrue.

Commercial Diets are "Processed" Junk Food

I think it is also important to address the concept of "processed" food, since this term is often misused. Obviously, anything not eaten raw and unwashed is "processed" to some extent, so the term is broad enough to be nearly mean-ingless. And despite the negative implications usually attached to the phrase, some kinds of processing clearly improve the safety and nutritional value of foods (washing and cooking, in particular). However, many critics of con-ventional pet nutrition use the term in an exclusively negative way, as a syn-onym for "unhealthy" and "toxic."

Most people probably hear the term "processed food" and think of snacks and convenience foods for humans: potato chips, packaged hot dogs, frozen chicken nuggets, and so on. There is some limited evidence that such foods may increase cancer risk in humans, which is a potential basis for con-cern.[36] Whether this is simply an association (e.g. people eating such foods are more likely to be overweight, exercise less, and have other risk factors for cancer), or a causal relationship (something in these foods increase cancer risk, directly or indirectly through something like increasing obesity) is unclear. In any case, no one thinks a diet of convenience foods and snacks alone is healthy, and mainstream dietary guidelines recommend plenty of fresh fruits and vegetables, whole grains, low-fat protein sources, and so on because there is evidence to support the health benefits of such a diet.[37] Therefore, it is reasonable to wonder how a packaged commercial diet could be safe or healthy for our pets.

One key difference between human convenience foods and pet food is that the former are designed primarily to appeal to consumers. Taste, appearance, mouth feel, packaging, price, and most other characteristics of packaged foods for humans are aimed at getting people to buy them. Nutritional considerations are a negligible factor, apart from those that can be used as marketing tools (e.g. calling a cookie full of sugar "low fat" or slapping a meaningless label like "All Natural" on something to fool people into imagining it is healthier).[38]

Pet foods, in contrast, are typically designed by nutritional experts to be complete and balanced, and support normal health. Sure, they have to be appealing to pets in terms of taste and smell, and to owners (which includes being affordable and which often leads to plenty of meaningless verbiage on packages). However, extensive research evidence exists demonstrating the nutritional needs of companion animals, and meeting these needs is a core requirement for a pet food from a reliable manufacturer.[39,40] Pet foods are intended to be the primary source of nutrition, and they are formulated and manufactured with this in mind.

Now most pet foods intended for adult maintenance or for growth in puppies and kittens have not been tested in large-scale, long-term clinical studies to demonstrate their impact on health. Some feeding trials are done for many diets, but these are foods, not medicines, so they are not required to meet that level of evidence. There are only a few commercial diets specifically intended for therapeutic medical uses that have been through extensive preclinical and clinical trial testing to validate medical claims made for them.

While it would be nice to have this kind of data for all commercial diets, it is false to suggest this means the health effects of feeding commercial foods haven't been studied. And it certainly makes no sense to suggest that alternative diets are healthier when there is even less evidence for the effects of those alternatives (a subject I will discuss in more detail shortly). Just because you buy your pets' food in a can or a bag doesn't mean it is the same as a bag of potato chips or a can of Spam.

Toxic Preservatives

A variety of synthetic antioxidants have been used in pet foods over the years to prevent spoilage and the risk of food poisoning that goes with it. These substances are sometimes feared as potential causes of cancer based on studies in rats or mice where enormous quantities are fed to the animals to evaluate potential risks. However, extensive research on these substances as they are actually used as preservatives in human and pet foods has failed to find such risks in the real world.[19,41,42] This is another example of the dangers in putting too much stock in the predictive value of laboratory studies.

Some companies have moved to using "natural" preservatives, such as vitamin E. These may be less effective, and there is no clear evidence that

327

they are safer, but the pet food industry is often forced to respond to the fears of consumers, stoked by claims from proponents of alternative diets, regardless of the evidence for or against the concerns.[43,44]

Genetically Modified Organisms (GMO)

This is a politically hot topic around the world and undoubtedly you have heard about health concerns associated with GMO foods eaten by humans. Such issues frequently spread from the domain of human health into the area of animal health, and concerns have been raised about the use of GMO ingredients in pet foods. As unpopular as it seems to be to say so right now, there is little evidence to support these fears, and a great deal of research suggesting the GMO ingredients currently in use are safe.[45–49]

There is always the potential, of course, that particular modifications of food crops and animals could lead to health risks. Tired yet of hearing that the devil is in the details? Talking about the safety of GMOs in general terms is like talking about the safety of herbal remedies or drugs or dietary supplements. All of these have potential benefits and risks that depend on their own characteristics as well as on the specific individuals and circumstances in which they are used.

Overall, however, the anxiety about genetically modified organisms is generally ideological and based on misconceptions or poor understanding of the relevant science. It is a form of the Appeal to Nature Fallacy I've already mentioned, in which something is feared to be harmful simply because humans had a hand in creating it. Each GMO has to be evaluated individually in terms of risks and benefits, but so far there is no real evidence to support concerns about negative health effects associated with GMO ingredients in pet foods.

By-Products

Critics of canned and dry pet foods will sometimes claim that they are nutritionally poor because they contain by-products. Most of us don't know precisely what this term means, but it sounds inherently second-rate. The folks who use the term to denigrate commercial foods often make wild claims about what it means, suggesting it includes inedible parts of animals, such as claws and feathers, or parts of diseased animals rejected for human consumption. Sounds pretty awful, eh?

The reality is more complicated and less shocking. Animal by-products are simply the parts of food animals that humans don't normally eat. Some of these may be low in nutritional quality (e.g. chicken feet), and most are at least as nutritious as the parts we do like to eat (internal organs, brains), while some contribute specific nutrients that may be more important for our carnivorous companions than for us (e.g. calcium from bone meal). These animal parts may be less aesthetically appealing to us, but they can be excellent nutrient sources if properly processed and used as part of a well-formulated diet.

Most countries have specific rules against using obviously unhealthy by-products in pet foods, such as diseased animals or those killed by some method other than the normal slaughter process. Pet food regulation also requires that all ingredients, including by-products, be free of infectious disease organisms.[40,50] This is why by-products are often not used raw but are rendered (cooked at high temperature) and then used as dry meals in pet foods since this process usually kills dangerous bacteria and parasites.

Once again, by-products are not inherently good or bad. Some are high-quality nutrient sources, others may be lower quality. They are not intended to be the sole nutrient source in pet foods, and improper processing can lead to some health risks, such as contamination with infectious organisms, just as can happen with any other animal ingredient in commercial or in homemade pet food. But the misleading claim that by-products are low quality and unsafe in pet foods is simply another scare tactic designed to drive people towards alternative feeding practices.[19,41,51]

Dead Pets in Pet Food

Soylent Green is…Rover? Probably not. This is perhaps the most extreme example of efforts to frighten pet owners about commercial diets. Promoters of this story take a few facts and weave them into an unlikely, but shocking narrative. Most countries have pretty strict regulations about the ingredients that can go into commercial pet foods, and these broad rules cover the use of euthanized animals as a food ingredient even if this is not explicitly mentioned in the law. Industry groups, as well as regulators, also have policies prohibiting this practice. Even apart from such rules and policies, though, the claim makes little sense for other reasons.

Food animals, such as cattle, pigs, sheep, and poultry, are the most common and economical source of animal ingredients for pet foods. These are mostly produced in large operations intended to produce food for humans. Apart from being an ethically terrible and unhealthy ingredient for pet foods, euthanized dogs and cats, presumably harvested from animal shelters or picked up by the roadside, would be an unreliable and expensive raw material compared to the ingredients produced by the food animal industry. And, of course, any company caught using dead pets in their pet food would be destroyed by public outrage and likely run out of business. What motivation these companies might have, then, for using such an ingredient is hard to fathom.

There have been several attempts to investigate commercial pet foods and look for evidence of dog or cat DNA, which might suggest there is some truth to this claim. So far, however, none of these investigations have found evidence that cats and dogs have been used as components of pet foods. The US Food and Drug Administration (FDA), for example, found no evidence of dog or cat DNA in pet foods it tested in 2002.[52] While this can't definitively prove this practice never happens, it is yet another piece of evidence against it.

So how did this idea get started? It's impossible to know for certain, but the evidence often cited in support of the claim that euthanized pets are used in pet food tends to be open to interpretation, and those inclined to be suspicious of commercial diets and the companies that produce them seem to take the darkest possible view of this evidence.

For example, most of the laws and regulations that would prohibit using euthanized pets in pet food don't actually address that issue directly. The law doesn't explicitly prohibit the practice precisely because there's little evidence it is actually occurring. Instead, the laws prohibit unsanitary and unsafe ingredients, potentially dangerous chemicals such as euthanasia drugs, and other general types of ingredients which would naturally include euthanized dogs and cats. Critics of commercial pet foods tend to claim that because the practice isn't named in the regulations it must actually be happening, which is not a particularly convincing claim.

Animals euthanized at shelters or killed by cars and not claimed are sometimes disposed of at rendering plants, where the bodies are broken down at high temperature into basic components, such as fats and simple proteins. These components are used in a variety of ways, from fats used as industrial lubricants to proteins being used in shrimp and fish farming. This is considered a more environmentally acceptable means of disposal than burning or burying the remains, but it is understandably disturbing to think about.

Because the parts of food animals not eaten by people are also rendered and are sometimes used in pet foods, there have been concerns that rendering products from euthanized dogs and cats might make their way into pet diets. This is prohibited, again by both regulations and industry policies, and there has not yet been any conclusive evidence that it occurs, but this may be one source of the belief that deceased pets are used as pet food ingredients.

Another very serious issue is that the drug pentobarbital, an anesthetic originally used for surgery but now most often used for euthanasia, does sometimes turn up as a contaminate in pet foods. In most of these instances, the amount has been too low to be considered a hazard, but there have been rare cases in which dogs have been sickened and even killed by pentobarbital in canned foods. Investigations into the source of this contamination have typically traced it to the accidental inclusion of euthanized cattle or horses in rendering products intended as pet food ingredients. Once again, no evidence has yet been found showing that euthanized dogs and cats have been the source of pentobarbital contamination of pet foods, but again this may be one source of the belief that this is happening.

Ultimately, like so many of the concerns raised by critics of science-based medicine and conventional nutrition, it is not possible to conclusively prove that the concern is never true under any circumstances. However, the consistent failure to find evidence for the claim despite repeated investigations over decades certainly makes it an unlikely occurrence and not a reason to fear commercial diets or choose untested alternatives with far less evidence for their safety and nutritional value.

So, Are Commercial Pet Foods Healthy?

The short answer is "Yes." The long answer is "Mostly yes, but it depends." There are hundreds of pet foods out there, and many companies with different approaches to formulating and manufacturing their products. There is undoubtedly variation in the quality of the foods themselves, and certainly differences in how each individual pet responds to different diets. I fed my 75-pound mixed-breed dog the same commercial diet for 16 happy, healthy years. When he passed away and I rescued a new, small-breed mutt from the local shelter, he had soft stools and trouble keeping on weight with the same diet. I tried a variety of other foods until I found one that kept him, and his poop, in good condition. All of the diets I tried met reasonable scientific standards for good nutrition, and my experiences don't justify condemning or excessively praising any of them. Health and nutrition are just complex, and some trial and error is always likely to be necessary.

The real question pet owners should ask is not so much whether commercial diets are good or bad but whether the alternatives to them have any real evidence that they are a better choice. So let's now take a look at a couple of popular alternative approaches to pet nutrition and see what claims are made for them and what evidence there is to judge these claims.

ORGANIC FOODS

The last forty years have seen a steady growth in the organic farming industry. Most developed nations now have extensive regulations dictating what "organic" means in the context of food production, but in general it refers to systems of agriculture than attempts to be more "natural" than conventional agriculture. Synthetic pesticides and fertilizers are replaced with chemicals found in nature or with biological pest control strategies, GMOs are avoided, and other practices are employed with the intent of minimizing the negative environmental impact of food production. There is some debate about how effective and successful organic methods are at achieving these goals,[53,54,55] but for our purposes the important question is whether the use of organic foods has any implications for the health of our pets.

People who choose organic foods for themselves are typically motivated by a belief that these foods are healthier, more nutritious, better tasting, and perhaps better for the environment than conventionally produced foods.[56,57,58] Similar beliefs underlie the desire to feed organic foods to our pets or to buy commercial diets that incorporate them.[59,60] Pet food companies do everything they can to take advantage of this desire, and many foods are aggressively marketed as organic or as containing organic ingredients.

You will likely not be shocked, however, to learn that there isn't much evidence that these foods are healthier or more nutritious than pet foods made from conventionally produced ingredients. There is no research comparing the health of pets fed organic and conventional foods, and there isn't likely to be in the future. Such studies are cumbersome and expensive, and it is easier and more profitable for pet food companies to simply cater to the positive associations most people have with the organic label rather than to generate research evidence which would not likely sway many consumers either way.

In this situation, we are forced to look at the evidence accumulated in studying organic foods intended for the human market, despite the inevitable problems with extrapolating from people to pets. While there is still vigorous debate and ongoing research on this subject, numerous reviews of many individual studies have been published evaluating the nutritional content and the potential health effects of organic foods. While there are sometimes small differences in the composition of foods produced organically or conventionally, there is no convincing evidence that these differences have any practical effect on the well-being of people eating these different foods.[61-65] Some studies have tried to look at associations between eating organic food and specific health risks, such as cancer, but the results have been inconsistent and are complicated by many other factors that affect such health risks.[66,67] Wealthy people, for example, are generally healthier and also eat more organic food than poor people, but there are many other differences in these groups that likely impact disease risk besides choosing organic or conventional produce.

Hopefully, even stronger evidence will be available in the future, but the data so far suggests there is no real advantage to organic foods in terms of health and nutrition for people, and there is no particular reason to expect the case would be different for our pets. There is also, however, no evidence that organic foods are any less nutritious or healthy than conventionally produced foods, so if the methods of organic farming appeal to you for other reasons and the costs are not prohibitive, organic diets are perfectly appropriate to feed your pets.

HOMEMADE PET FOOD

For most of us, memories of our parents or grandparents cooking for us are a powerful symbol of their love and care. If food is love, then preparing food for someone we care about is an expression of this love. Many of us feel a kind of affection for our pets that is similar in many ways to our feelings for our children, and the idea of cooking for them is quite appealing. Most pet owners, of course, do not have the time to prepare their pets' food, or they may not feel sure what kind of food would be healthy for their animal family members, and surveys show that the majority still rely on commercial foods. However, homemade diets are growing in popularity. There are many sources of recipes for cooking your pets' food, and of course many proponents of such diets who will tell you this is safer and healthier than feeding a commercial diet.

Until fairly recently, mostly dogs in affluent countries were fed table scraps, whatever was left over after the people in the family finished eating. It is generally recognized now, however, that this is an unreliable feeding strategy. While our canine friends may enjoy a bit of our leftovers now and again, table scraps are not nutritionally complete or appropriate for our pets, and they often contain ingredients that can be harmful (e.g. raisins, onions, some spices, etc.).

Cats have historically been left mostly to their own devices, being expected to hunt their own food and to be happy with a bit of milk or leftover meat from time to time. However, most cat owners today, and certainly those who keep their cats exclusively indoors, now feel responsible for providing a healthy diet for their feline companions.

What Is It?

The term "homemade diet" is pretty vague, and it encompasses a variety of feeding approaches. Few pet owners rely primarily on table scraps, though there are some who consider this an appropriate homemade diet. Numerous websites and books now provide recipes for preparing pet foods at home. These include a wide range of ingredients including meat from many different kinds of animals, plants, and often vitamin and mineral supplements. It is also possible to prepare some basic ingredients, such as meat and a carbohydrate source like rice or pasta, at home and then mix these with a commercial product intended to provide all the other essential nutrients for your pet.

Some companies have even started producing commercial "homemade" diets. These generally include meats, vegetables, and cereals mixed with micronutrient supplements and then cooked and delivered in small quantities frozen or refrigerated for immediate use. These are not technically "homemade," of course, and they are often referred to as "fresh food diets" or "whole food diets," to distinguish them from kibble and canned pet foods.

Truly homemade and commercial fresh-food diets are typically marketed with health claims. Making your own pet food or having regular deliveries of small quantities of freshly prepared food is always more expensive and often less convenient than feeding traditional commercial diets, so advocates of these strategies promote them by claiming that they are healthier for your pet than conventional pet food.

This marketing often makes use of some of the scare tactics and misinformation about commercial diets that I have just discussed. It also frequently refers to scientific evidence purporting to show that fresh foods are healthier for humans than processed foods and implying the same is true for our pets. In fact, a major tool for promoting homemade and other fresh-food involves likening them to human food and trying to take advantage of all the positive associates we have with cooking for and sharing food with other people.

Does It Work?

By "work" here I mean is there evidence that homemade or fresh-food diets have health benefits for dogs and cats? Do these diets prevent or treat disease, and do pets fed this way live longer or better-quality lives?

The main source of evidence cited to support the health benefits of fresh and homemade diets are studies in humans suggesting people who consume more fresh food, especially a variety of fruits and vegetables, may have generally better health and be at lower risk of some specific diseases than people who eat less of these foods or more processed and "fast" food.[36,68-70] There is good evidence suggesting that fresh foods have health benefits for humans compared with more highly processed foods, so it is understandable to wonder if the same might be true for our pets.

Placebos for Pets?

Unfortunately, this is where, once again, it gets complicated. First of all, we don't really know why people who report eating more fruits and vegetables in observational studies seem healthier in some ways than people who say they eat less of these foods. Are there protective elements in fresh foods that directly reduce the risk of disease? Or are there harmful things in processed or convenience foods that promote disease? Is the difference even due to the foods themselves or to other associated variables? For example, people who eat more fruits and vegetables may also exercise more, and they tend to be more affluent and have better access to healthcare and education than people who eat more fast food. Diet may be more of a marker of a healthy lifestyle than the actual reason for some people to be healthier than others.[71,72]

The best way to sort out these different possibilities would be a controlled research study. Randomly assigning large numbers of people to eat different diets, keeping everything else in their lives the same, and then comparing their health over many years would help determine the true effect of diet on health. For obvious practical and ethical reasons, such a study can't be done, and so we have to be cautious in interpreting the results of less controlled, observational studies.

We also have to be cautious about extrapolating from diet research in humans to our dogs and cats. Eating more fruits and vegetables might well be good for you or me, but our pets have rather different nutritional needs, and the same might well not be true for them. And we should bear in mind the difference between commercial pet foods and the "processed" convenience foods humans often eat. The hamburgers and crisps and canned meat people are often substituting for fruits and vegetables and whole grains in

339

diet studies are not the same as the deliberately formulated balanced diets commercial pet food makers provide.

There is little direct research into the relative health effects of home-made and commercial diets in pets. I do believe the evidence in humans is at least strongly suggestive that fresh foods have some true health benefits for us, and I think the hypothesis that this might also be true for our pets is plausible and worth exploring. The kinds of studies that cannot easily be done in people might actually be possible in dogs and cats, and it would be possible and ethical to compare the health of pets or research animals fed existing commercial diets and balanced, properly produced homemade diets. Such studies could potentially change the way we feed our pets quite dra-matically, but so far they have not been conducted, so the purported benefits of homemade diets are hypothetical and unproven.

Is It Safe?

What could be safer than cooking for your pet at home just like you cook for yourself? Well, it turns out there are some potential risks to homemade diets. Just as people sometimes fall ill due to bacteria or other organisms that con-taminate fresh meat and produce, our pets can be affected by these as well. Proper food handling is just as important for our pets as it is for us. There is a tendency to believe that because our pets don't know any better and often seem to get away with eating rotten food, trash, or even their own waste, they must be immune to food-borne illness. This is absolutely not true, so any homemade diet should meet the same health and safety standards as human foods. This increases the cost[73] and the trouble of making such a diet, which is likely one reason why a majority of pet owners still prefer to feed prepared commercial diets.

Multiple research studies have been done looking at the nutritional content of homemade diets.[74-79] Recipes for homemade pet food from the Internet or books aimed at pet owners often turn out to be unbalanced, lacking some micronutrients or having an excess of others. This is true even of recipes published by veterinarians who are educated about nutrition but who are not board-certified specialists in the subject. The mountains of data about the nutritional requirements of dogs and cats and the nutritional content of thousands of different food ingredients is challenging to wade through and distill into a simple, reliable recipe. Large companies with nutrition specialists on staff and rigorous quality control systems can often do a better job of producing a nutritionally complete and consistent food.

The consequences of these formulation problems aren't entirely clear. As I mentioned previously, micronutrient deficiencies or excesses often take a long time to develop and can be subtle and variable between individuals. Even dramatic deficiencies, such as the lack of taurine in commercial foods that was causing heart disease in cats prior to the 1980s, can be hard to identify and solve without deliberate and ongoing research.[80] People feeding homemade diets to their individual pets are not likely to be able to detect most negative health effects, and unfortunately there has not yet been long-term controlled research to determine whether or not the common problems in the recipes available to most of us are serious health risks. There have been some individual case reports of pets made ill by improperly formulated homemade diets, but the extent of this risk is not known.

One way to mitigate the risk of feeding an unbalanced homemade diet is to employ the services of a veterinary nutrition specialist in formulating the diet. While this also adds to the cost and work of making food for your pet, it has the advantages of not only reducing the risk that the diet you make will be nutritionally flawed, but it allows the nutritionist to tailor the food to the needs of your particular pet. Pets who are overweight or underweight, or those who have specific medical conditions which can be impacted by nutrition may benefit from a homemade diet designed by a nutritionist specifically for their needs.

Bottom Line

There is a plausible theoretical argument that fresh foods may be healthier than commercial diets, but so far there is little evidence investigating this idea. Commercial diets may actually be better for our pets than homemade diets due to the common nutritional deficiencies or excesses of most homemade diets and the hazards of making it improperly rather than the fresh nature of the food itself. Definitive comparisons between these types of diet have not been made.

For the majority of us, commercial cat and dog food remains a safe, healthy, convenient, and affordable diet for our pets. For those who like the idea of making food for their pets, the best option is to get help from a board-certified veterinary nutrition specialist in designing the diet for your particular pet. Feeding a commercial fresh food diet from a company with nutritionists on staff and effective, transparent safety and quality control procedures is also a reasonable option.

RAW DIETS

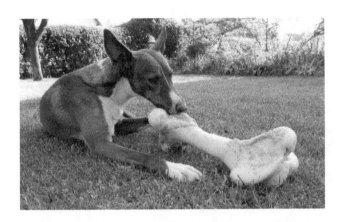

What Is It?

Perhaps the most controversial alternative feeding strategy right now is the practice of feeding raw meat, often with bones, vegetables, and other ingredient, to pet dogs and cats. Raw feeding has continued to grow in popularity over the last decade despite resistance from most vets and public health authorities.[81-84] As with most alternative health practices, there are a variety of theories and specific beliefs behind raw feeding, but there are several consistent themes that most proponents of the approach adhere to and use in promoting it.

The first we have already discussed, which is the claim that commercial diets are nutritionally inappropriate and unhealthy. All of the criticisms of conventional diets I have addressed are put to the service of convincing people raw diets are a better choice. Once again, while commercial pet foods are not perfect or without risks, the evidence clearly shows they are healthy and nutritionally appropriate for the vast majority of dogs and cats, and millions of pets live long and healthy lives eating these foods.

The other main theoretical argument for raw diets is our old friend the Appeal to Nature Fallacy. The argument runs something like this: Dogs and cats are carnivores and they, or their ancestors, ate whole prey in the wild. Evolution has adapted carnivores to this diet, so it is the optimal diet for them. Our pet dogs and cats are essentially the same in their nutritional needs as their wild cousins or ancestors, so a diet as much like raw, whole prey as possible is the healthiest diet for them.

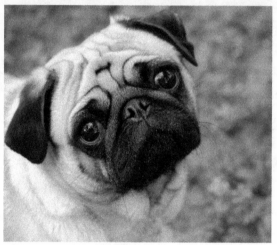

Is this a predator? 2012 by DodosD under Creative Commons by SA 3.0

Hopefully, after all that has come before this chapter, you are already picking out the flaws in this line of reasoning. To begin with, dogs are classified by scientists in the order of mammals known as the Carnivora for evolutionary reasons. Not all animals in this group necessarily eat meat, however. The giant panda, for example, is classified as a carnivore in the same family as bears, yet it is a completely vegetarian species. Evolutionary relationships are useful in many ways, but they do not dictate the dietary needs of a species.

Wild canines, like wolves and foxes, have a variety of dietary habits. Some are primarily carnivorous whilst others eat a fair amount of plant material. Dogs have been living with human beings for tens of thousands of years, and they have been domesticated and altered extensively by us in that time. Try imaging a pack of savage feral Welsh corgis chasing down an elk and stripping the flesh from its bones. It should be pretty clear from that image that whatever their evolutionary heritage, dogs are not wolves anymore!

Studies have shown significant anatomic and functional differences between wolves and the domestic dog, and many of these involve systems for eating and digesting food. For all the millennia dogs have lived with humans, they have scavenged our leftovers and shared our food, and evolution has adapted them to a much more varied and less meat-centered diet than wolves or many other wild canids.[85-91]

Cats, on the other hand, have generally been altered far less by their association with humans than dogs. While dogs are most properly classified as omnivores, or facultative carnivores, cats are true carnivores in terms of their anatomy and physiology. Domestic cats do likely have nutritional needs very similar to wild felines. So does this mean they are better off if fed a raw diet?

Well, as you know now the Appeal to Nature Fallacy is a fallacy precisely because what happens in nature doesn't predict what is good or bad in terms of health. The diet wild animals eat is not the perfect diet designed for their long-term health and happiness; it is simply the diet that is available to them. Evolution works by an impersonal process in which animals do their best to meet their physical needs with what is available in their environment and then reproduce. The individuals who are best at meeting these needs leave more offspring and genes behind, and over time the population comes to be more like the more successful individuals because their genes become more common. Species and their environments are always interacting and changing, and there is never an ideal moment in which a species is optimally suited for its environment and every individual is perfectly happy and healthy.

Animals typically live longer, healthier lives in captivity compared to their wild relatives.[92] Wild carnivores frequently suffer from malnutrition, often starving when they can't catch sufficient prey to meet their calorie and other needs. They also suffer from parasites, infectious diseases, and injuries from catching and consuming whole prey, and they endure this either suffering or die from it.[93-104] This is not a perfect, blissful state of nature our pets should aspire to, it is simply the way things are in nature.

Humans no longer live like our stone age ancestors, and we have altered our homes, our clothes, and our diets significantly from that "natural" state. As a result, we suffer less and live longer, healthier lives because of "artificial" practices such as washing and cooking and refrigerating our feed and providing ourselves with nutrients that were once hard to come by. The reduction of scurvy and rickets in modern children compared to those of our ancestors is a good thing, and similarly the reduction in parasites and malnutrition in our pets thanks to "artificial" feeding practices is a positive change.

Placebos for Pets?

Raw feeding is often associated with other alternative medicine beliefs and practices. Surveys show that pet owners who feed raw diets are less likely to trust nutrition advice from veterinarians and are also less likely to adhere to other recommendations, such as vaccination and parasite prevention, than owners who feed traditional commercial diets.[105,106] Veterinarians who promote raw feeding and condemn conventional diets are also often suspicious of vaccines and other science-based medical therapies and frequently advocate alternative medical practices.[35,107,108]

It is not surprising, then, that theories and beliefs which underlie other alternative practices are also found in arguments for raw diets. Vitalism, the belief that health and disease involve not only the physical body but the quality of our spiritual being as well, is sometimes used as an argument for feeding raw. Cooked or otherwise processed foods are claimed to be "dead" or lacking in some vital life force that is still present in raw foods, and consuming this life force in food is thought to be essential to good health for our pets. As is always the case with vitalist theories, this is essentially a tenet of faith and so cannot be scientifically evaluated in a way that proves or disproves it to anyone's satisfaction.

None of these basic theoretical justifications for a raw diet, that commercial diets are unhealthy, that our pets are essentially identical to wild carnivores, that a diet as close as possible to that they would eat in nature is best for their health, or that raw food contains some intangible but essential spiritual nutrient lacking in cooked food, hold up very well to logical scrutiny. There are, however, other claims about the health benefits of raw diets that we can examine. Proponents will argue that pets fed raw diets are healthier in specific ways than those eating commercial pet food. Better stool and coat quality, more energy, less susceptibility to disease, and longer life are all pro-posed benefits to feeding raw to our pets. So what evidence is there for these claims?

Does It Work?

The practical benefits of raw diets, like any other approach to fostering health, can only be determined accurately by rigorous scientific research. Stories about good individual experiences with raw diets, or bad experiences with conventional foods, are simply anecdotes, subject to all the error and bias and uncertainty that makes anecdotal evidence so unreliable. Unfortu-nately, the majority of the evidence raw feeding advocates present to make their case is nothing more than such anecdotes and stories. When we get past the theoretical claims, we find little in the way of real evidence.

Some of the same arguments made for fresh-food diets generally are made in support of raw diets. As I discussed earlier, there is some suggestion that eating more fresh foods may have some health advantages for humans, but the issue is complicated and unresolved. The same arguments and un-certainties apply to raw diets, with the added question of whether the lack of cooking itself provides additional benefits. There are no strong, definitive clinical studies looking at long-term feeding of raw vs commercial diets that can tell us with any confidence whether there are health advantages to one or the other.

A few small and short-term studies have been done in which dogs and cats have been fed raw foods. These show some interesting changes in the bacteria living in the guts of these subjects, in stool, and in metabolism and other variables.[109–113] However, these studies simply show that some small

348

things change when the diet is changed, not that raw diets have meaningful health effects or that whatever effects are seen are due primarily to the lack of cooking. One study has suggested some possible benefits for dental health in dogs fed a raw diet, but another study identified dental disease and broken teeth caused by such diets.[114,115]

Overall, there is no convincing research evidence to support the theories and claims for why raw diets should be better for our pets than cooked home-made or conventional commercial diets.[106,116,117]

Is It Safe?

Unlike the benefits of raw diets, which are theoretical and unproven, the risks are well documented. Commercial raw diets which meet industry standards are likely to be nutritionally complete, but many raw advocates feed home-prepared diets, and just like other homemade foods, these diets are frequently nutritionally unbalanced and incomplete.[116,118–123] There is even one report of a whole-prey diet (whole ground rabbit) which was studied in cats as a representative of a "natural" diet but which turned out to generate severe heart disease due to taurine deficiency in the cats eating it.[124] So much for "natural" meaning "healthy!"

The widespread use of bones in raw diets also presents a significant risk of tooth fractures and injury to the gastrointestinal tract.[115,125–128] Even wild carnivores are at risk for acute dental and gastrointestinal trauma from bones, as well as chronic tooth wear, and this can lead to the "natural" outcomes of suffering or death.[129,130,131] Pet dogs and cats are at least as susceptible to this risk as wild carnivores, and the natural outcomes are clearly unacceptable to owners.

The most significant risk of raw diets is from food-borne infectious disease. Numerous studies have shown raw diets to be frequently contaminated with potentially dangerous bacteria. While such pathogens can contaminate cooked diets as well, the risk is significantly higher for raw foods.[132] Other studies have shown that animals eating these diets often shed these dangerous organisms in their feces, which exposes humans and other animals to the risk of infection.

Most importantly, serious illness and death in cats and dogs, and in their owners, have been caused by pathogens found in raw pet diets.[84,116,133–137] While the number of confirmed cases of pets and humans suffering or dying from food-borne illness caused by raw diets is small, this is a very serious health hazard. While healthy adult pets may be able to resist these organisms to some extent, there is no absolute immunity in dogs and cats to food-borne illness. Very young, old, and sick animals, and their human caregivers, are at even higher risk.

Bottom Line

The theories behind why raw diets might have health benefits are not very plausible or logically sound. None of the purported benefits have been demonstrated in controlled scientific studies, so specific health claims rest only on the weak pillars of these dubious theories and anecdotal evidence. The little research that has been done on raw foods has yet to show any compelling evidence of meaningful health effects.

There are, however, clear risks to feeding raw, including nutritional deficiencies or excesses, risk of injury from bones, and risk of severe infection and death in both pets and humans. While properly formulated raw diets can be nutritionally appropriate and the risks of infectious disease can be mitigated by scrupulous food handling, the established risks of raw diets and the complete lack of compelling evidence for any health benefits makes the use of such diets a choice based on ideology or personal belief, not sound scientific evidence.

Ultimately, by feeding raw you are choosing to take a small but potentially severe risk with your health and that of your pets in exchange for unproven and unlikely benefits. Those interested in feeding raw despite this should be very careful about doing everything possible to reduce the risks, including feeding a commercial product, avoiding feeding bones, and paying strict attention to food handling safety rules.

SO HOW DO I DECIDE WHAT TO FEED MY PETS?

Having hopefully dispelled some of the more common myths and misconceptions about pet nutrition, and given you a little context and a science-based approach to the subject, I want to finish by pointing you in the direction of some resources and strategies for making good choices about feeding your own pets.

Step 1: Relax

As I said at the beginning, we have learned a great deal since the days when our dogs ate our trash or table scraps and our cats had to catch their own food or starve. Most of the feeding options out there, from the commercial diets that the vast majority of pet owner use to some of the homemade or fresh-food alternatives, are perfectly reasonable, healthy diets to use. Our pets are resilient and can have long, healthy, happy lives on a wide variety of different diets so long as we avoid the most extreme deficiencies or excesses, which most foods do. While the choice of a food for our animal friends is important and does matter to their well-being, there are no magical perfect foods that will guarantee a life free from all illness, and there are very few awful dangerous foods that will directly harm our pets. Most of the options typical, reasonable pet owners choose are fine for most pets most of the time. So relax.

Step 2: Be Skeptical

The pet food industry, including alternative commercial products and the advice sold by proponents of unconventional feeding practices, is a desperate competition for your belief and your money. The most honest and reputable individuals and companies have to work to convince you that their product is better than everyone else's, even if there is no research evidence to prove this (as there virtually never is). Outright lying is uncommon, and illegal, in the mainstream commercial pet food market, but exaggeration, implication, innuendo, and all manner of "spin" is fair game and widely employed. And outright falsehoods, even if genuinely believed by their purveyors, are rampant online and in the marketing of alternative dietary approaches.

In this maelstrom of information and misinformation, it pays to take much of what you hear with a grain or two of salt. In particular, be skeptical of information from folks trying to sell you something, especially when that information appears to be leading you in the direction of what they are selling. Also be wary of anyone making extreme and unsubstantiated claims. Remember, there are no miracle foods and most of the horror stories about pet food are exaggerated or simply untrue, so if someone is telling you these horror stories or promising miracles, they are likely not a reliable source of information. If it sounds too good (or too bad) to be true, it probably is.

Try to apply what you have learned about making reasonable, science-based decisions to the process of evaluating diets and marketing claims. Look for research evidence rather than anecdote, for reasonable and measured claims, not promises of miracles, and for an honest admission of the complexity and uncertainty that is inevitably part of any nutrition claims. Consider the credentials and biases of sources. A board-certified veterinary nutritionist is likely to be a better source of information than the guy working at the local pet food store. Someone working for a specific pet food company might be expected to have more bias in favor of that company's products than a nutritionist who consults for many companies or works independently or at a university. And anyone promoting alternative medicine along with an unconventional or unusual approach to nutrition is likely going to have many of the biases and beliefs we've seen turn up repeatedly in looking at alternative therapies, so if you are skeptical of these you may want to look at such a person's claims about nutrition especially closely.

Step 3: Think Scientifically

If you decide you want to feed a commercial pet food, I would strongly recommend taking a look at *Dog Food Logic* by Linda Case.[17] This book takes a balanced, open-minded, and science-based look at the pet food industry, marketing claims, pet food labels, and many other issues surrounding choosing a commercial diet. I would also recommend finding a veterinary nutrition specialist near you to consult for advice.

If you are dedicated to feeding a fresh food diet for your pets, cooked or raw, again I would strongly recommend consulting with a nutritionist to ensure the diet you make is as nutritionally appropriate for your individual pets as possible and as safe as possible for them and for you.

Food is love, and because love is such a powerful emotion it can sometimes lead us to make poor decisions. Because we love our pets and want the best for them, we need to include reason and science in making choices about what we feed them. Understanding the basics of nutrition, the common myths and misconceptions about nutrition you will run across, the warning signs of unreliable, unscientific information, and the resources and choices available to you, now you are in a position to enjoy the excitement of feeding time with the confidence that your choices are sound and well-informed.

For what a man more likes to be true, he more readily believes.
Man prefers to believe what he prefers to be true.

- Francis Bacon

Placebos for Pets?

[1] Schürks M, Glynn RJ, Rist PM, Tzourio C, Kurth T. Effects of vitamin E on stroke subtypes: meta-analysis of randomised controlled trials. *BMJ*. 2010;341:c5702. doi:10.1136/BMJ.C5702

[2] Klein EA, Thompson IM, Tangen CM, et al. Vitamin E and the risk of prostate cancer. *JAMA*. 2011;306(14):1549. doi:10.1001/jama.2011.1437

[3] Bjelakovic G, Nikolova D, Gluud C. Antioxidant supplements and mortality. *Curr Opin Clin Nutr Metab Care*. 2013;17(1):1. doi:10.1097/MCO.0000000000000009

[4] Brown AC. Kidney toxicity related to herbs and dietary supplements: Online table of case reports. Part 3 of 5 series. *Food Chem Toxicol*. 2017;107(Pt A):502-519. doi:10.1016/j.fct.2016.07.024

[5] Ebbing M, Bønaa KH, Nygård O, et al. Cancer incidence and mortality after treatment with folic acid and Vitamin B. *JAMA*. 2009;302(19):2119. doi:10.1001/jama.2009.1622

[6] Brasky TM, White E, Chen C-L. Long-term, supplemental, one-carbon metabolism-related Vitamin B use in relation to lung cancer risk in the Vitamins and Lifestyle (VITAL) Cohort. *J Clin Oncol*. 2017;35(30):3440-3448. doi:10.1200/JCO.2017.72.7735

[7] Wu Q-J, Xiang Y-B, Yang G, et al. Vitamin E intake and the lung cancer risk among female nonsmokers: a report from the Shanghai Women's Health Study. *Int J cancer*. 2015;136(3):610-617. doi:10.1002/ijc.29016

[8] Klein EA, Thompson IM, Tangen CM, et al. Vitamin E and the risk of prostate cancer: the Selenium and Vitamin E Cancer Prevention Trial (SELECT). *JAMA*. 2011;306(14):1549-1556. doi:10.1001/jama.2011.1437

[9] Vogiatzi MG, Jacobson-Dickman E, DeBoer MD, Drugs, and Therapeutics Committee of The Pediatric Endocrine Society. Vitamin D supplementation and risk of toxicity in pediatrics: A review of current literature. *J Clin Endocrinol Metab*. 2014;99(4):1132-1141. doi:10.1210/jc.2013-3655

[10] Geller AI, Shehab N, Weidle NJ, et al. Emergency department visits for adverse events related to dietary supplements. *N Engl J Med*. 2015;373(16):1531-1540. doi:10.1056/NEJMsa1504267

[11] Neuhouser ML, Wassertheil-Smoller S, Thomson C, et al. Multivitamin use and risk of cancer and cardiovascular disease in the Women's Health Initiative cohorts. *Arch Intern Med*. 2009;169(3):294. doi:10.1001/archinternmed.2008.540

[12] Russell RM. The enigma of β-carotene in carcinogenesis: what can be learned from animal studies. *J Nutr*. 2004;134(1):262S-268S. doi:10.1093/jn/134.1.262S

[13] Khan SA. Multivitamins and Iron (Toxicity). In: *Merck Veterinary Manual*. Kenilworth, NJ; 2018.

[14] Nakamura Y, Gotoh M, Fukuo Y, et al. Severe calcification of mucocutaneous and gastrointestinal tissues induced by high dose administration of vitamin D in a puppy. *J Vet Med Sci*. 2004;66(9):1133-1135.

[15] Valimaki E. Vitamin D intoxication in a. cat- case report. *Suom Eläinlääkäril*. 2018;124(7):371-374..

[16] Davies M. Veterinary clinical nutrition: success stories: an overview. *Proc Nutr Soc.* 2016;75(03):392-397. doi:10.1017/S002966511600029X

[17] Case LP. *Dog Food Logic : Making Smart Decisions for Your Dog in an Age of Too Many Choices.* Wenatchee, WA; Dogwise Publishing: 2014.

[18]Laflamme D, Izquierdo O, Eirmann L, Binder S. Myths and misperceptions about ingredients used in commercial pet foods. *Vet Clin North Am Small Anim Pract.* 2014;44(4):689-698. doi:10.1016/j.cvsm.2014.03.002

[19] Laflammme D. Focus on Nutrition: Cats and carbohydrates: implications for health and disease. *Compend Contin Educ Vet.* 2010;32(1):E1-3.

[20] Murray SM, Fahey GC, Merchen NR, Sunvold GD, Reinhart GA. Evaluation of selected high-starch flours as ingredients in canine diets. *J Anim Sci.* 1999;77(8):2180-2186.

[21] Bazolli RS, Vasconcellos RS, de-Oliveira LD, Sá FC, Pereira GT, Carciofi AC. Effect of the particle size of maize, rice, and sorghum in extruded diets for dogs on starch gelatinization, digestibility, and the fecal concentration of fermentation products1. *J Anim Sci.* 2015;93(6):2956-2966. doi:10.2527/jas.2014-8409

[22] de-Oliveira LD, Carciofi AC, Oliveira MCC, et al. Effects of six carbohydrate sources on diet digestibility and postprandial glucose and insulin responses in cats1. *J Anim Sci.* 2008;86(9):2237-2246. doi:10.2527/jas.2007-0354

[23] Carciofi AC, Takakura FS, de-Oliveira LD, et al. Effects of six carbohydrate sources on dog diet digestibility and post-prandial glucose and insulin response. *J Anim Physiol Anim Nutr (Berl).* 2008;92(3):326-336. doi:10.1111/j.1439-0396.2007.00794.x

[24] Laflame D. Cats and carbohydrates: Why is this still controversial? In: *Proceedings of the 2018 ACVIM Forum.* Seattle, WA; 2018.

[25] de Godoy MRC, Kerr KR, Fahey GC, Jr. Alternative dietary fiber sources in companion animal nutrition. *Nutrients.* 2013;5(8):3099-3117. doi:10.3390/nu5083099

[26] Adin D, DeFrancesco TC, Keene B, et al. Echocardiographic phenotype of canine dilated cardiomyopathy differs based on diet type. *J Vet Cardiol.* 2019;21:1-9. doi:10.1016/J.JVC.2018.11.002

[27] Kaplan JL, Stern JA, Fascetti AJ, et al. Taurine deficiency and dilated cardiomyopathy in golden retrievers fed commercial diets. Loor JJ, ed. *PLoS One.* 2018;13(12):e0209112. doi:10.1371/journal.pone.0209112

[28] Freeman LM, Stern JA, Fries R, Adin DB, Rush JE. Diet-associated dilated cardiomyopathy in dogs: what do we know? *J Am Vet Med Assoc.* 2018;253(11):1390-1394. doi:10.2460/javma.253.11.1390

[29] Shmalberg J. Carbs and cancer: Should you worry? In: *Small Animal and Exotics Proceedings. North American Veterinary Conference.* Orlando, FL; 2013.

[30] Pemberton PW, Lobley RW, Holmes R, Sørensen SH, Batt RM. Gluten-sensitive enteropathy in Irish setter dogs: characterisation of jejunal microvillar membrane proteins by two-dimensional electrophoresis. *Res Vet Sci.* 62(2):191-193.

[31] Lowrie M, Garden OA, Hadjivassiliou M, et al. The clinical and serological effect of a gluten-free diet in border terriers with epileptoid cramping syndrome. *J Vet Intern Med*. 2015;29(6):1564-1568. doi:10.1111/jvim.13643

[32] Niland B, Cash BD. Health benefits and adverse effects of a gluten-free diet in non-celiac disease patients. *Gastroenterol Hepatol (N Y)*. 2018;14(2):82-91

[33] Palmieri B, Vadala' M, Laurino C. A review of the gluten-free diet in non-celiac patients: beliefs, truths, advantages and disadvantages. *Minerva Gastroenterol Dietol*. December 2018. doi:10.23736/S1121-421X.18.02519-9

[34] Dodds WJ, Laverdure D. *Canine Nutrigenomics : The New Science of Feeding Your Dog for Optimum Health*.; Wenatchee, WA; Dogwise Publishing: 2015

[35] Fiolet T, Srour B, Sellem L, et al. Consumption of ultra-processed foods and cancer risk: results from NutriNet-Santé prospective cohort. *BMJ*. 2018;360:k322. doi:10.1136/bmj.k322

[36] DeSalvo KB, Olson R, Casavale KO. Dietary guidelines for Americans. *JAMA*. 2016;315(5):457. doi:10.1001/jama.2015.18396

[37] Peloza J, Montford W. The health halo: how good PR is misleading shoppers. *The Guardian*. March 11, 2015

[38] Council NR. *Nutrient Requirements of Dogs and Cats*. Washington, D.C.: National Academies Press; 2006. doi:10.17226/10668

[39] Association of American Feed Control Officials. *2018 Official Publication : Association of American Feed Control Officials*. Champaign, IL: Association of American Feed Control Officials (AAFCO); 2018

[40] Case LP, Daristotle L, Hayek MG, et al. Common nutrition myths and feeding practices. *Canine Feline Nutr*. January 2011:277-294. doi:10.1016/B978-0-323-06619-8.10026-X

[41] Błaszczyk A, Augustyniak A, Skolimowski J. Ethoxyquin: An antioxidant used in animal feed. *Int J Food Sci*. 2013;2013:1-12. doi:10.1155/2013/585931

[42] Gross KL, Bollinger R, Thawnghmung P, Collings GF. Effect of three different preservative systems on the stability of extruded dog food subjected to ambient and high temperature storage. *J Nutr*. 1994;124(suppl_12):2638S-2642S. doi:10.1093/jn/124.suppl_12.2638S

[43] Hilton JW. Antioxidants: function, types and necessity of inclusion in pet foods. *Can Vet J = La Rev Vet Can*. 1989;30(8):682-684

[44] Landrum AR, Hallman WK, Jamieson KH. Examining the impact of expert voices: communicating the scientific consensus on genetically-modified organisms. *Environ Commun*. August 2018:1-20. doi:10.1080/17524032.2018.1502201

[45] National Academies of Sciences E and M. *Genetically Engineered Crops*. Washington, D.C.: National Academies Press; 2016. doi:10.17226/23395

[46] Van Eenennaam AL, Young AE. Prevalence and impacts of genetically engineered feedstuffs on livestock populations1. *J Anim Sci.* 2014;92(10):4255-4278. doi:10.2527/jas.2014-8124

[47] Nicolia A, Manzo A, Veronesi F, Rosellini D. An overview of the last 10 years of genetically engineered crop safety research. *Crit Rev Biotechnol.* 2014;34(1):77-88. doi:10.3109/07388551.2013.823595

[48] Na KI. *A Decade of EU-Funded GMO Research.*; 2001. Available at: http://ec.europa.eu/research/research-eu. Accessed December 19, 2018

[49] Food and Drug Administration H. *Current Good Manufacturing Practice, Hazard Analysis, and Risk-Based Preventive Controls for Food for Animals; Final Rule.* Federal Register 80 (180); 2015

[50] Wortinger A. Nutritional myths. *J Am Anim Hosp Assoc.* 2005;41(4):273-276. doi:10.5326/0410273

[51] Center for Veterinary Medicine United States Food and Drug Administration. *Food and Drug Administration/Center for Veterinary Medicine Report on the Risk from Pentobarbital in Dog Food.* Silver Springs, MD; 2002

[52] Treu H, Nordborg M, Cederberg C, et al. Carbon footprints and land use of conventional and organic diets in Germany. *J Clean Prod.* 2017;161:127-142. doi:10.1016/J.JCLEPRO.2017.05.041

[53] Balmford A, Amano T, Bartlett H, et al. The environmental costs and benefits of high-yield farming. *Nat Sustain.* 2018;1(9):477-485. doi:10.1038/s41893-018-0138-5

[54] Searchinger TD, Wirsenius S, Beringer T, Dumas P. Assessing the efficiency of changes in land use for mitigating climate change. *Nature.* 2018;564(7735):249-253. doi:10.1038/s41586-018-0757-z

[55] Funk C, Kennedy B. The new food fights: U.S. public divides over food science. Pew Research; Washington, D.C.: 2016. Available at: https://www.pewresearch.org/science/2016/12/01/the-new-food-fights/. Accessed June 23, 2019.

[56] Shaw Hughner R, McDonagh P, Prothero A, Shultz II CJ, Stanton J. Who are organic food consumers? A compilation and review of why people purchase organic food. *J Cons Behav. 2007;6(2-3):94-110.* doi:10.1002/cb.210

[57] Baudry J, Péneau S, Allès B, et al. food choice motives when purchasing in organic and conventional consumer clusters: Focus on sustainable concerns (The NutriNet-Santé Cohort Study). *Nutrients.* 2017;9(2). doi:10.3390/nu9020088

[58] Miller N. *Pet Food in the U.S., 13th Edition: How Millennials Are Rapidly Changing The Organic Pet Food Industry.* Rockville, MD; 2017. Available at: https://www.packagedfacts.com/Content/Blog/2017/02/07/1-in-3-US-Pet-Owners-Millennials-What-it-Means-for-the-Pet-Food-Market. Accessed December 20, 2018

[59] Walet E. Are trends in human food reflected in pet food purchase? Master's Thesis; Opebn Univ. of the Netherlands. 2015. Available at: https://dspace.ou.nl/bitstream/1820/6538/1/Walet%20E%20scriptie.pdf Accessed December 20, 2018

[60] Średnicka-Tober D, Barański M, Seal CJ, et al. Higher PUFA and n-3 PUFA, conjugated linoleic acid, α-tocopherol and iron, but lower iodine and selenium concentrations in organic milk: a systematic literature review and meta- and redundancy analyses. *Br J Nutr*. 2016;115(06):1043-1060. doi:10.1017/S0007114516000349

[61] Barański M, Średnicka-Tober D, Volakakis N, et al. Higher antioxidant and lower cadmium concentrations and lower incidence of pesticide residues in organically grown crops: a systematic literature review and meta-analyses. *Br J Nutr*. 2014;112(05):794-811. doi:10.1017/S0007114514001366

[62] Dangour AD, Dodhia SK, Hayter A, Allen E, Lock K, Uauy R. Nutritional quality of organic foods: a systematic review. *Am J Clin Nutr*. 2009;90(3):680-685. doi:10.3945/ajcn.2009.28041

[63] Mie A, Andersen HR, Gunnarsson S, et al. Human health implications of organic food and organic agriculture: a comprehensive review. *Environ Health*. 2017;16(1):111. doi:10.1186/s12940-017-0315-4

[64] Smith-Spangler C, Brandeau ML, Hunter GE, et al. Are Organic Foods Safer or Healthier Than Conventional Alternatives? *Ann Intern Med*. 2012;157(5):348. doi:10.7326/0003-4819-157-5-201209040-00007

[65] Baudry J, Assmann KE, Touvier M, et al. Association of Frequency of Organic Food Consumption With Cancer Risk. *JAMA Intern Med*. 2018;178(12):1597. doi:10.1001/jamainternmed.2018.4357

[66] Bradbury KE, Balkwill A, Spencer EA, et al. Organic food consumption and the incidence of cancer in a large prospective study of women in the United Kingdom. *Br J Cancer*. 2014;110(9):2321-2326. doi:10.1038/bjc.2014.148

[67] ATS Statement. *Am J Respir Crit Care Med*. 2002;166(1):111-117. doi:10.1164/ajrccm.166.1.at1102

[68] Guidelines for the management of adults with hospital-acquired, ventilator-associated, and healthcare-associated pneumonia. *Am J Respir Crit Care Med*. 2005;171(4):388-416. doi:10.1164/rccm.200405-644ST

[69] Weaver CM, Dwyer J, Fulgoni VL, et al. Processed foods: contributions to nutrition. *Am J Clin Nutr*. 2014;99(6):1525-1542. doi:10.3945/ajcn.114.089284

[70] Weaver CM, Miller JW. Challenges in conducting clinical nutrition research. *Nutr Rev*. 2017;75(7):491-499. doi:10.1093/nutrit/nux026

[71] Michels KB. Nutritional epidemiology—past, present, future. *Int J Epidemiol*. 2003;32(4):486-488. doi:10.1093/ije/dyg216

[72] Casna BR, Shepherd ML DS. Cost of homemade versus commercial adult maintenance canine diets. In: *NAVC Clinician's BriefAAVN Clinical Nutrition & Research Symposium*. Oxon Hill, MD: Educational Concepts; 2017. Available at: https://files.brief.vet/migration/article/45821/sym-caps_2017-aavn-45821-article.pdf. Accessed December 28, 2018

[73] Johnson LN, Linder DE, Heinze CR, Kehs RL, Freeman LM. Evaluation of owner experiences and adherence to home-cooked diet recipes for dogs. *J Small Anim Pract*. 2016;57(1):23-27. doi:10.1111/jsap.12412

[74] Larsen JA, Parks EM, Heinze CR, Fascetti AJ. Evaluation of recipes for home-prepared diets for dogs and cats with chronic kidney disease. *J Am Vet Med Assoc*. 2012;240(5):532-538. doi:10.2460/javma.240.5.532

[75] Stockman J, Fascetti AJ, Kass PH, Larsen JA. Evaluation of recipes of home-prepared maintenance diets for dogs. *J Am Vet Med Assoc*. 2013;242(11):1500-1505. doi:10.2460/javma.242.11.1500

[76] Heinze CR, Gomez FC, Freeman LM. Assessment of commercial diets and recipes for home-prepared diets recommended for dogs with cancer. *J Am Vet Med Assoc*. 2012;241(11):1453-1460. doi:10.2460/javma.241.11.1453

[77] Pedrinelli V, Gomes M de OS, Carciofi AC. Analysis of recipes of home-prepared diets for dogs and cats published in Portuguese. *J Nutr Sci*. 2017;6:e33. doi:10.1017/jns.2017.31

[78] Remillard RL. Homemade diets: Attributes, pitfalls, and a call for action. *Top Companion Anim Med*. 2008;23(3):137-142. doi:10.1053/j.tcam.2008.04.006

[79] Pion PD, Kittleson MD, Rogers QR, Morris JG. Myocardial failure in cats associated with low plasma taurine: a reversible cardiomyopathy. *Science*. 1987;237(4816):764-768

[80] American Veterinary Medical Association (AVMA). Raw or Undercooked Animal-Source Protein in Cat and Dog Diets. https://www.avma.org/KB/Policies/Pages/Raw-or-Undercooked-Animal-Source-Protein-in-Cat-and-Dog-Diets.aspx. Published 2012. Accessed December 28, 2018

[81] Center for Veterinary Medicine USF and DA. Animal Health Literacy - Get the Facts! Raw Pet Food Diets can be Dangerous to You and Your Pet. https://www.fda.gov/animalveterinary/resourcesforyou/animalhealthliteracy/ucm373757.htm. Published 2018. Accessed December 28, 2018

[82] Freeman LM, Chandler ML, Hamper BA, Weeth LP. Current knowledge about the risks and benefits of raw meat-based diets for dogs and cats. *J Am Vet Med Assoc*. 2013;243(11):1549-1558. doi:10.2460/javma.243.11.1549

[83] Schlesinger DP, Joffe DJ. Raw food diets in companion animals: a critical review. *Can Vet J = La Rev Vet Can*. 2011;52(1):50-54

[84] Serpell J. *The Domestic Dog: Its Evolution, Behavior and Interactions with People*. 2nd ed. (Serpell J, ed.). Cambridge University Press; 2017

[85] Sturgeon A, Jardine CM, Weese JS. Comparison of the fecal microbiota of wild wolves, dogs fed commercial dry diets and dogs fed raw meat diets. In: *Proceedings 2014 ACVIM Research Forum*. Vol 28. John Wiley & Sons, Ltd (10.1111); 2014:1346-1374. doi:10.1111/jvim.12375

[86] Axelsson E, Ratnakumar A, Arendt M-L, et al. The genomic signature of dog domestication reveals adaptation to a starch-rich diet. *Nature*. 2013;495(7441):360-364. doi:10.1038/nature11837

[87] Ziesenis A, Wissdorf H. [The ligaments and menisci of the femorotibial joint of the wolf (Canis lupus L., 1758)--anatomic and functional analysis in comparison with the domestic dog (Canis lupus f. familiaris)]. *Gegenbaurs Morphol Jahrb*. 1990;136(6):759-773

[88] Wayne RK. Molecular evolution of the dog family. *Trends Genet*. 1993;9(6):218-224

[89] Vilà C, Maldonado JE, Wayne RK. Phylogenetic relationships, evolution, and genetic diversity of the domestic dog. *J Hered*. 90(1):71-77

[90] Reiter T, Jagoda E, Capellini TD. Dietary variation and evolution of gene copy number among dog breeds. *PLOS One*. 2016. doi:10.1371/journal.pone.0148899

[91] Tidière M, Gaillard J-M, Berger V, et al. Comparative analyses of longevity and senescence reveal variable survival benefits of living in zoos across mammals. *Sci Rep*. 2016;6:36361. doi:10.1038/srep36361

[92] Mukherjee S, Heithaus MR. Dangerous prey and daring predators: a review. *Biol Rev*. 2013;88(3):550-563. doi:10.1111/brv.12014

[93] Holmes JC, Podesta R. The helminths of wolves and coyotes from the forested regions of Alberta. *Can J Zool*. 1968;46(6):1193-1204. doi:10.1139/z68-169

[94] Young TP. Natural die-offs of large mammals: implications for conservation. *Conserv Biol*. 1994;8(2):410-418. doi:10.1046/j.1523-1739.1994.08020410.x

[95] Bosch G, Hagen-Plantinga EA, Hendriks WH. Dietary nutrient profiles of wild wolves: insights for optimal dog nutrition? *Br J Nutr*. 2015;113(S1):S40-S54. doi:10.1017/S0007114514002311

[96] Choquette LPE, Gibson GG, Kuyt E, Pearson AM. Helminths of wolves, *Canis lupus* L., in the Yukon and Northwest Territories. *Can J Zool*. 1973;51(10):1087-1091. doi:10.1139/z73-158

[97] Amanda A. Parasites of the African painted dog (Lycaon pictus) in captive and wild populations: Implications for conservation. 2011. http://researchrepository.murdoch.edu.au/id/eprint/10519/2/02Whole.pdf

[98] Berentsen AR, Becker MS, Stockdale-Walden H, Matandiko W, McRobb R, Dunbar MR. Survey of gastrointestinal parasite infection in African lion (*Panthera leo*), African wild dog (*Lycaon pictus*) and spotted hyaena (*Crocuta crocuta*) in the Luangwa Valley, Zambia. *African Zool*. 2012;47(2):363-368. doi:10.1080/15627020.2012.11407561

[99] Fuchs B. Sarcoptic mange in the Scandinavian wolf population. *BMC Vet Res.* 2014;12(1):156

[100] Benson JF, Mills KJ, Loveless KM, Patterson BR. Genetic and environmental influences on pup mortality risk for wolves and coyotes within a Canis hybrid zone. *Biol Conserv.* 2013;166:133-141. doi:10.1016/J.BIOCON.2013.06.018

[101] Mech LD, Nelson ME. Evidence of Prey-caused Mortality in Three Wolves. *Am Midl Nat.* 1990;123(1):207. doi:10.2307/2425775

[102] Mech LD. Productivity, mortality, and population trends of wolves in northeastern Minnesota. *J Mammal.* 1977;58(4):559-574. doi:10.2307/1380004

[103] Woodroffe R, Davies-Mostert H, Ginsberg J, et al. Rates and causes of mortality in Endangered African wild dogs Lycaon pictus: lessons for management and monitoring. *Oryx.* 2007;41(02):215. doi:10.1017/S0030605307001809

[104] Morgan SK, Willis S, Shepherd ML. Survey of owner motivations and veterinary input of owners feeding diets containing raw animal products. *PeerJ.* 2017;5:e3031. doi:10.7717/peerj.3031

[105] Gyles C. Raw food diets for pets. *Can Vet J.* 2017;58(6):537-539

[106] Billinghurst I. *Give Your Dog a Bone.* Bathurst, N.S.W. Warrigal Publishing; 1993

[107] Pitcairn RH, Pitcairn SH. *Dr. Pitcairn's Complete Guide to Natural Health for Dogs & Cats.* Emmaus, PA. Rodale; 2017

[108] Schmidt M, Unterer S, Suchodolski JS, et al. The fecal microbiome and metabolome differs between dogs fed Bones and Raw Food (BARF) diets and dogs fed commercial diets. Loor JJ, ed. *PLoS One.* 2018;13(8):e0201279. doi:10.1371/journal.pone.0201279

[109] Kim J, An J-U, Kim W, Lee S, Cho S. Differences in the gut microbiota of dogs (Canis lupus familiaris) fed a natural diet or a commercial feed revealed by the Illumina MiSeq platform. *Gut Pathog.* 2017;9:68. doi:10.1186/s13099-017-0218-5

[110] Araújo, I. C. S.; Furtado, A. P.; Araújo, G. C. P.; Rocha CG. Effect of the diet of healthy dogs on clinical analysis and behavioral aspects. *Arq Bras Med Veterinária e Zootec.* 2018;70(3):689-698

[111] Kerr KR, Vester Boler BM, Morris CL, Liu KJ, Swanson KS. Apparent total tract energy and macronutrient digestibility and fecal fermentative end-product concentrations of domestic cats fed extruded, raw beef-based, and cooked beef-based diets. *J Anim Sci.* 2012;90(2):515-522. doi:10.2527/jas.2010-3266

[112] Kerr KR, Dowd SE, Swanson KS. Faecal microbiota of domestic cats fed raw whole chicks v. an extruded chicken-based diet. *J Nutr Sci.* 2014;3:e22. doi:10.1017/jns.2014.21

[113] Marx F, Machado G, Pezzali J, et al. Raw beef bones as chewing items to reduce dental calculus in Beagle dogs. *Aust Vet J.* 2016;94(1-2):18-23. doi:10.1111/avj.12394

[114] Robinson J, Gorrel C. The oral status of a pack of foxhounds fed a "natural" diet. In: *Proceedings. Fifth World Veterinary Dental Congress.* Birmingham, England; 1997

[115] Freeman LM, Chandler ML, Hamper BA, Weeth LP. Current knowledge about the risks and benefits of raw meat-based diets for dogs and cats. *J Am Vet Med Assoc.* 2013;243(11):1549-1558. doi:10.2460/javma.243.11.1549

[116] Schlesinger DP, Joffe DJ. Raw food diets in companion animals: a critical review. *Can Vet J = La Rev Vet Can.* 2011;52(1):50-54

[117] Taylor MB, Geiger DA, Saker KE, Larson MM. Diffuse osteopenia and myelopathy in a puppy fed a diet composed of an organic premix and raw ground beef. *J Am Vet Med Assoc.* 2009;234(8):1041-1048. doi:10.2460/javma.234.8.1041

[118] Freeman LM, Michel KE. Veterinary Medicine Today: Timely Topics in Nutrition-Evaluation of raw food diets for dogs. *J Am Vet Med Assoc.* 2001;218(5):705-709. doi:10.2460/javma.2001.218.705

[119] Lauten SD, Smith TM, Kirk CA, Bartges JW, Adams A WS. Computer analysis of nutrient sufficiency of published home-cooked diets for dogs and cats. In: *Proceedings of the American College of Veterinary Internal Medicine Forum.* Baltimore, MD; 2005

[120] Stockman J, Fascetti AJ, Kass PH, Larsen JA. Evaluation of recipes of home-prepared maintenance diets for dogs. *J Am Vet Med Assoc.* 2013;242(11):1500-1505. doi:10.2460/javma.242.11.1500

[121] Larsen JA, Parks EM, Heinze CR, Fascetti AJ. Evaluation of recipes for home-prepared diets for dogs and cats with chronic kidney disease. *J Am Vet Med Assoc.* 2012;240(5):532-538. doi:10.2460/javma.240.5.532

[122] Remillard RL. Homemade diets: Attributes, pitfalls, and a call for action. *Top Companion Anim Med.* 2008;23(3):137-142. doi:10.1053/j.tcam.2008.04.006

[123] Glasgow A, Caver N, Marks S, Pedersen N. *Role of Diet in the Health of the Feline Intestinal Tract and in Inflammatory Bowel Disease.* Center for Companion Animal Health, School of Veterinary Medicine, UC Davis; 2002

[124] Rousseau A, Prittie J, Broussard JD, Fox PR, Hoskinson J. Incidence and characterization of esophagitis following esophageal foreign body removal in dogs: 60 cases (1999?2003). *J Vet Emerg Crit Care.* 2007;17(2):159-163. doi:10.1111/j.1476-4431.2007.00227.x

[125] Gianella P, Pfammatter NS, Burgener IA. Oesophageal and gastric endoscopic foreign body removal: complications and follow-up of 102 dogs. *J Small Anim Pract.* 2009;50(12):649-654. doi:10.1111/j.1748-5827.2009.00845.x

[126] Frowde PE, Battersby IA, Whitley NT, Elwood CM. Oesophageal disease in 33 cats. *J Feline Med Surg.* 2011;13(8):564-569. doi:10.1016/j.jfms.2011.04.004

[127] Thompson HC, Cortes Y, Gannon K, Bailey D, Freer S. Esophageal foreign bodies in dogs: 34 cases (2004-2009). *J Vet Emerg Crit Care.* 2012;22(2):253-261. doi:10.1111/j.1476-4431.2011.00700.x

[128] Steenkamp G, Gorrel C. Oral and dental conditions in adult african wild dog skulls: A preliminary report. *J Vet Dent.* 1999;16(2):65-68. doi:10.1177/089875649901600201

[129] Van Valkenburgh B. Incidence of tooth breakage among large, predatory mammals. *Am Nat.* 1988;131(2):291-302. doi:10.1086/284790

[130] VanValkenburgh B, Hertel F. Tough times at la brea: tooth breakage in large carnivores of the late Pleistocene. *Science (80-).* 1993;261(5120):456-459. doi:10.1126/science.261.5120.456

[131] Nemser SM, Doran T, Grabenstein M, et al. Investigation of Listeria, Salmonella, and toxigenic Escherichia coli in various pet foods. *Foodborne Pathog Dis.* 2014;11(9):706-709. doi:10.1089/fpd.2014.1748

[132] *Investigation into an Outbreak of Shiga Toxin Producing Escherichia Coli (STEC) O157 PT 21/28 Stx2 in England.*; 2017. Available at: https://assets.publishing.service.gov.uk/government/uploads/system/uploads/attachment_data/file/765498/STEC_O157_PT21.28_Outbreak_Report.pdf"

[133] Chengappa MM, Staats J, Oberst RD, Gabbert NH, McVey S. Prevalence of *Salmonella* in raw meat used in diets of racing greyhounds. *J Vet Diagnostic Investig.* 1993;5(3):372-377. doi:10.1177/104063879300500312

[134] Finley R, Ribble C, Aramini J, et al. The risk of salmonellae shedding by dogs fed Salmonella-contaminated commercial raw food diets. *Can Vet J.* 2007;48(1):69-75

[135] Joffe DJ, Schlesinger DP. Preliminary assessment of the risk of Salmonella infection in dogs fed raw chicken diets. *Can Vet J.* 2002;43(6):441-442

[136] Weese JS, Rousseau J, Arroyo L. Bacteriological evaluation of commercial canine and feline raw diets. *Can Vet J.* 2005;46(6):513-516

[137] Strohmeyer RA, Morley PS, Hyatt DR, Dargatz DA, Scorza AV, Lappin MR. Evaluation of bacterial and protozoal contamination of commercially available raw meat diets for dogs. *J Am Vet Med Assoc.* 2006;228(4):537-542. doi:10.2460/javma.228.4.537

9|
A Quick Guide to Other CAM Practices

The purpose of science in medicine is to attempt to get at the truth.
Why should falsehood and ignorance be warm, while truth and
knowledge should be cold? Only more and better science will
perform the humane function of eliminating the errors encouraged
by warm emotion.

- D. F. Horrobin

Introduction

My purpose in this chapter is to provide very brief assessments of some of the important treatments and issues I have not covered elsewhere. There is an enormous number of alternative treatments recommended for dogs and cats, and it would be impossible for me to evaluate more than a tiny fraction of them. A book devoted to this alone would be enormous, rapidly out of date, and filled with assessments that said little more than, "There is insufficient evidence to evaluate this product." I have included a few supplements and herbal products that are very commonly used and concerning which there is sufficient research evidence to at least make a tentative guess at whether they are safe and effective or not.

I have also discussed vaccines, neutering, and some other issues that are not CAM but that are often part of the information CAM practitioners provide to pet owners, and which I believe is often misleading.

I do not suggest that this chapter is in any way comprehensive, but hopefully it will be useful in two ways. First, the treatments I cover are widely used and marketed, so these assessments may help you in making decisions about them in the care of your own pets. Second, as always, they are meant to serve as a template for the methods you can use yourself to evaluate therapies I do not discuss. The pattern should be clear at this point, and I will make the steps even more explicit in Chapter 10. If you try to answer the same questions for each treatment you encounter that I answer for those discussed here, using the same standards of scientific reasoning and evidence, you will be well on your way to providing the best, science-based pet care possible.

ANIMAL COMMUNICATORS/PET PSYCHICS

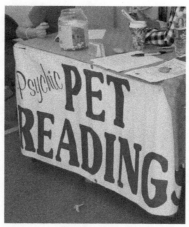

Psychic Pet Reading 2009 by Erik Fitzpatrick under Creative Commons by SA 2.0

Placebos for Pets?

What Is It?

There are individuals who claim that they have some direct mental connection to the thoughts of dogs and cats and can intuitively understand what they want or fear and relay this to the animals' owners. Like most types of psychic phenomena, this is based on the principle that there is some nonphysical force or energy associated with the thoughts of humans and animals and that this can be detected and interpreted from a distance by individuals with a special ability or training. This is distinctly different from legitimate behavioral science, which interprets the behavior of animals in ways that allow some understanding, prediction, and manipulation of their subsequent behavior and may involve postulating internal mental states that cannot be directly observed.

Animal communicators are sometimes involved in pet healthcare when they are consulted by owners trying to make decisions about their pets' treatment. Most commonly, we encounter this when owners are struggling with the end of a pet's life and trying to assess the quality of life for their friend and decide whether further treatment or euthanasia is in their pet's best interests. This is a deeply emotional and difficult experience, and some owners feel they can better make such decisions if they have direct evidence for how their pet feels and what he or she may want.

Does It Work?

The basic principle of psychic communication with animals is inconsistent with a scientific understanding of how mental phenomena work. No force that transmits thoughts directly from an animal to a person, or vice versa, over a distance has even been identified.

367

There has been extensive research in humans into purported psychic phenomena of many kinds, including telepathy. Most studies do not meet the standards of high-quality scientific experimentation, and alternative explanations for the findings based on cognitive error and bias are more plausible than the theoretical concept of telepathy. Consistent, repeatable, reliable evidence for these phenomena has never been found, and belief in them continues to rest primarily on faith and personal, anecdotal experiences.[1-5]

I have found no controlled research evidence investigating the subject of whether some people can communicate telepathically with dogs and cats. However, there is a published report of an informal experiment in which a skeptic borrowed a neighbor's cat and then invited a pet psychic to "read" the cat and tell her about it. The psychic was consistently incorrect about many known details of the cat's life. However, she demonstrated many of the specific techniques, known as cold reading, which psychics, magicians, and con artists are known to use to appear to have information that could only have been acquired through supernatural means. The references for this article include some excellent descriptions of how such techniques create the appearance of telepathy.[6]

Is It Safe?

There are no obvious, direct physical risks from interaction with an animal communicator. However, many psychics seem to perform something of an informal counseling role for pet owners, and owners sometimes rely on their interpretation of the pet's feelings to help make medical decisions. Reliance on fabricated information about your pet's thoughts and desires to decide whether to pursue medical treatment or to euthanize your pet steals your power as the caregiver to decide for yourself what is in the best interests of your pet. Pet psychics are invested in appearing effective and in satisfying their clients, not necessarily in the interests of the animals they purport to communicate with. I have seen several owners persist in uncomfortable and fruitless treatment of animals who were suffering because a psychic told them the pet had said it was "not ready to go yet," and I consider this a form of harm to these animals.

Bottom Line

Complete nonsense.

AROMATHERAPY AND ESSENTIAL OILS

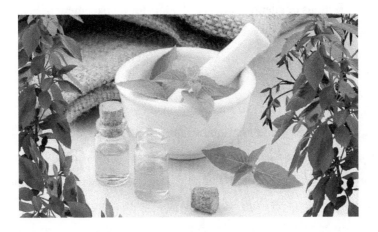

What Is It?

Essential oils are chemicals extracted and purified from plants that typically have distinctive odors.[7] Aromatherapy is a practice in which such oils are used in a variety of ways, from exposing patients to the odor to applying the oils, topically or internally, in order to have beneficial effects.[8] Though scattered references to historical use of plant oils for medical purposes have been found, there is no consistent historical tradition or theoretical explanation for the proposed therapeutic value of these chemicals. Aromatherapy as currently practiced is a twentieth-century invention.[8,9] Proponents of aromatherapy put forward a variety of explanations for the therapeutic potential of essential oils, from suggested physiologic effects on brain chemistry and the immune system to vitalist explanations focusing on the effects of these chemicals on the spiritual well-being of patients.

Proposed uses of essential oils in humans vary from reduction of stress or other manipulations of mood to treatment of serious illness. In dog and cat patients, practitioners using essential oils most often recommend topical use for infections or allergies and use of odors for management of behavioral problems.

Does It Work?

The theories proposed to explain the action of essential oils range from vague and not consistent with established scientific knowledge to plausible. There are many *in vitro* and lab animal studies of essential oils showing that they can have a wide variety of effects on microorganisms and animal cells in test tubes and on the physiology of rodents and other animal models. Some of these findings suggest potential uses for these compounds, others highlight potential risks.[1,10-12]

There are numerous systematic reviews of many clinical trials in humans involving essential oils. The majority of these trials are of low quality (unblinded, uncontrolled, etc.), and most systematic reviews conclude that the evidence is not definitive for meaningful clinical benefits.[7,8,13-16] The most convincing research suggests that topical use of some essential oils may have antiseptic properties that can be useful in the treatment of superficial infections and dental disease.[17,18] Mouthwashes with essential oils have been shown to reduce plaque buildup, for example, and topical tea tree oil has been shown to be helpful for some types of acne and other skin infections. There is also some evidence that subjective psychological outcomes can be affected by the use of essential oils, though it is difficult to distinguish true physiologic effects from placebo effects for these sorts of symptoms.[8,13,15,19]

There are numerous *in vitro* studies suggesting some essential oils have antimicrobial properties for bacteria and yeast that commonly infect dogs and cats.[20,21] A few clinical trials have been conducted to investigate the topical use of essential oils to treat infections and allergic skin conditions.[22,23,24] Many of these are difficult to interpret since the essential oils are mixed with other ingredients and so the effect of each component cannot be determined. The existing evidence is suggestive that some products may have some clinical benefit, though the details (which oils, which conditions, how these compare with conventional treatments, and so on) are unclear.

There is less literature looking at the potential behavioral effects of essential oil aromas, and the results are not conclusive.[25-31] While it is possible these odors may have beneficial effects, it is also possible that they may be unpleasant for species with far greater sensitivity to smells than humans, and this is very difficult to determine since our pets cannot tell us directly about their responses to such stimuli.

Is It Safe?

In humans, allergic reactions to inhaled and topical essential oils are reported. More severe, even fatal, responses have also occurred though these are rare.[1,32] In dogs and cats, similar allergic reactions are known to occur. Several specific oils have been reported to cause serious toxic effects, including tea tree oil, pennyroyal, wintergreen, cinnamon, pine, sweet birch, and others.[33-37] The risk from diffusers is unclear, but direct topical application of some oils, especially tea tree oil, has been associated with severe local and systemic toxic reaction.

Cats appear more sensitive than dogs to most essential oils, and the risk of accidental ingestion through self-grooming or attempting to eat an aromatherapy product directly makes the risks in dogs and cats greater than in adult humans (though similar cases of accidental overdose and toxicity do occur in children). Deaths have been reported, though these are rare.

Bottom Line

Might have some uses, especially applied topically for infections, but uncertain and some significant risks.

COLD/LOW-LEVEL LASER THERAPY

What Is It?

At its simplest, laser therapy is the application of light to living organisms to improve health. However, there is a bewildering amount of detail behind this simple idea. The wavelength and power of the laser, the location and duration of exposure, the number of treatments, and many other variables are crucial to the effects achieved.

Generally, low-level lasers utilize wavelengths between 600-1000nm and power levels from 5-500mW. More powerful lasers are used in surgery, but these function primarily to cut or cauterize tissue or otherwise cause controlled damage. Low-level lasers are intended to have biological effects on tissue without causing damage.[38]

The US Food and Drug Administration classifies lasers, from Class 1 to Class 4, based primarily on their potential to harm the user or the patient. Low-level laser therapy typically involves Class 3 lasers, though more powerful Class 4 devices are becoming more popular.[1,39]

The most common recommended uses of low-level laser therapy are to facilitate wound healing, reduce inflammation, and treat musculoskeletal pain. However, proponents of laser therapy, and companies selling lasers, often suggest that this tool can treat many other medical conditions. Lasers have been promoted for specific clinical problems (e.g. allergic skin disease, gingivitis, bacterial and viral infections, envenomation), vaguely defined general health improvement (e.g. enhancing immune function, normalizing metabolic function), and unscientific nonsense (e.g. fixing "Qi-stagnation" and "energizing" cells).[1,40,41,42]

Does It Work?

There is an enormous body of *in vitro* evidence showing effects of laser light on various tissues. It is clear that the laser has significant biological effects in such models, and some of the effects seen could potentially have clinical benefits in living patients.[1]

373

Multiple systematic reviews of lab animal studies are available. One found that there were some potentially beneficial effects in bone healing models, though there were few studies to review.[43] Another reviewed *in vitro* and animal model studies relevant to wound healing and concluded there was insufficient evidence to justify clinical trials in humans.[44] In contrast, a more recent review of animal wound-healing models concluded that there is good evidence for benefits from low-level laser treatment, though not all protocols are effective for all types of wounds, so the details of indication and technique matter.[45]

There have been many preclinical studies of laser therapy for a variety of conditions in veterinary species, and again the quality is variable and the results are mixed. Some studies of wound healing, for example, show possible benefits[46] while many others do not.[47–51] Some studies looking at lasers for skin disease have found a beneficial effect[52] and others no apparent effect at all.[53]

In the human literature, there are hundreds of systematic reviews available for specific conditions, often with several different reviews of the same studies. But there is great inconsistency in the results. Many reviews conclude that the evidence is not strong enough to support definitive statements about efficacy. Some reviews do show results supporting benefit for particular conditions, though in some cases other reviews of the same evidence reach different conclusions.

For example, there have been three systematic reviews in the last ten years of studies investigating laser therapy for osteoarthritis of the knee. Each sorted through hundreds of studies and selected a different subset as the highest quality studies to assess. One review concluded there was good evidence for beneficial effects.[54] Another determined there were some positive findings but insufficient evidence on important therapeutic variables to conclusively demonstrate a benefit.[55] The third review concluded there was no good evidence that laser therapy is useful in treatment of knee osteoarthritis.[56] This is representative of the pattern seen in reviews of this treatment for all conditions.

There are a few clinical trials in dogs and cats, but they have significant limitations and often inconsistent findings. For example, a pilot study adding laser therapy to standard treatment for dogs with acute intervertebral disk rupture suggested laser treatment might have shortened time to walking after surgery.[57] However, the absence of randomization, blinding, and placebo controls limit the strength of this conclusion. Another similar study did not report any clinical benefit.[58] A very small study of laser therapy and physical therapy for dogs with disk disease also failed to find any benefit.[59]

Similarly, a recent study of laser therapy as an adjunctive treatment for dogs undergoing surgery for a ruptured ligament in the knee found no effect on comfort or the healing of soft tissue or bone. Some effect on gait was seen, though it was small and of doubtful clinical significance.[5] An earlier study of pre-operative laser treatment in dogs having the same surgery showed a similar pattern, finding no significant differences in most outcomes evaluated but a small difference in one measure of weight-bearing.[6] A number of recent studies of laser therapy for dogs undergoing knee surgery have been similarly inconsistent.[60,61,62]

Overall, the clinical trial literature in veterinary medicine is sparse and has many methodological limitations. Some positive effects have been reported, but no consistent pattern of meaningful clinical benefit has yet emerged.

Is It Safe?

Experimental and clinical studies of low-level laser therapy have found few adverse effects.[1,17,19,63] Inappropriate use of higher-power lasers or excessive duration of treatment can result in thermal tissue damage. There are also potential risks to operators of laser equipment. In the absence of research evaluating the long-term effects of ongoing laser treatment, the potential for harm is unknown. Safety guidelines, from government agencies, manufacturers, and the medical literature, are available and should be scrupulously followed.

Bottom Line

Might help for some conditions but evidence is weak

COLLOIDAL SILVER

What Is It?

Silver has a history of mainstream medical use based on tradition and theory, but it has been abandoned by science-based medicine in favor of safer and more effective treatments. There are a few legitimate uses of silver-containing compounds,[64-67] but unfortunately these are often misrepresented as supporting inappropriate uses of other silver-containing substances. There is virtually no research on colloidal silver in actual patients, and what there is fails to meet basic standards of quality. There are, however, lots of anecdotes which people wrongly believe can be used to support treatment with this substance.

Oral colloidal silver remedies contain a liquid, usually water, with microscopic particles of silver suspended in it. Some topical products contain the silver particles suspended in a cream or ointment. Proponents recommend this remedy for many conditions, including infections, metabolic diseases such as diabetes or thyroid disease, and even cancer.[3]

Does It Work?

While some medical uses of silver are legitimate, none involve oral colloidal silver. Silver has some antiseptic properties, so it can kill some infectious organisms that come in contact with it. Topical use of ointments for burns and to prevent eye infections in newborns, and impregnation of catheters and other medical equipment with silver, are effective uses of silver for this purpose.[1-4,68] However, taking colloidal silver orally is an entirely different thing, and there are no proven benefits from this practice. There are absolutely no clinical trials in humans showing oral colloidal silver has any health benefits.[69]

One study has been published looking at colloidal silver in dogs.[70] This was not actually published in a veterinary journal but in a journal devoted to nanotechnology. The reason for this is obvious when reading the article. The study has none of the expected mechanisms for controlling bias or error in a clinical study and amounts to little more than a complicated collection of anecdotes. The authors claim that the use of colloidal silver in this study

377

saved the lives of some dogs with canine distemper, a serious viral infection. This would be fantastic if it were true, but the deficiencies in the study make the results nothing more than unreliable guesswork.

Is It Safe?

The medical use of colloidal silver has actually been banned in the US by the Food and Drug Administration,[71] though it is still legal to sell some kinds of colloidal silver as dietary supplements without claims of any medical benefits. The reason for this is that there is no reason to believe oral silver has medical benefits, and it can have risks when used orally.[3,6,72–74] The most obvious of these is argyria, a permanent discoloration of the entire body.

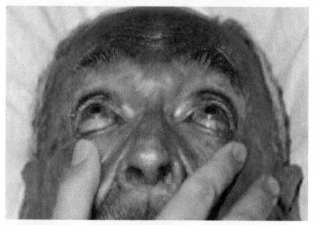

© 2008 Herbert L. Fred, Hendrik A. van Dijk. Textbook is licensed under CCY by 2.0

Less visually dramatic but potentially more serious risks include kidney disease and neurologic disorders. Taking silver orally can also interfere with the effectiveness of several medications, from antibiotics to thyroid hormone supplements.

Bottom Line

Colloidal silver has been abandoned as a medical treatment by mainstream medicine because there is no reason to believe it works and it is clear it has significant risks. There is no reliable clinical research evidence to justify using colloidal silver in humans or veterinary species.

CRANBERRY

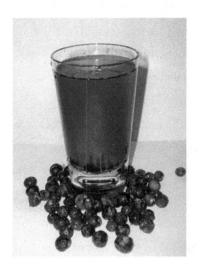

What Is It?

Like most herbal remedies, cranberry has traditionally been thought helpful for a wide variety of unrelated disorders, but it is now pretty firmly established in most people's minds as useful for urinary tract infections (UTIs). The question of whether cranberries, in some form, have value in treating or preventing UTIs is a pretty old one. There are scientific references on the subject going back to the 1960s.[75]

Unfortunately, as usual the subject is more complicated than is generally realized. The theoretical justification for using cranberry to treat UTIs used to be that it acidified urine and made it less hospitable for bacteria. However, that is no longer believed to be true. The more popular theory today is that chemicals in cranberry, called proanthocyanidins, interfere with the attachment of bacteria to the bladder wall, making it easier for the body to eliminate these bacteria and harder for infections to get started.[76]

As with all herbal remedies, of course, even if this turns out to be true, it isn't always a guarantee that the cranberry products you buy will actually work for you, or your pets. Limited regulation and poor quality control for herbal products means that even if there are specific compounds found to be useful in research studies, these may not be present in a sufficient amount or in a usable form in commercial products. Herbal medicine is very much a "buyer beware" market.[77–80]

Does It Work?

The current proposed mechanism is certainly plausible and supported by the results of *in vitro* studies. There are numerous systematic reviews of dozens of clinical studies in humans.[76,81–86] The conclusions of these reviews vary, some suggesting a possible benefit in reducing the occurrence of UTIs and others judging the evidence to be inconclusive. The different conclusions may be related to the variety of forms and doses of cranberry extract used in different studies, differences between the cause and characteristics of UTIs in different groups (children, adult women, people with underlying bladder or immune system diseases, etc.), and differences in data analysis methods.[76,81,84,87] Overall, the best we can say is that some cranberry supplements may help with prevention of UTIs in some people, but the evidence is far from strong and consistent.

As in humans, there is some preclinical research in dogs and cats which suggests cranberry supplements might be useful for prevention of UTIs in some cases.[88] However, as always there is far less research evidence on actual patients. The very few clinical studies that have been done so far are mixed and inconclusive (sorry, once again no cat clinical trials are available).[89,90]

In the face of suggestive preclinical research, inconclusive clinical studies in humans, and few clinical studies in dogs, the best we can say is that we cannot be certain, but there is not yet much reason to expect cranberry supplements are useful in preventing urinary tract infections in our pets.

Is It Safe?

No clear and significant safety concerns have been seen with those cranberry supplements or juices studied in clinical trials. There is some potential for large amounts of cranberry to upset the stomach, and there may be some increased risk of bladder stones in humans with long-term use, but overall the risks appear to be small.[91,92]

Bottom Line

There is some evidence that cranberry might be helpful in preventing urinary tract infections in humans but given that we've been trying to prove that for fifty years, the evidence is not impressive. The scant research so far in dogs is not more compelling.

CUPPING

What Is It?

Cupping is the practice of placing a glass or plastic container on the skin and creating a partial vacuum, with heat or a suction pump. Sometimes, the skin under the cups is cut or scarified (so-called "wet cupping") to induce bleeding. This leaves a visible bruise, which is often impressive, and is supposed to prevent or treat injury by increasing blood flow, expelling toxins, moving Qi, or any of a number of other purported mechanisms.[93] The treatment has roots in several folk medicine traditions, including Traditional Chinese Medicine, but modern alternative practitioners often employ it outside of these traditions.[94]

Cupping is pretty uncommon in animals, partly due to the difficulty of performing the procedure on animals with hair, and potentially because people report it can be quite uncomfortable and it is likely most dogs and cats would not tolerate it.

Does It Work?

There is no convincing evidence to support the various theoretical rationales for why cupping should be helpful in people. There are quite a few reviews of clinical trials in humans, but they are typically inconclusive because the clinical trial evidence is weak and rife with uncontrolled bias. Most reviews are in dedicated alternative medicine journals, and even such sympathetic sources usually acknowledge that the evidence is weak and inconsistent. Well-controlled studies typically find no objective benefits, but because of the subjective nature of pain and the difficulty in completely controlling for placebo effects, studies sometimes show improvements in discomfort reported by patients.[1,95–106]

There are no published clinical trials evaluating cupping in dogs and cats.

Is It Safe?

Serious injuries, including burns and infections, have been reported in humans due to cupping.[1,107–113]

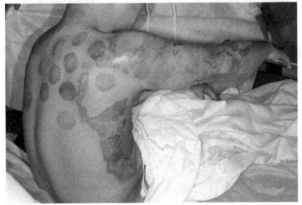

Image from Seifman MA, Alexander KS, Lo CH, et al. Cupping: the risk of burns. Med J Aust. 2017;206(11):500.[21]

Bottom Line

There is no reliable evidence that cupping has any benefits in dogs and cats, and it is painful and has significant risks, so it should not be used.

Brennen McKenzie

FISH OILS

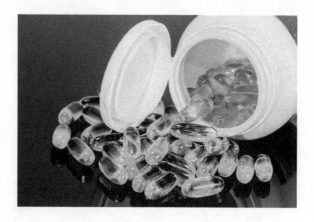

What Is It?

The main components of fish and other marine oils that are thought useful in medicine are two essential fatty acids, eicosapentaenoic acid (EPA) and docosahexaenoic acid (DHA). These are hypothesized to affect inflammation, fat metabolism, and numerous other physiologic activities in a wide variety of ways. The effects EPA and DHA have in the body, and the potential medical implications of these, are numerous and complex.

Almost as numerous are the medical problems in humans fish oils have been suggested to impact. Increasing one's intake of EPA and DHA, either through eating more fish or through the use of supplements, has been suggested to prevent or help treat cardiovascular disease, dementia and other mental health disorders, inflammatory bowel disease, arthritis, skin allergies, dry eye, and many others.[114–129] In dogs and cats, fish oil has been recommended for skin allergies, arthritis, age-related behavioral changes analogous to dementia in humans, and many other conditions.[130–147]

Does It Work?

There is extensive *in vitro*, lab animal, and other preclinical research, including many studies looking at the effects of EPA and DHA in various quantities and ratios on the health of humans, cats, and dogs. This literature demonstrates significant and complex biological effects, many of which have the potential to influence health in positive and negative ways.[17,27,148–154]

The clinical trial literature in humans is enormous, with hundreds of reviews evaluating several thousand clinical studies. Unfortunately, there is still significant uncertainty about the true effects of fish oil supplements on most health conditions. They are most widely used for the prevention of cardiovascular diseases, such as stroke and heart attacks, but this use is controversial, and some recent reviews suggest they provide no real benefit.[8,16] In any case, since these diseases are uncommon in dogs and cats, it's not clear how relevant this research is to the veterinary use of fish oil supplements.

There are, however, many other conditions in humans for which fish oils have been studied, from arthritis to asthma, from diabetes to dementia, from allergies to cancer. The evidence is complex and nearly always conflicting, with some studies showing benefits and others not.[1–15,155,156] This human research suggests there may be benefits to the use of fish oil in dogs and cats, but confidence in this can only come from appropriate studies in these species.

The clinical trial literature in dogs and cats is, of course, smaller and lower quality than in humans, but there are a fair number of studies and a few reviews that have been published.[17–26,157] Some of these employ fish oils in combination with other interventions, so it is sometimes difficult to know what exactly the fish oil aspect of the overall treatment contributes to the results seen.

More studies have evaluated fish oils for management of arthritis in dogs than any other use. All of these studies show effects by some measures but not by others, and all have methodological limitations, so the evidence suggests a possible benefit, but it is by no means consistent or conclusive.[17,21–26,34,41]

There are also several studies that show some benefits in dogs with allergic skin disease, usually in conjunction with other therapies rather than as a sole treatment.[17,33,34] A couple of trials suggest more unusual uses, such as reducing the rate of abnormal heart rhythms in boxers with a specific kind of heart disease,[158] but there is very little data on these topics. Most recommended uses for cats and dogs are based on anecdote or extrapolation from preclinical or human clinical studies.

Is It Safe?

In humans, the most common side effects of fish oil are mild gastrointestinal disturbances.[43] There is some theoretical concern for an increased risk of bleeding, but this doesn't seem to be a significant problem in real-world use.[159] The research in pets is very similar, with quite a few potential risks but little real harm other than nausea, diarrhea, and other gastrointestinal symptoms seen in clinical studies.[17,35,36,44]

Bottom Line

Probably has some small benefit for allergic skin disease and possibly arthritis. Most other uses in dogs and cats haven't been clearly established through clinical studies.

LYSINE

What Is It?

In medicine, there is something like a life cycle for medical treatments. The popular conception of this life cycle is the story of effective treatments. An insight or accident leads to a hypothesis, which is tested at various levels from *in vitro* to animal model to clinical use, and ultimately we validate the hypothesis and conquer the original problem.

Unfortunately, this is the exception rather than the rule. Far more often, the life cycle of medical therapies involves an insight or accident leading to a hypothesis which early, flawed evidence appears to support but which ultimately turns out to be wrong. This is a well-established phenomenon of the clinical trial literature, often called the Decline Effect or the Proteus Effect.[160,161]

Treatments based on such hypotheses are eventually abandoned in most cases, though some prove quite tenacious. Anecdote and personal experience frequently lend ineffective interventions a prolonged postmortem existence, therapeutic zombies that stagger on long after the scientific evidence should have put them to rest. A great example of the life cycle of an ineffective treatment is the use of L-lysine for the prevention and management of feline herpesvirus (FHV-1).

Brennen McKenzie

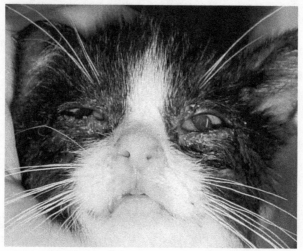

Cat with Herpesvirus URI 2005 by Kalumet under Creative Commons by SA 3.90

FHV-1 is a ubiquitous virus that causes upper respiratory symptoms (sneezing, runny nose and red runny eyes) in kittens. The majority of cats harbor the virus for life, and their immune systems keep it from causing trouble most of the time. Sometimes, during another illness or period of stress, or when a cat with latent FHV-1 (that is, with the virus being held in check by the immune system) is exposed to a cat actively shedding the virus, then the latent infection can break out of the control of the immune system and cause symptoms. In most cases, this resurgence is short-lived, and the immune system eventually gets the upper hand on its own. Lysine is a supplement intended to prevent such recurrences or make them go away faster.

Lysine is a common amino acid, a component of proteins, found in food. The theory behind how it could help cats with FHV-1 has to do with the idea that lysine could reduce the levels of another amino acid in the body, arginine, and that without enough arginine, a herpesvirus could not reproduce or cause illness.

388

Does It Work?

Early *in vitro* work on human herpesvirus (HHV-1) suggesting lysine might inhibit reproduction of the virus and could potentially have clinical benefits first appeared in the mid-1960s.[162] This was followed by the first clinical studies of lysine for HHV-1 about ten years later.[163] By the 1980s, the literature on lysine and HHV was glowing, and it seemed a safe and effective therapy had been found.[164]

Veterinary medicine caught the coattails of this process in the 1990s, with the first published *in vitro* study of lysine for FHV-1 appearing in 1995.[165] Clinical studies followed in the early 2000s, and lysine quickly became a widely available supplement used for FHV-1 management.[166]

However, the scientific process rolled on, and despite the enthusiasm of clinicians and researchers, cracks in the lysine narrative soon appeared. Limitations and potential sources of bias in the early literature were addressed in subsequent studies, and the apparent benefits melted away. The most recent reviews in human medicine have concluded that there is no reliable evidence to support the use of lysine for herpesvirus management, and it is not included in current treatment guidelines.[167,168,169] Lysine supplements are still available and marketed for this use, of course, because patients and some clinicians cling to their belief in the efficacy of this treatment despite the evidence, based predominantly on anecdotal experience.

The story has played out in a similar way in veterinary medicine, with the usual time lag. The initial theoretical rationale for use of lysine, for example, has not held up to subsequent study. Research in cats has failed to validate the basic theory of how lysine is supposed to work. Oral lysine does not appear to inhibit FHV-1 replication under normal physiologic conditions.[7]

A similar fate has befallen the initial claims for clinical effects of lysine in cats. Early studies, with small numbers of patients and methodological limitations, produced some positive results which could not be reproduced in larger, better-controlled research.[7]

The most recent comprehensive reviews of the evidence for lysine in FHV-1 patients are not encouraging.[7,170] The more optimistic of the two states that "there is considerable variability" in the research results and that while "data from these studies suggest that lysine...may reduce viral shedding in latently infected cats...the stress of...administration in shelter situations may well negate its effects and data do not support dietary supplementation."[11]

Another comprehensive systematic review of the subject is considerably more blunt, systematically rejecting every aspect of the rationale for lysine use: "Based on the complete lack of scientific evidence for the efficacy of lysine supplementation, we recommend an immediate stop of lysine supplementation for cats."[7]

The accumulation of evidence against the use of lysine for FHV-1 cases has had an impact. Some shelter medicine specialists, for example, now recommend against this practice.[171,172,173] However, there has also been resistance to abandoning this treatment despite the evidence. Unfortunately, such resistance has not been based so much on any substantive dispute about the science but instead on the seductive power of anecdotal evidence.

Is It Safe?

There is some limited evidence suggesting lysine could actually exacerbate FHV-1 symptoms, which would certainly make abandoning it the right choice.[7] Most studies, however, do not show any sign of undesirable effects, so it is probably harmless. However, wasting resources on treatment that has been through the scientific vetting process for over fifty years and has still failed to show convincing evidence of benefits really doesn't seem like an effective way to practice medicine

Bottom Line

Despite being widely used for many years, it seems very unlikely that lysine supplements have any benefits in cats with herpesvirus infections.

Brennen McKenzie

MUSIC THERAPY

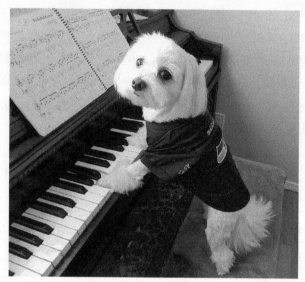

2015 by Ron Clausen under Creative Commons by SA 3.0

What Is It?

It has become quite popular to play music for dogs and cats in shelters or hospitals with the intent of reducing the inevitable stress and anxiety they are likely to experience in such environments. Given the profound effect music has on human emotions, it is reasonable to ask the question, could animals experience the same kind of emotional effects and could music help soothe them in times of stress? As a veterinarian, a musician (well, I play mandolin and guitar a bit), and a former primatologist working in environmental enrichment, I find this an intriguing idea.

However, I know from my own behavior research work and clinical veterinary practice that it is extremely difficult to consistently and objectively

392

define and measure stress in non-human animals. I also know that it is all too easy to assume that the world seems much the same to our animal companions as it seems to us, and that they share our likes and dislikes. Finally, I also know that nothing in medicine is free, and if music has meaningful benefits for our pets and patients, it likely has some risks as well (remember McKenzie's Law!).

Humans are unique in the extent to which they deliberately create patterns of sounds, often using tools made for that purpose, with the specific intent of inducing emotional responses in others of our species. Arguably, many species create music of a sort. Birds, humpback whales, and others can create quite complex and engaging sound patterns. I think it is fair to say that these differ in many ways from the type of music humans create and the purposes these sounds serve, so I also think it is a good idea to be cautious about assuming other animals will perceive or respond to human music as we do.

And as we all know, music is incredible in its variety, with dramatic differences in musical styles and tastes between cultures, generations, and individuals. What I find energizing or entertaining, my wife may find grating and annoying. So again, we should be careful in making confident generalizations about what other animals may like or dislike, or whether music will have the kinds of effects on them we anticipate.

Does It Work?

The short, most accurate answer is "We aren't sure." A wide variety of physiologic and behavioral responses to various types of musical stimuli have been observed, and they seem to vary not only from species to species but with the type of music and even with the particular study.[174-177] And while many of the results are consistent with the investigator's expectations, there are plenty of findings that were surprising. Music can have effects that might be beneficial or harmful or, in some cases, it might have no measurable effects at all. While some measures of stress and anxiety may seem to improve in some studies, other measures don't. And there is little consistency from one study to the next in the pattern of responses seen, suggesting that whatever effects playing music may have on dogs and cats, it is not predictable and reliable in different individuals or different settings.[1-3,178-182]

In general, "quieter" types of music, such as classical or "New Age" music, seem to reduce physiologic and behavioral responses associated with stress, and other genres either have no effect or may even worsen these measures. However, some studies looking at classical music find no effects, or effects for some composers and not others, and other studies find positive effects from other genres, or even white noise.[1-9] One study has even created music based on the acoustic features of cat vocalizations and seems to show cats prefer this to music written for humans.[6]

Apart from the variety in results of different studies, there are serious problems with the way the effects of music are measured and interpreted. Most of the studies in dogs, for example, contain few of the usual controls for bias and error so important in making scientific research results reliable. Subjects are often chosen and allocated to different groups by convenience rather than randomly, and the investigators observing and recording behaviors are rarely blinded to the music condition.

The lack of blinding and other controls complicates this research by making it impossible to rule out that we are seeing changes based on our own expectations more than our animals' behavior. If you think classical music is more likely to calm dogs than country music and you watch dogs and note their behavior while you and they listen to each kind of music, it is quite likely you will unconsciously interpret what you see and what you think it means through the filter of your own expectations. This is a variety of the caregiver placebo effect[183,184] I have discussed previously, in which we see what we hope and expect to see in our pets' responses to the things we do for them.

Is It Safe?

No evidence of serious harm has been seen in studies of music as a behavioral therapy for dogs and cats. Some studies have shown an increase in measures of stress and anxiety, however, which is as unpredictable as the apparent beneficial effects that have been seen. It is possible some animals may feel better when music is played for them, but there is always the chance some might actually feel worse.[1,2,4,5,9]

Bottom Line

Some studies suggest that playing quiet music may reduce signs of stress in dogs and cats, but the results are very inconsistent, and the studies are often flawed and difficult to interpret. There are probably no significant risks, but it is possible that music could actually increase anxiety in some animals.

NATUROPATHY

What Is It?

Naturopathy is a pleasant-sounding term for an approach to health and disease that is quite different from that of science-based medicine. It is an example of an alternative philosophy that has great appeal from a certain perspective but which, when examined closely, has little real substance. Naturopathy is an inconsistent conglomeration of treatments based on vague, vitalist philosophical principles and an extreme dedication to the Appeal to Nature fallacy.[185]

According to the American Council of Animal Naturopathy (ACAN), "The philosophy of naturopathy has been in existence since the beginning of time," and "The definition of naturopathy is a philosophy and system of following the laws of health that God mandated in nature to keep the body balanced."[186] According to more skeptical sources, it took shape in Europe in the late nineteenth century and grew in popularity with the counterculture and New Age movements of the 1960s and 1980s.[1,187,188] ACAN defines naturopathy as "A philosophy and system of prevention of disease first and then treatment of disease that avoids drugs and surgery and emphasizes the use of nature or natural agents such as exercise, water, herbs, etc. to assist the body in bringing its self back into balance and health."[2]

The Six Principles of Naturopathy listed by ACAN,[2] identical to those espoused by human naturopathic organizations such as the American Association of Naturopathic Physicians (AANP),[189] describe the philosophy in more detail. Some key points are:

- The body has the inherent ability to heal itself.

- This healing process is intelligent and ordered.

- Every illness has a cause. Causes may occur on the physical, mental or emotional level.

- Symptoms are expressions of the body's attempt to heal but are not the cause of illness.

- Animal Naturopaths use nature's methods that minimize the risk of harmful side effects. Methods designed to suppress symptoms but not remove the underlying cause are usually harmful, their use is always avoided. [By which they mean most scientific medical therapies.]

- All aspects of that animal (physical, mental and emotional) are taken into account.

- Illness is due to improper diet, habits, exposure to toxins and general lifestyle.

The assumptions upon which naturopathy is based are dubious. As I've discussed several times, the distinction between "natural" and "unnatural," and the suggestion that the former is equivalent to "healthy" and the latter to "unhealthy," is an appealing but ultimately empty idea. Even if we could distinguish wholly "natural" from wholly "artificial" medical treatments, there is no reason to believe one would be inherently safer or more effective than the other.

Because the philosophical basis for naturopathy is so vague and ill-defined, the actual practice of naturopaths encompasses almost any form of alternative therapy. Among the practitioners listed on the ACAN website as Certified Animal Naturopaths are practitioners of homeopathy, Traditional

Chinese Veterinary Medicine, and several other therapies that are question-able or completely lacking in any validity. Whatever a particular practitioner chooses to define as "natural" is apparently acceptable within a naturopathic approach apart from vaccines, pharmaceutical medicine, and many other conventional therapies.

It is important to point out that the "board certification" in naturopathy offered by ACAN and other such groups is not recognized by the various official organizations which regulate veterinary medical specialties. It is equivalent to similar certifications for homeopaths,[190] psychics,[191] and as-trologers[192] in that it is invented by naturopaths to legitimize themselves and is not recognized by mainstream veterinary medicine. In fact, there is no requirement that those who take the various certification courses the ACAN offers be veterinarians, so "certified naturopaths" may not even be trained healthcare professionals.

Does It Work?

Answering this question is challenging because of the vague and inconsistent definitions for naturopathy. I have written elsewhere in this book about in-dividual treatments naturopaths often use, such as homeopathy, TCVM, herbal medicine, massage, and others. Many of these are unproven or clearly ineffective. Others, like herbal remedies, probiotics, and some dietary sup-plements may have some benefit. Categorizing them all as "natural" tells us nothing about which are helpful and which aren't.

Interestingly, some of the recommendations naturopaths give, espe-cially for humans, are identical to those given by conventional doctors. No one disagrees with the idea that clean, healthy food is essential for life,

398

though what exactly this means may be open to dispute. Similarly, clean fresh air and water, appropriate exercise, and a positive attitude are undoubtedly good for everyone, though they may not be the key to perfect health or immortality. The fact is that much of what naturopaths recommend may be perfectly reasonable, or even supported by good scientific evidence despite the fact that they are recommending it regardless of the evidence and based on a philosophy largely incompatible with science.

Like many alternative medicine proponents, naturopaths are happy to cite scientific research when it supports their beliefs and claims, but they are likely to dismiss any which does not. Several studies have found that the bulk of the diagnoses and treatment recommendations made by naturopaths are not supported by reliable scientific evidence.[4,193,194] In addition, naturopathy is difficult to study in a controlled manner due to the inconsistency and variation in practices employed, so there is relatively little research on the general approach. A recent attempt at a systematic review of human naturopathy found twelve studies that met the inclusion criteria, and while they appeared to show some benefits, they all had significant weaknesses and limitations that made it impossible to draw reliable conclusions.[195] There also appears to be absolutely no controlled clinical research on naturopathy in veterinary species.

That leaves only the inevitable testimonials as evidence, which you now understand prove nothing.

Is It Safe?

Again, it is difficult to comment on the safety of naturopathy as a general approach because it is so ill-defined and specific therapies are not consistent between practitioners. I have discussed the risks of particular practices, such as homeopathy, herbal medicine, TCVM, and other alternative therapies employed by naturopaths elsewhere. The biggest risk of the philosophy itself is that it often involves counseling people against seeking and using conventional medical diagnostics and treatments. Naturopaths are frequently opposed to vaccination,[196–201] for example, which is a position that clearly places people and animals at unnecessary risk of illness and death from preventable diseases. Naturopathy, like any other prescientific and unproven medical practice, is not a safe or reliable substitute for scientific medical care, and eschewing conventional care in favor of naturopathy risks losing the opportunity to receive effective therapy in a timely way.

Naturopaths often present themselves as appropriate substitutes for primary care doctors, for humans and animals, despite the fact that many of them lack of any real scientific or medical training. Even in those instances when the therapy they recommend is reasonable (such as diet and exercise advice) or harmless in itself (such as homeopathy), these individuals are not qualified to detect and respond to serious health problems.

Bottom Line

Lots of theoretical nonsense and a wide variety of specific treatments that range from reasonable to worthless. Overall, naturopaths are not a reliable source of healthcare information, and they do harm in discouraging science-based medical treatment.

NEUTERING

Along with vaccination, neutering is one of the first and most common medical treatments we apply to our pets. Like all such treatments, there are risks and benefits, and the balance between these has to be evaluated in light of the best available scientific evidence and the specific, unique circumstances and characteristics of our individual pets. Neutering practices have changed over time, as both cultural views and the available scientific evidence have changed. Neutering is also approached very differently in different countries, based primarily on societal attitudes and values. As always, decisions about if, when, and how to neuter your pet require you to understand the evidence for potential risks and benefits as well as the uncertainty about these, and to integrate this evidence with your personal values in communication with your veterinarian. My purpose here is not to tell you what the right decision is but to give you information to help you make a thoughtful, informed decision for yourself.

What Is It?

Neutering is the removal of the main source of the sex hormones, androgens for males and estrogens for females. This is usually accomplished by surgically removing the testes in males and the ovaries in females, though various other techniques can also reduce or eliminate the effects of these hormones. Lots of different terms are used for these procedures, with "spaying" most commonly used for females and "castration" for males, but neutering refers to any procedure which removes most of the sex hormones in an individual.

The primary purpose for neutering a dog or cat is to prevent reproduction. One of the primary reasons neutering become commonplace in many countries in the twentieth century was a recognition that it could help reduce the number of stray and unwanted dogs and cats that had to be put to death by animal control authorities, as well as the public health risks stray animals can present for humans.[202–206]

There are also many potential effects of neutering on the health and behavior of individual dogs and cats.[207,208] Some of these benefit the animal, such as the reduction in the risk of diseases such as mammary cancer or uterine infections in neutered females. Others benefit owners, such as the reduced tendency for neutered male dogs to roam and fight and the reduced odor and indiscriminate spraying of urine in neutered male cats. With such potential benefits, of course, come some possible risks, from the neutering procedures themselves and from biological changes caused by the removal of sex hormones.

The short- and long-term effects of neutering have been intensively studied. They are many and incredibly complex, and the exact effect on any individual pet is nearly impossible to predict. Neutering practices are often changing based on changes in how people view their animal companions and in how scientists understand the potential effects of neutering. Comprehensive reviews of the risks and benefits of neutering are long and filled with uncertainty, and they must be updated often as the evidence grows. No universal or lasting recommendation for all animals is possible. My goal here is to give you a brief overview of the issues as we currently understand them, as well as to highlight the significant uncertainty we must accept. I hope this will help you appreciate that there is no single, simple "right answer" on this subject and the decisions you make must simply be the best decisions possible for your pet given your goals and the most up-to-date, yet inevitably imperfect, scientific knowledge on the subject.

I have included a couple of tables in this section which summarize some of the effects of neutering in males and females. These look complicated, but they are actually a simpler way to give a general sense of the evidence than discussing each condition and the effects of neutering in detail. I have listed conditions thought to be associated with neutering, how common these are, how serious they are, and what effect neutering might have on each condition. Again, this is not an exhaustive or eternal list, but it should give you some useful information about some of the more important conditions neutering might affect and the ways in which neutering can benefit or harm dogs and cats. Much more detail about these topics can be found in the articles listed in the references for this section.

Benefits of Neutering

I have altered the usual questions here to consider benefits and risks rather than effectiveness and safety because I believe this structure works better for understanding this complex subject. I have written a couple of scientific reviews on this subject, and they tend to be as long as some entire chapters in this book. You probably won't need that level of detail in making decisions about neutering your pets (though if you do or you are just interested, you can find much more information in some of the references).

Apart from benefits to the population as a whole, neutering can have specific benefits for individual dogs and cats. There is some evidence, for example, that neutered animals live longer than intact animals, though it is not completely clear why this is or even if it is a direct effect of neutering.[7,209] The risks associated with reproduction are also obviously eliminated if we neuter our pets. Infections, some serious metabolic diseases, and serious injury are potential risks of reproduction, especially for females. The risk of some diseases not specifically associated with reproduction is also lower in neutered animals. These differ significantly for males and females, so I will list them separately.

Females

Two of the most common and most serious diseases that occur in intact females are cancer of the mammary glands (breast cancer, as it is called in humans) and pyometra, a severe infection of the uterus. Both of these conditions are very common, and both can be difficult to treat and potentially fatal. Pyometra can be completely prevented by removal of the ovaries, and this is much easier and safer in healthy dogs and cats than removing an infected uterus in a female who has this condition.[7,210] It is almost certainly true that neutering prevents mammary cancer in females, though the direct evidence for this is not entirely without limitations.[211,212]

Some other diseases prevented by neutering include cancers of the ovaries and other parts of the reproductive system, however these are not nearly as common as breast cancer.[7] This is an important distinction since the potential effect of neutering, for good or ill, on a specific condition matters more if that condition is common and serious than if it is rare or mild. If neutering, for example, dramatically reduces the risk of a serious and common disease like breast cancer, it may still be the right choice for a female dog even if it turns out to increase the risk for other cancers which are rare or for non-cancerous diseases that are easily treated. This sort of consideration of not only what effect neutering has on particular diseases but the overall balance of risks and benefits is complicated and challenging, but it leads to much better decisions that simplistic assessments based on looking only at some of the effects of neutering and ignoring the relative frequency and seriousness of the various conditions it can influence.

Neutering also reduces the behaviors associated with estrus or "heat" cycles in female dogs and cats. While it is unclear how this impacts the well-being of the animals themselves, such behaviors are often very disturbing for owners. This is more than an issue of human convenience since unacceptable behaviors are the most common reason people abandon or relinquish their pets, so this can obviously have a negative impact on the welfare of these animals.[213,214,215] Neutered female dogs and cats are considered more acceptable as pets by most people.

Males

The benefits of neutering in males are less dramatic than in females. Behavioral benefits are often the most obvious for owners. Intact male cats are often challenging to keep as pets due to aggression and urine spraying, though many cat breeders manage these animals perfectly well.[216,217,218] Similarly, intact male dogs tend to be more aggressive towards other dogs, which complicates taking them out in public. They are also more likely than neutered males to roam and chase after females in heat, which can increase their chances of being hit by cars and running into other hazards.[15, 219-225]

The specific diseases that are reduced by neutering in males are typically less common and serious than breast cancer and pyometra in females. Non-cancerous disease of the prostate is effectively eliminated by neutering, though this can often be effectively managed with medication or by neutering in those dogs in which it occurs.[226,227,228] Overall, it is not clear that there are significant individual health benefits from neutering in male dogs and cats.

Risks of Neutering

The most obvious potential risk of neutering is the risk associated with the surgery and anesthesia required for the procedure. However, in practice these are very common procedures that have extremely low rates of serious complications.[5,229–233]

As you will see in the tables, there are plenty of diseases that *may* be more common in neutered animals than in intact pets. However, assessment of this is extremely challenging, and though there are many studies, they all have significant limitations and often conflict with one another. Breed, age, the timing of neutering, and many other factors also influence disease risk, so it is almost never appropriate to say that neutering is the cause of a particular disease, only that it may be one of several risk factors.

An example of a health risk that is clearly greater in neutered animals is obesity.[7,234] The removal of sex hormones alters appetite and eating behavior in ways that predisposes neutered animals to eat more and gain weight. Being overweight, in turn, is an important factor in many diseases, from diabetes, to arthritis, to cancer. However, neutering is only one factor in the development of this problem. Another factor that we, as pet owners, have total control over in most cases is how much we feed our pets. Neutered pets can be maintained at a healthy weight just as easily as intact animals if we simply feed them appropriately.

A much more complicated issue is whether neutering increases the risk for cancer. There are many studies showing differences in the occurrence of particular cancers in intact and neutered dogs (as always, there is far less evidence for cats). However, the results are wildly inconsistent. In one study,[235] for example, the risk of mast cell tumors was greater in female golden retrievers neutered at less than six months of age or more than one year of age than in intact females. However, there was no difference in risk for male golden retrievers, and there was no effect on the risk of this cancer for males or females of the closely related Labrador retriever breed.

In another study, the risk of a different cancer, lymphosarcoma, seemed to increase with neutering in females but decrease with neutering in males.[236] Several other studies looking at the same cancer, however, have found different results.[34,35,237,238]

Deciding what significance, if any, this kind of evidence has on your decision to neuter your pet is very difficult. If your pet is the same age and breed as the dogs in a particular study, then the results of that study might seem a reasonable guide to the potential risk or benefit of neutering. However, an apparent increased risk of one kind of rare cancer in female golden retrievers who are neutered tells you little or nothing about the risk of a different cancer in a different breed neutered at a different age, or even about the risk in male golden retrievers!

The best I can say about the overall evidence regarding neutering and cancer is that the procedure *might* increase the risk of some cancers in some breeds of dog, but that is still a very tenuous conclusion. We have to be very cautious about how we use this kind of information. It is perfectly reasonable to look at the existing data and consider delaying neutering your female golden retriever until after she is a year old since a few studies suggest that may help diminish the effect of neutering on the risk of some cancers that this breed gets more often than other breeds. However, it is not reasonable to look at these studies and decide your female golden, or your male border collie for that matter, is better off not neutered at all because of the cancer risk. The evidence isn't nearly strong enough to make confident generalizations.

Bottom Line

Overall, like everything else we do in medicine, neutering has both risks and benefits. The balance between these is unusually complex and difficult to determine, so universal, one-size-fits-all rules about neutering simply aren't appropriate. And there are arguments for and against neutering besides the health effects. At this point, my own interpretation is that male dogs are likely to be equally healthy overall whether neutered or not, though there is some slim case to be made for waiting until they are fully grown to neuter them if they are a large breed. Female dogs are almost certainly going to be better off if neutered in terms of overall health, though again some case can be tentatively made that large breed females might benefit from waiting to neuter after full growth.

It is critical, though, to recognize that these general guidelines are not strict rules and are based on weak and contradictory evidence. My assessment would have been different five years ago, and it might be different in the future as more evidence develops. There is no single right answer here and claiming there is ignores the nuances and complexity of the issue.

It is equally critical to remember that we are talking about small differences in risk for most conditions, not dramatic differences. With a few exceptions (such as pyometra and mammary cancer), most of the diseases influenced by neutering are also influenced much more so by genetics and other factors. Just as there is no clear right answer, there is no devastatingly wrong answer, and pet owners shouldn't feel as if they made the wrong decision if their pet develops a health problem that might or might not be affected to some degree by neutering. The precise balance of risks and benefits is unknowable for each individual, and reasonable arguments can be made for a variety of decisions.

Table 1: Effects of Neutering on Females

Condition	How Common?	How Serious?	Effect of Spaying	Species	Comments
Unwanted litters	Very Common	Very	Prevents	dog, cat	significant pet overpopulation and associated euthanasia
Risks of reproduction	Uncommon	Variable	Prevents	dog, cat	dystocia, brucellosis, diabetes, others; risk of dystocia can be high for certain breeds
Mammary neoplasia	Very Common	Very	Probably ↓	dog, cat	generally poor prognosis
Pyometra	Very Common	Very	Prevents	dog, cat	
Uterine neoplasia	Rare	Variable	Prevents	dog, cat	some benign/removable, some malignant
Ovarian neoplasia	Uncommon	Variable	Prevents	dog, cat	

Vaginal/Vulvar neoplasia	Uncommon	Moderate	↓ Dramatically	dog	
Osteosarcoma	Uncommon	Very	Possibly ↑	dog	risk variable by breed
Hemangiosarcoma	Uncommon	Very	Probably ↑	dog	risk variable by breed
Lymphosarcoma	Uncommon	Very	Possibly ↑	dog	risk variable by breed
Mast Cell Neoplasia	Common	Moderate	Probably ↑	dog	risk variable by breed, often curable
Transitional cell carcinoma	Uncommon	Very	↑	dog	risk variable by breed
Cruciate ligament disease	Common	Moderate	↑	dog	risk variable by breed, surgically treatable
Hip dysplasia	Common	Moderate	Probably ↑	dog	risk variable by breed
Aggressive behavior	Common	Very	Possibly ↑	dog, cat	
Urinary incontinence	Very Common	Mild	Possibly ↑	dog	medically controllable in 65-75% of cases
Urinary tract infection	Common	Mild	Possibly ↑	dog	easily treatable
Hypothyroidism	Uncommon	Moderate	Possibly ↑	dog	easily treatable
Diabetes mellitus	Uncommon	Very	Possibly ↑	dog, cat	risk variable by breed
Acute pancreatitis	Uncommon	Very	Possibly ↑	dog	
Obesity	Common	Very	↑	dog, cat	easily prevented by calorie restriction
Longevity	--	--	Possibly ↑	dog, cat	neutering influences causes of death

↓=decreases/reduces, ↑=increase/exacerbates

Table 2: Effects of Neutering on Males

Condition	How Common?	How Serious?	Effect of Castration	Species	Comments
Unwanted litters	Very Common	Very	Prevents	dog, cat	significant pet overpopulation population and associated euthanasia
Testicular neoplasia	Uncommon	Moderate	Prevents	dog	most benign and surgically removable
Prostate disease	Very Common	Variable	↓ dramatically	dog	some have few symptoms others have severe, chronic disease
Behavior problems	Common	Variable	Variable	dog, cat	conflicting studies; most report less aggression, roaming, urine marking
Perineal hernias	Uncommon	Moderate	↓	dog	can often be repaired surgically
Perianal fistulas	Uncommon	Moderate	↓	dog	incidence varies by breed, some respond well to treatment others are serious chronic problem
Prostatic neoplasia	Uncommon	Very	Probably ↑	dog	poor prognosis
Osteosarcoma	Uncommon	Very	Possibly ↑	dog	risk variable by breed
Hemangiosarcoma	Uncommon	Very	Probably no effect	dog	risk variable by breed
Lymphosarcoma	Uncommon	Very	Unclear	dog	risk variable by breed
Mast Cell Neoplasia	Common	Moderate	Probably no effect	dog	risk variable by breed, often curable
Cruciate Ligament Disease	Common	Moderate	↑	dog	risk variable by breed, surgically treatable

411

Hip dysplasia	Common	Moderate	Probably ↑	dog	risk variable by breed, common in a few breeds
Femoral physeal fracture	Uncommon	Moderate	Possibly ↑	cat	obesity may be confounding factor
Hypothyroidism	Uncommon	Moderate	Possibly ↑	dog	easily treatable
Diabetes mellitus	Uncommon	Very	Possibly ↑	dog, cat	risk variable by breed
Acute pancreatitis	Uncommon	Very	Possibly ↑	dog	
Obesity	Common	Very	↑	dog, cat	easily prevented by calorie restriction
Longevity	--	--	Possibly ↑	dog, cat	neutering influences causes of death

↓=*decreases/reduces,* ↑=*increase/exacerbates*

ORTHOMOLECULAR MEDICINE

What Is It?

One of the most impressive-sounding labels for an unproven therapy is Orthomolecular Medicine. The origin of the term, coined by Nobel laureate Linus Pauling, gives it added gravitas. As it turns out, though, it's mostly just a fancy way of claiming that there are medical benefits to giving high doses of vitamins above and beyond the ordinary, and quite small amounts necessary for normal health.

Proponents of this concept argue that many diseases are due to undetected vitamin or mineral deficiencies, usually attributed to the unspecified evils of modern life or industrial agriculture. They also seem to follow the philosophy that if a little is good, more is better, arguing that extremely high doses of essential micronutrients can treat or prevent illness.[239]

Practitioners of orthomolecular medicine do, however, employ a variety of tests and treatment methods, and there is little consistency to the field beyond the use of high doses of vitamins. Many will employ unproven diagnostic tests, such as hair analysis or blood tests not proven to have any relevance to health. Many will also use a variety of supplements besides vitamins, as well as using other CAM treatments. Like much of CAM, it seems that orthomolecular medicine often means whatever any individual practitioner chooses for it to mean.

As I discussed in the chapter on dietary supplements, it is culturally difficult to argue against the benefits of vitamins, or to suggest they might cause harm. The memory of a time in which people in Western societies were routinely deficient in micronutrients, and when supplementation provided seemingly miraculous benefits, is still accessible. And there are still places in the world in which the poor not only do not have our nutrient-excess health problems but in which vitamin deficiencies are still common, and supplementation can be beneficial. Recent surveys suggest vitamins are seen as generally benign even by doctors, who often knowingly use them as placebo therapies.[240]

Does It Work?

The grand claims made in the 1970s by Pauling and others about the benefits of megadoses of vitamins have had a long time to prove themselves, and they have so far failed to do so. While there are certainly studies showing benefits to targeted vitamin supplementation, the general principles, unconventional diagnostic tests, and specific claims for megadoses of vitamins as preventatives or cures for disease are mostly unproven or simply untrue.[241–246]

In veterinary medicine, as usual, there is little research evidence. There are some case reports and papers from the 1970s that are long on theorizing and short on hard data. These are balanced by a number of *in vitro* and animal model studies showing the implausibility or potential dangers of megadoses of vitamins, as well as clinical trials in humans which have so far failed to demonstrate consistent, meaningful benefits.[1,3–7,247–250] Despite claims by some CAM veterinarians about the value of high doses of vitamins, there are no clinical trials showing that the principles or practices of orthomolecular medicine have any benefits in dogs and cats.

Is It Safe?

There is ample and growing evidence in humans, as well as in lab animals, that high doses of vitamins can have significant health risks, from increasing the risk of cancer and other diseases to increased mortality.[1,9,11,251–260] The specific risk varies with the particular vitamin, with fat soluble vitamins such as Vitamin A and D being the easiest to overdose, but even water-soluble vitamins such as the B vitamins, which we used to believe could be given in high doses without risk because any excess would simply be excreted, have turned out to have potential dangers in people.[261] In the absence of compelling evidence for health benefits, the high doses of these substances recommended under the label of orthomolecular medicine should be avoided.

Bottom Line

Unlikely to be any significant benefits and some serious possible risks.

PHEROMONES

What Is It?

Pheromones are chemical compounds produced by an animal which have predictable physiologic and behavioral effects on other animals of the same species.[262] They are a form of social signaling that can influence behavior related to reproduction, aggression, feeding, social coordination, and many other areas.[1] The chemical nature and effects of specific pheromones have been well characterized in some species, particularly insects.[263] In other species, such as humans, there is great debate about whether pheromones exist or, if they do, how significant their effects may be.[264]

In small animal veterinary medicine, there has been considerable interest over the last couple of decades in the therapeutic use of pheromones.[265,266,267] Several companies have produced products based on purported dog and cat pheromones and marketed to address various behavioral problems, including various forms of fear and anxiety, aggression, stress-related illness, and undesirable urine marking or destructive behaviors.

Does It Work?

Given the marketing and widespread use of pheromone products, it might be assumed that there is a robust evidence base for the plausibility and clinical benefits of these products. However, as is often the case in veterinary medicine, the market is well ahead of the science, and there is surprisingly little data characterizing the composition, physiologic and behavioral effects, and clinical benefits of dog and cat pheromone products.

The exact composition of most cat and dog pheromones, and the composition of the synthetic versions used in commercial products, are very difficult to determine from published sources. There is virtually no published peer-reviewed research characterizing the discovery, composition, variability, and physiologic effects of dog and cat pheromones.[268-272] The general principle that mammalian pheromones can affect behavior is well supported by basic science. However, the claims made for the composition and actions of specific dog and cat pheromones do not have a robust preclinical research literature to support them.

There is a moderate amount of published clinical research evidence concerning dog and cat pheromone products. A systematic review of clinical studies prior to 2010 has been conducted.[273] After eliminating studies that did not meet minimum quality criteria, the authors analyzed seven studies in dogs and seven in cats involving pheromone products (Adaptil for dogs and Feliway for cats) and various behavioral problems. None of the cat studies provided convincing evidence of a benefit, and only one study in dogs found some benefit in reducing anxiety in puppies during training.[12]

Since this review was published, several additional clinical studies of pheromone products in dogs and cats have appeared. Each has its own strengths and limitations. Negative findings outnumber positive ones. Most evaluate numerous variables and find that only a few differ between treated animals and the control group. Strong, consistent evidence of clinically significant benefits has not been found, though some small positive effects are sometimes seen for some variables. [274-278]

Is It Safe?

No evidence of any significant harm has been seen in any of the studies of dog and cat pheromones, so the risk of using them is very low.

Bottom Line

There are reasons to think pheromones could be useful, but their value has not been consistently demonstrated in clinical studies.

PROLOTHERAPY

What Is It?

Prolotherapy is a treatment for joint, connective tissue, and other musculo-skeletal pain and dysfunction pain. The practice consists of injecting various substances into painful or dysfunctional joints and connective tissue. There is a wide range of substances that are used with much variation among practitioners of prolotherapy. Examples of these substances include dextrose or other sugars, vitamin B12, local anesthetic agents, a wide variety of herbal products, homeopathic remedies, zinc sulfate, the patient's own blood, and hundreds of others. Often, cocktails of multiple substances are used based on the individual preferences of the practitioner.

The theoretical rationale for the practice is that the substances injected into damaged joints or connective tissue will cause inflammation and chemical or cellular activity that will lead to repair of the affected tissues. There are also theoretical explanations involving the stimulation of cells involved in healing, such as fibroblasts, or the release of growth factors and other substances that are associated with tissue repair, which might plausibly explain how prolotherapy could be beneficial. The precise mechanisms are not well understood for any of the proposed theories, but these range from plausible and science based to highly implausible.[279,280,281]

Does It Work?

The evidence for the theoretical rationales behind prolotherapy varies, but the principle that substances which induce inflammation and those which stimulate tissue proliferation directly may reduce clinical symptoms does have some support in preclinical research.

There have been many clinical trials in humans, most involving arthritis of various joints and a few investigating prolotherapy for other conditions. Systematic reviews of these studies are mixed, but there is a growing consensus that some types of prolotherapy, such as injecting dextrose (a sugar) into arthritic joints likely do have real symptomatic benefits for people. Evidence for other uses of prolotherapy is still inconclusive.[2,3,282–289]

One small but high-quality clinical trial of dextrose prolotherapy for elbow and knee arthritis has been performed in dogs.[290] The dogs receiving the placebo treatment did as well or better on all measures of response, so this trial did not suggest any benefit from prolotherapy for dogs with this condition. There are no published studies in cats. All strong claims for the effectiveness of prolotherapy in pets rely entirely on theoretical arguments, extrapolation from research in humans, and anecdote.[291]

Is It Safe?

In the human research, the only commonly reported side effects are local pain, inflammation, and bleeding. Infections can happen with any joint injection, but these are uncommon if proper technique is used. Serious injuries have rarely been reported in people, often involving the injection of substances not widely used for this therapy.[2-11] The limited studies in dogs have reported no significant safety concerns.

Bottom Line

There are some possible benefits for arthritis but no direct evidence yet in dogs and cats. There is also some small chance of serious risks.

PULSED ELECTROMAGNETIC FIELD THERAPY (PEMF)

What Is It?

PEMF is the application of electrical fields, and the magnetic fields they create, to the tissues of patients with the purpose of treating various health conditions. Typically, an antenna of some type is placed over the skin of patients and an electrical current is passed through it to generate electric and magnetic fields in the tissues below the skin. There is tremendous variety in the specific nature of PEMF treatment based on technical variables, such as the size, shape, and position of the antennae used, the strength of the current employed, the frequency and wavelength of the electromagnetic energy applied to the patient, the timing and duration of treatment, and many others.

This means that it is not easy to extrapolate results from one study to the use of devices that may function very differently.

In general, the theoretical principles underlying PEMF are plausible and based on well-established basic science. Claims made for specific devices vary from soundly science based to mystical and pseudoscientific, but the general idea that such devices could have medical benefits is a reasonable one.

Does It Work?

Given the variety of specific PEMF devices and treatment protocols, as well as the differences between species and conditions for which PEMF is used, this is not a simple question to answer. There is *in vitro* and lab animal research indicating significant biologic effects from PEMF on cells and tissues.[292-295] Electromagnetic fields can cause some cells to grow faster and others to self-destruct. It can influence gene expression, the production of signaling molecules, and the release of inflammatory mediators. This research also provides support for some potential clinical uses, particularly involved in the healing of fractured bones and soft tissue wounds, and possibly in the treatment of some cancers. Such research cannot reliably predict the effects on real-world patients, but it is consistent and strong enough to justify focused clinical studies of specific treatment protocols in particular conditions.

There are quite a few such clinical trials in humans. Reviews of these trials are not always consistent in their conclusions, and this may have to do with the variation in PEMF treatment practices used in the clinical trials that are evaluated. There is some evidence to support the use of PEMF in improving the healing of broken bones, though not all reviews agree that the results are strong enough to be conclusive.[293,296,297] Similarly, there is clinical trial evidence in humans suggesting PEMF can reduce pain from arthritis and can improve wound healing, but again not all reviews agree the evidence is conclusive.[298–302]

A recent narrative review of veterinary uses for PEMF highlights the supporting evidence but largely ignores negative studies or systematic reviews which consider the evidence inconclusive.[295] The authors appear to be convinced of the value of PEMF (indeed, two of the three are consultants for a company manufacturing a PEMF device), which illustrates how narrative reviews can be shaped by the existing beliefs of the authors and are less explicitly objective than systematic reviews.

In terms of clinical trial research, very little has yet been done in veterinary species. A few small, low-quality studies suggest benefits for post-surgical pain, arthritis, and for prostate disease in dogs. One study in horses found no benefit for back pain. A recently published trial in dogs having surgery for ruptured disks in the spine and severe neurologic disease found no effect greater than placebo in the main outcome measures evaluated. An unpublished study in dogs with the same condition, however, reports beneficial effects on pain and wound healing. This limited and inconsistent research does not yet allow a definitive judgement on whether or not PEMF is a useful clinical therapy for dogs and cats. Unfortunately, this has not stopped the therapy from being widely adopted by veterinarians and pet owners.[303–309]

Is It Safe?

The extensive research done so far on lab animals and humans has found very little indication of any short-term harm to PEMF treatment. There is not enough evidence to determine if there are any potential long-term risks.[302]

Bottom Line

Some possible benefits, though evidence is still uncertain, and little risk. Should not be substituted for established therapies.

REIKI

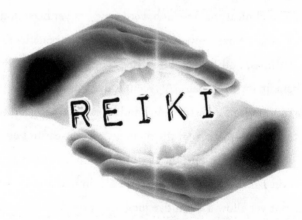

2016 by queeselreiki under Creative Commons by SA 4.0

What Is It?

Reiki is a form of "energy medicine," a disparate collection of therapies based on the idea that health and disease are determined, wholly or in part, by nonphysical or spiritual energies that cannot be scientifically detected or studied but that can be sensed intuitively and manipulated by believers to affect health. There are many other forms of faith healing or energy medicine which differ in the theoretical explanations for their actions and in the degree of connection to particular religious traditions, including various styles of Christian faith healing, healing touch, therapeutic touch, Qigong, Tellington Touch, and others.

Many forms of alternative medicine claim some or all of their effects to be due to manipulation of spiritual or energetic forces (vitalism), and there are not always clear distinctions between different varieties, but Reiki and several others are characterized by an emphasis on using touch or hand movements to channel and manipulate energy for healing purposes.

Reiki was invented (or discovered, depending on your point of view) by a Japanese monk named Mikao Usui in the early twentieth century. Supposedly, he had been looking for a long time for a form of spiritual healing and had a vision during a long period of solitary meditation and fasting that led to his development of Reiki. Subsequent Reiki Masters have modified and developed the technique and spread it to other countries.[310,311,312]

Does It Work?

Like all vitalist treatments, the underlying principles of Reiki cannot be scientifically studied and must be taken on faith. The notion that nonphysical forces which cannot be seen or scientifically studied can nevertheless be intuitively sensed and manipulated with significant impact on physical diseases is scientifically implausible.

Despite the inherent difficulty in studying a therapy based on undetectable forces, many clinical trials have been conducted on Reiki, and on other types of energy medicine. Most are methodologically flawed and subject to placebo effects and other forms of bias and error. No convincing research evidence has emerged that Reiki, therapeutic touch, or other similar practices have any objective or significant impact on physical disease in humans or in veterinary species.[313-318] Several studies have suggested that despite claims to the contrary, practitioners cannot reliably sense the presence of a patient or their "energy" when effectively blinded, which begs the question of how they can be channeling this mysterious force intentionally if they cannot detect it.[319]

As I discussed when talking about massage therapy, however, studies do suggest that the attention and human contact associated with Reiki and similar therapies is comforting to many human patients and can lead to improvement in subjective symptoms or the patients' experience of their illness and their medical care. There is reason to believe that many domestic animals, including dogs and cats, may also experience comfort and positive physiologic responses to human contact, so Reiki may induce these responses regardless of the existence of any putative spiritual forces.[320-327] This may have some mild clinical benefits, but it is unlikely to significantly affect the outcome of serious illness.

Is It Safe?

No direct harm has been seen in studies of Reiki. The major risk of Reiki and other forms of energy healing is the delay or rejection of appropriate diagnosis and effective treatment that may occur if people mistakenly believe these therapies offer real hope of improving their pets' condition.

Bottom Line

Complete nonsense.

YUNNAN BAIYAO

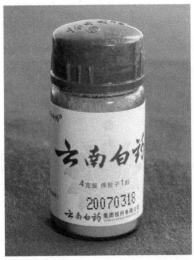

Yunnan Baiyao 2007 by Yongxinge under Creative Commons by SA 3.0

What Is It?

I don't intend to cover many specific herbal remedies since there are thousands, and most do not have sufficient research evidence to say much about them. However, Yunnan Baiyao is one of the most widely used, even by vets not otherwise interested in alternative therapies, so I think it is worth talking a bit about.

There are many issues owners and veterinarians should consider before using herbal remedies for pets, and Yunnan Baiyao (YB) illustrates several of these. It is a Chinese Medicine remedy sometimes recommended for patients with hemorrhage or cancer (though some sources list dozens of unrelated medical applications).[328,22]

The precise ingredients in YB are proprietary. Several lists of possible constituents have appeared online, but these are inconsistent, and there is no standardization or accurate disclosure of how much of each ingredient is present. This makes any rigorous evaluation of efficacy and safety nearly impossible, and it raises serious ethical questions about a company selling, and veterinarians recommending, a product with undisclosed ingredients. Many of the proponents of herbal medicine, who recommend YB regularly, would be horrified at the idea of the rest of us using a drug from a pharmaceutical company if that company refused to say exactly what it contained or how it was made and had not done any research to show it was safe or effective, so YB illustrates the double standard associated with the evaluation of scientific and alternative treatments.

Since the chemical composition of plants vary with many factors, herbal remedies often have different compositions with every batch, which can affect both safety and efficacy. It is well documented that herbal products can be contaminated with undisclosed toxins and even pharmaceuticals.[15–20] Batches of YB, for example, have been found to contain lead, and some sources report that it contains progesterone.[21] Serious injury and death in humans have been linked to such adulteration of herbal remedies.[23]

Voluntary industry self-regulation has been proposed to mitigate these concerns.[24] However, such self-regulation is not an approach most of us would consider acceptable for pharmaceutical medicines, and the rationale for lower standards for herbal remedies is unclear.

Does It Work?

In the case of Yunnan Baiyao, as for many herbal remedies, rationales and proposed mechanisms vary from highly implausible to moderately plausible. Many proponents of this remedy use the system of Traditional Chinese Medicine (TCM) to guide selection and use of YB and other Chinese herbal products. As I discussed in detail in Chapter 6, this is a prescientific set of philosophical concepts and folk beliefs involving balancing vital humors and spiritual forces to prevent and treat disease. Herbal remedies are chosen according to supposed relationships between the taste or physical appearance of plants or other ingredients and these humors or energies.[329]

As an example, in this model, one of the plant constituents of YB, *Panax notoginseng*, is judged sweet and slightly bitter in taste and so should "Transform Stasis, Resolve Stagnation, Tonify Qi, Invigorate Blood, and Clear Heat."[328] Such unscientific folk medicine practices do not provide a plausible or rational basis for herbal prescribing.

There are also more scientific proposed rationales for the claimed effects of YB. Preclinical studies of some of the ingredients indicate a variety of biological effects *in vitro* and in animal models. Some of these effects might support the purported pro-coagulant activity,[330–333] but other studies do not show such effects.[334–339,27] Overall, the *in vitro* and lab animal studies are varied and conflicting, and the body of evidence does not provide a clear plausible rationale for the many, often incompatible, clinical effects claimed.[340–350]

A recent systematic review of studies done in humans involving YB found some evidence of possible beneficial effects but also found that 1) most of the published research was of low quality and high risk of bias, 2) for some conditions the apparent effect disappears when lower quality studies are excluded, and 3) there is evidence of publication bias, in which negative studies remain unpublished, creating an inaccurate impression of the true state of the evidence. Overall, the authors stated that the variation in how studies have been done and the concern that negative evidence is being suppressed "preclude certain conclusions."[351]

There have been some veterinary studies of YB, both in lab animals and in actual clinical patients. Table 3 summarizes these studies and indicates the extent to which they did or did not use key controls for bias such as randomization (assigning subjects to the test treatment or another treatment, such as a placebo, by chance), blinding (making sure the folks evaluating the effect don't know which group is getting which treatment, so they cannot intentionally or unconsciously bias the results), and the use of a control group (a group getting a placebo or something other than the YB being studied).

Table 3. In vivo studies of Yunnan Baiyao in veterinary species

Study	N=	Rand	Blind	Con-trols	Effect	Comments
Ogle, 1976[5]	54 (rats) 10 rabbits	N	N	Y	Y	YB reduced subjective bleeding time in cut rat livers and *in vitro* clotting time of rabbit blood more than saline or starch (applied topically

						or mixed w/ blood)
Ogle, 1977[6]	? (Rats) ? (Rabbits)	N	N	Y	Y	YB reduced subjective bleeding time in cut rat livers and *in vitro* clotting time of rabbit blood more than starch solution (given by orogastric tube)
Graham, 2002[7]	6 (ponies)	?	?	Y	Mixed	TBT-yes ACT-no 247 vs 318 seconds in TBT (oral use)
Epp, 2005[9]	5 (horses)	Y	Y	Y	No	Many lab measures and clinical EIPH evaluated (oral use)
Fan, 2005[8]	17 (rats)	Y	Y	Y	Y	Bleeding time cut tail tips 10.53-16.81min wheat flour vs 7.1-14.13min YB (topical use)
Murphy, 2017[352]	67 (dogs)	N	N	Y	No	Retrospective, YB +/- aminocaproic acid with right atrial hemangiosarcoma, no difference in symptoms or survival (oral use)
Lee, 2017[10]	8 (dogs)	Y	Y	Y	No	No change in lab measures of clotting (oral use)
Frederick, 2017[11]	8 (dogs)	Y	Y	Y	No	No change in BMBT or lab measures of clotting (oral use)

MacRae, 2017[12]	6 (dogs)	N	N	N	No	No effect on lab measures of clotting (oral use)
Adelman, 2017[13]	19 (dogs)	Y	Y	Y	Mixed	Bleeding time after Bx (300+/- 12 sec YB: 367+/- 9 sec placebo) BMBT - no difference TEG (lab measure of clotting) - no difference Total blood loss - no difference
Ness, 2017[14]	12 (horses)	Y	Y	Y	No	No effect on any *in vitro* measure of hemostasis

Of these eleven studies, six found no effect at all, and two others showed mixed results. Of the three positive studies, two did not report any of the key methods for limiting bias and other errors. Several of the studies did not find any effect on measures of blood clotting, which undermines the basic plausibility for the product.

Is It Safe?

While no serious adverse events have been reported for YB, no study has specifically evaluated safety, and the inconsistency in composition and usage for YB makes it difficult to ascertain what risks it may present. Any drug which encourages blood to clot could reduce bleeding, but it could also increase the risk of strokes and other harm caused by excessive blood clotting, and proponents for YB have never explained how it is supposed to only have the desired effect without any risk or undesirable effects.

YB is often used in animals with active bleeding from incurable cancers. The rationale for this is the usual idea that even if it doesn't work, it can't

430

hurt. As I will discuss in the next chapter, using the example of the Gonzalez Protocol for people with terminal cancer, it is actually possible to make life worse even for patients who will die soon no matter what we do. And grasping at straws makes it harder for us, as pet owners, to find a necessary acceptance of the impending loss of a beloved companion.

Bottom Line

Yunnan Baiyao seems very unlikely to have significant benefits in light of the mostly negative research evidence, and it is unclear if it is safe.

CONCLUSIONS

There are an almost uncountable number of other alternative therapies I could have included in this chapter. With the number of new and resurrected CAM practices appearing all the time, reviewing them all is an impossible task. In this chapter, I have tried to demonstrate the application of the principles and techniques of science-based medicine to those therapies I discuss, both to generate a resource for considering these treatments and also as an illustration of the approach I have tried to teach throughout this book. As a dedicated pet owner or veterinary professional, you can use the same approach to evaluate any therapy you might consider using in your animal companions or your patients.

In the next chapter, I will review the basic principles underlying science-based pet care and provide some final examples and strategies to help you make the best possible decisions about the treatment of the animals in your care.

Brennen McKenzie

Science . . . warns me to be careful how I adopt a view which jumps with my preconceptions, and to require stronger evidence for such belief than for one to which I was previously hostile. My business is to teach my aspirations to conform themselves to fact, not to try and make facts harmonize with my aspirations.

- Thomas Huxley

Placebos for Pets?

[1] Shermer M. Psychic drift. Why most scientists do not believe in ESP and psi phenomena. *Sci Am*. 2003;288(2):31.

[2] Hines T. *Pseudoscience and the Paranormal*. Prometheus Books. Amherst, NY; 2003..

[3] Kurtz P. *A Skeptic's Handbook of Parapsychology*. Prometheus Books. Amherst, NY; 1985.

[4] Wiseman R. 'Heads I Win, Tails You Lose': How Parapsychologists Nullify Null Results - CSI. *Skept Inq*. January 2010..

[5] Hyman R. Psi experiments: Do the best parapsychological experiments justify the claims for psi? *Experientia*. 1988;44(4):315-322. doi:10.1007/BF01961269

[6] Stollznow K. The Ballad of Jed (and the Pet Psychic). *Skept Inq*. March 2009.

[7] Vigan M. Essential oils: renewal of interest and toxicity. *Eur J Dermatol*. 20(6):685-692. doi:10.1684/ejd.2010.1066

[8] Herz RS. Aromatherapy facts and fictions: A scientific analysis of olfactory effects on mood, physiology and behavior. *Int J Neurosci*. 2009;119(2):263-290. doi:10.1080/00207450802333953

[9] Gattefossé R-M, Tisserand R, Davies L. *Gattefossé's Aromatherapy*. C.W. Daniel. New York, NY; 1993..

[10] Freires I, Denny C, Benso B, de Alencar S, Rosalen P. Antibacterial activity of essential oils and their isolated constituents against cariogenic bacteria: A systematic review. *Molecules*. 2015;20(4):7329-7358. doi:10.3390/molecules20047329

[11] de Sousa D, Hocayen P, Andrade L, Andreatini R. A systematic review of the anxiolytic-like effects of essential oils in animal models. *Molecules*. 2015;20(10):18620-18660. doi:10.3390/molecules201018620

[12] Tsang HWH, Ho TYC. A systematic review on the anxiolytic effects of aromatherapy on rodents under experimentally induced anxiety models. *Rev Neurosci*. 2010;21(2):141-152.

[13] Forrester LT, Maayan N, Orrell M, Spector AE, Buchan LD, Soares-Weiser K. Aromatherapy for dementia. *Cochrane Database Syst Rev*. February 2014. doi:10.1002/14651858.CD003150.pub2

[14] Hines S, Steels E, Chang A, Gibbons K. Aromatherapy for treatment of postoperative nausea and vomiting. *Cochrane Database Syst Rev*. March 2018. doi:10.1002/14651858.CD007598.pub3

[15] Cooke B, Ernst E. Aromatherapy: a systematic review. *Br J Gen Pract*. 2000;50(455):493-496.

[16] Smith CA, Collins CT, Crowther CA. Aromatherapy for pain management in labour. *Cochrane Database Syst Rev*. 2011;(7):CD009215. doi:10.1002/14651858.CD009215

[17] Stoeken JE, Paraskevas S, van der Weijden GA. The long-term effect of a mouthrinse containing essential oils on dental plaque and gingivitis: A systematic review. *J Periodontol*. 2007;78(7):1218-1228. doi:10.1902/jop.2007.060269

[18] Van Leeuwen M, Slot D, Van der Weijden G. The effect of an essential-oils mouthrinse as compared to a vehicle solution on plaque and gingival inflammation: A systematic review and meta-analysis. *Int J Dent Hyg*. 2014;12(3):160-167. doi:10.1111/idh.12069

[19] Lee Y-L, Wu Y, Tsang HWH, Leung AY, Cheung WM. A Systematic review on the anxiolytic effects of aromatherapy in people with anxiety symptoms. *J Altern Complement Med*. 2011;17(2):101-108. doi:10.1089/acm.2009.0277

[20] Perrucci S, Mancianti F, Cioni P, Flamini G, Morelli I, Macchioni G. *In vitro* antifungal activity of essential oils against some isolates of *Microsporum canis* and *Microsporum gypseum*. *Planta Med*. 1994;60(02):184-186. doi:10.1055/s-2006-959448

[21] Ebani V, Nardoni S, Bertelloni F, Najar B, Pistelli L, Mancianti F. Antibacterial and antifungal activity of essential oils against pathogens responsible for otitis externa in dogs and cats. *Medicines*. 2017;4(2):21. doi:10.3390/medicines4020021

[22] Bond R, Lloyd DH. A double-blind comparison of olive oil and a combination of evening primrose oil and fish oil in the management of canine atopy. *Vet Rec*. 1992;131(24):558-560.

[23] Low SB, Peak RM, Smithson CW, Perrone J, Gaddis B, Kontogiorgos E. Evaluation of a topical gel containing a novel combination of essential oils and antioxidants for reducing oral malodor in dogs. *Am J Vet Res*. 2014;75(7):653-657. doi:10.2460/ajvr.75.7.653

[24] Blaskovic M, Rosenkrantz W, Neuber A, Sauter-Louis C, Mueller RS. The effect of a spot-on formulation containing polyunsaturated fatty acids and essential oils on dogs with atopic dermatitis. *Vet J*. 2014;199(1):39-43. doi:10.1016/j.tvjl.2013.10.024

[25] Goodwin S, Reynolds H. Can aromatherapy be used to reduce anxiety in hospitalised felines. *Vet Nurse*. 2018;9(3):167.

[26] Komiya M, Sugiyama A, Tanabe K, Uchino T, Takeuchi T. Evaluation of the effect of topical application of lavender oil on autonomic nerve activity in dogs. *Am J Vet Res*. 2009;70(6):764-769. doi:10.2460/ajvr.70.6.764

[27] Wells DL. Aromatherapy for travel-induced excitement in dogs. *J Am Vet Med Assoc*. 2006;229(6):964-967. doi:10.2460/javma.229.6.964

[28] ELLSE L, WALL R. The use of essential oils in veterinary ectoparasite control: a review. *Med Vet Entomol*. 2014;28(3):233-243. doi:10.1111/mve.12033

[29] Nardoni S, Mugnaini L, Pistelli L, et al. Clinical and mycological evaluation of an herbal antifungal formulation in canine Malassezia dermatitis. *J Mycol Med*. 2014;24(3):234-240. doi:10.1016/j.mycmed.2014.02.005

[30] Nardoni S, Costanzo AG, Mugnaini L, et al. Open-field study comparing an essential oil-based shampoo with miconazole/chlorhexidine for haircoat disinfection in cats with spontaneous microsporiasis. *J Feline Med Surg*. 2017;19(6):697-701. doi:10.1177/1098612X15625709

[31] Graham L, Wells DL, Hepper PG. The influence of olfactory stimulation on the behaviour of dogs housed in a rescue shelter. *Appl Anim Behav Sci.* 2005;91(1-2):143-153. doi:10.1016/j.applanim.2004.08.024

[32] Posadzki P, Alotaibi A, Ernst E. Adverse effects of aromatherapy: a systematic review of case reports and case series. *Int J Risk Saf Med.* 2012;24(3):147-161. doi:10.3233/JRS-2012-0568

[33] Marshall J. Essential Oils and Dogs. Pet Poison Helpline. Available at: https://www.petpoisonhelpline.com/pet-safety-tips/essential-oils-dogs/ Accessed June 26, 2019.

[34] Benson K. Essential Oils and Cats. Pet Poison Helpline. Available at: https://www.petpoisonhelpline.com/blog/essential-oils-cats/ Accessed June 26, 2019.

[35] Genovese AG, McLean MK, Khan SA. Adverse reactions from essential oil-containing natural flea products exempted from Environmental Protection Agency regulations in dogs and cats. *J Vet Emerg Crit Care.* 2012;22(4):470-475. doi:10.1111/j.1476-4431.2012.00780.x

[36] Khan SA, McLean MK, Slater MR. Concentrated tea tree oil toxicosis in dogs and cats: 443 cases (2002–2012). *J Am Vet Med Assoc.* 2014;244(1):95-99. doi:10.2460/javma.244.1.95

[37] Villar D, Knight MJ, Hansen SR, Buck WB. Toxicity of melaleuca oil and related essential oils applied topically on dogs and cats. *Vet Hum Toxicol.* 1994;36(2):139-142.

[38] Pryor B. Therapeutic laser in veterinary medicine. *Vet Clin North Am Small Anim Pract.* 2015;45(1):45-56. doi:10.1016/J.CVSM.2014.09.003

[39] Food and Drug Administration (FDA). *Performance Standards for Light-Emitting Products.* 21CFR1040.10; 2018. Available at: https://www.accessdata.fda.gov/scripts/cdrh/cfdocs/cfcfr/CFRSearch.cfm?fr=1040.10&SearchTerm=laser. Accessed December 29, 2018.

[40] Petermann U. Die lokale Lasertherapie in der Veterinärmedizin. *Zeitschrift für Ganzheitliche Tiermedizin.* 2016;30(04):113-122. doi:10.1055/s-0042-117301

[41] Downing R. Laser therapy in veterinary medicine. *Innov Vet Care.* February 2017. doi:10.1002/lsm.22212

[42] Petermann U. Pulse laser as ATP-generator: the use of low level laser-therapy in alleviating Qi-shortcomings. *Zeitschrift für Ganzheitliche Tiermedizin.* 2012;26(1):8-14.

[43] Bashardoust Tajali S, Macdermid JC, Houghton P, Grewal R. Effects of low power laser irradiation on bone healing in animals: a meta-analysis. *J Orthop Surg Res.* 2010;5:1. doi:10.1186/1749-799X-5-1

[44] Lucas C, Criens-Poublon LJ, Cockrell CT, de Haan RJ. Wound healing in cell studies and animal model experiments by Low Level Laser Therapy; were clinical studies justified? A systematic review. *Lasers Med Sci.* 2002;17(2):110-134.

[45] Gál P, Stausholm MB, Kováč I, et al. Should open excisions and sutured incisions be treated differently? A review and meta-analysis of animal wound models following low-level laser therapy. *Lasers Med Sci.* 2018;33(6):1351-1362. doi:10.1007/s10103-018-2496-7

[46] Singh M, Bhargava M, Sahi A, Jawre S. Efficacy of low level LASER therapy on wound healing in dogs. *Indian J Vet Surg.* 2011;32(2):103-106.

[47] Cole GL, Lux CN, Schumacher JP, et al. Effect of laser treatment on first-intention incisional wound healing in ball pythons (*Python regius*). *Am J Vet Res.* 2015;76(10):904-912. doi:10.2460/ajvr.76.10.904

[48] In de Braekt MM, van Alphen FA, Kuijpers-Jagtman AM, Maltha JC. Effect of low level laser therapy on wound healing after palatal surgery in beagle dogs. *Lasers Surg Med.* 1991;11(5):462-470.

[49] Kurach LM, Stanley BJ, Gazzola KM, et al. The effect of low-level laser therapy on the healing of open wounds in dogs. *Vet Surg.* 2015;44(8):988-996. doi:10.1111/vsu.12407

[50] Petersen SL, Botes C, Olivier A, Guthrie AJ. The effect of low level laser therapy (LLLT) on wound healing in horses. *Equine Vet J.* 1999;31(3):228-231.

[51] Bharti B, Pandey S, Garg UK, Shukla BP. Low level laser therapy for the healing of contaminated wounds in dogs: histopathological changes. *Indian J Vet Surg.* 2013;34(1):57-58.

[52] Olivieri L, Cavina D, Radicchi G, Miragliotta V, Abramo F. Efficacy of low-level laser therapy on hair regrowth in dogs with noninflammatory alopecia: a pilot study. *Vet Dermatol.* 2015;26(1):35-e11. doi:10.1111/vde.12170

[53] Stich AN, Rosenkrantz WS, Griffin CE. Clinical efficacy of low-level laser therapy on localized canine atopic dermatitis severity score and localized pruritic visual analog score in pedal pruritus due to canine atopic dermatitis. *Vet Dermatol.* 2014;25(5):464-e74. doi:10.1111/vde.12144

[54] Wyszyńska J, Bal-Bocheńska M. efficacy of high-intensity laser therapy in treating knee osteoarthritis: A first systematic review. *Photomed Laser Surg.* 2018;36(7):343-353. doi:10.1089/pho.2017.4425

[55] Rayegani SM, Raeissadat SA, Heidari S, Moradi-Joo M. Safety and effectiveness of low-level laser therapy in patients with knee osteoarthritis: A systematic review and meta-analysis. *J lasers Med Sci.* 2017;8(Suppl 1):S12-S19. doi:10.15171/jlms.2017.s3

[56] Huang Z, Chen J, Ma J, Shen B, Pei F, Kraus VB. Effectiveness of low-level laser therapy in patients with knee osteoarthritis: a systematic review and meta-analysis. *Osteoarthr Cartil.* 2015;23(9):1437-1444. doi:10.1016/j.joca.2015.04.005

[57] Draper WE, Schubert TA, Clemmons RM, Miles SA. Low-level laser therapy reduces time to ambulation in dogs after hemilaminectomy: a preliminary study. *J Small Anim Pract.* 2012;53(8):465-469. doi:10.1111/j.1748-5827.2012.01242.x

[58] Williams C, Barone. Is low level laser therapy an effective adjunctive treatment to hemilaminectomy in dogs with acute onset parapleglia secondary to intervertebral disc disease?. In: *Profeedings of the 2010 Americam College of Veterinary Internal Medicine Forum*. Denver, CO.

[59] Bennaim M, Porato M, Jarleton A, et al. Preliminary evaluation of the effects of photobiomodulation therapy and physical rehabilitation on early postoperative recovery of dogs undergoing hemilaminectomy for treatment of thoracolumbar intervertebral disk disease. *Am J Vet Res*. 2017;78(2):195-206. doi:10.2460/ajvr.78.2.195

[60] Rogatko C, Baltzer W, Tennant R. Preoperative low level laser therapy in dogs undergoing tibial plateau levelling osteotomy: A blinded, prospective, randomized clinical trial. *Vet Comp Orthop Traumatol*. 2017;30(01):46-53. doi:10.3415/VCOT-15-12-0198

[61] Renwick SM, Renwick AI, Brodbelt DC, Ferguson J, Abreu H. Influence of class IV laser therapy on the outcomes of tibial plateau leveling osteotomy in dogs. *Vet Surg*. 2018;47(4):507-515. doi:10.1111/vsu.12794

[62] Kennedy KC, Martinez SA, Martinez SE, Tucker RL, Davies NM. Effects of low-level laser therapy on bone healing and signs of pain in dogs following tibial plateau leveling osteotomy. *Am J Vet Res*. 2018;79(8):893-904. doi:10.2460/ajvr.79.8.893

[63] Rayegani SM, Raeissadat SA, Heidari S, Moradi-Joo M. Safety and effectiveness of low-level laser therapy in patients with knee osteoarthritis: A systematic review and meta-analysis. *J lasers Med Sci*. 2017;8(Suppl 1):S12-S19. doi:10.15171/jlms.2017.s3

[64] Tran PL, Huynh E, Hamood AN, et al. The ability of a colloidal silver gel wound dressing to kill bacteria *in vitro* and *in vivo*. *J Wound Care*. 2017;26(sup4):S16-S24. doi:10.12968/jowc.2017.26.Sup4.S16

[65] Richter K, Facal P, Thomas N, et al. Taking the silver bullet: Colloidal silver particles for the topical treatment of biofilm-related infections. *ACS Appl Mater Interfaces*. 2017;9(26):21631-21638. doi:10.1021/acsami.7b03672

[66] Fung MC, Bowen DL. Silver products for medical indications: risk-benefit assessment. *J Toxicol Clin Toxicol*. 1996;34(1):119-126.

[67] Lansdown ABG. Silver in health care: Antimicrobial effects and safety in use. *Biofunctional Text Ski*. 2006;33:17-34. doi:10.1159/000093928

[68] Scott JR, Krishnan R, Rotenberg BW, Sowerby LJ. The effectiveness of topical colloidal silver in recalcitrant chronic rhinosinusitis: a randomized crossover control trial. *J Otolaryngol - Head Neck Surg*. 2017;46(1):64. doi:10.1186/s40463-017-0241-z

[69] National Center for Complementary and Integrative Health (NCCIH). Colloidal Silver. NCCIH Pub No. D209. Available at: https://nccih.nih.gov/health/colloidalsilver. Published 2017. Accessed December 29, 2018.

[70] Bogdanchikova N, Muñoz RV, Saquero AH, et al. Silver nanoparticles composition for treatment of distemper in dogs. *Int J Nanotechnol.* 2016;13(1/2/3):227. doi:10.1504/IJNT.2016.074536

[71] Food and Drug Administration (FDA). *Drug Products Containing Colloidal Silver Ingredients or Silver Salts Offered Over-the-Counter (OTC) for the Treatment and/or Prevention of Disease.*; 2028. Available at: https://www.accessdata.fda.gov/scripts/cdrh/cfdocs/cfcfr/CFRSearch.cfm?fr=310.548. Accessed December 29, 2018.

[72] Wadhera A, Fung M. Systemic argyria associated with ingestion of colloidal silver. *Dermatol Online J.* 2005;11(1):12.

[73] Hadrup N, Lam HR. Oral toxicity of silver ions, silver nanoparticles and colloidal silver – A review. *Regul Toxicol Pharmacol.* 2014;68(1):1-7. doi:10.1016/j.yrtph.2013.11.002

[74] Sterling JP. Silver-resistance, allergy, and blue skin: Truth or urban legend? *Burns.* 2014;40:S19-S23. doi:10.1016/j.burns.2014.10.007

[75] MOEN D V. Observations on the effectiveness of cranberry juice in urinary infections. *Wis Med J.* 1962;61:282-283.

[76] Wang C-H, Fang C-C, Chen N-C, et al. Cranberry-Containing Products for Prevention of Urinary Tract Infections in Susceptible Populations. *Arch Intern Med.* 2012;172(13):988-996. doi:10.1001/archinternmed.2012.3004

[77] Blacksell L, Byard RW, Musgrave IF. Forensic problems with the composition and content of herbal medicines. *J Forensic Leg Med.* 2014;23:19-21. doi:10.1016/J.JFLM.2014.01.008

[78] Byard RW, Musgrave I, Maker G, Bunce M. What risks do herbal products pose to the Australian community? *Med J Aust.* 2017;206(2):86-90.

[79] Kosalec I, Cvek J, Tomić S. Contaminants of Medicinal Herbs and Herbal Products. *Arch Ind Hyg Toxicol.* 2009;60(4):485-501. doi:10.2478/10004-1254-60-2009-2005

[80] de Carvalho LM, Moreira AP, Martini M, Falcão T. The illegal use of synthetic pharmaceuticals in herbal formulations: An overview of adulteration practices and analytical investigations. *Forensic Sci Rev.* 2011;23(2):73-89.

[81] Vasileiou I, Katsargyris A, Theocharis S, Giaginis C. Current clinical status on the preventive effects of cranberry consumption against urinary tract infections. *Nutr Res.* 2013;33(8):595-607. doi:10.1016/j.nutres.2013.05.018

[82] Micali S, Isgro G, Bianchi G, Miceli N, Calapai G, Navarra M. Cranberry and recurrent cystitis: More than marketing? *Crit Rev Food Sci Nutr.* 2014;54(8):1063-1075. doi:10.1080/10408398.2011.625574

[83] Ghouri F, Hollywood A, Ryan K. A systematic review of non-antibiotic measures for the prevention of urinary tract infections in pregnancy. *BMC Pregnancy Childbirth.* 2018;18(1):99. doi:10.1186/s12884-018-1732-2

[84] Luís Â, Domingues F, Pereira L. Can cranberries contribute to reduce the incidence of urinary tract infections? A systematic review with meta-analysis and trial sequential analysis of clinical trials. *J Urol*. 2017;198(3):614-621. doi:10.1016/j.juro.2017.03.078

[85] Jepson RG, Williams G, Craig JC. Cranberries for preventing urinary tract infections. *Cochrane Database Syst Rev*. 2012;10:CD001321. doi:10.1002/14651858.CD001321.pub5

[86] Fu Z, Liska D, Talan D, Chung M. Cranberry reduces the risk of urinary tract infection recurrence in otherwise healthy women: A systematic review and meta-Analysis. *J Nutr*. 2017;147(12):2282-2288. doi:10.3945/jn.117.254961

[87] Liska DJ, Kern HJ, Maki KC. Cranberries and urinary tract infections: How can the same evidence lead to conflicting advice? *Adv Nutr*. 2016;7(3):498-506. doi:10.3945/an.115.011197

[88] Howell A. The science behind cranberry for urinary tract health. In: *Small Animal and Exotics. Proceedings of the North American Veterinary Conference*. Gainesville, FL; 2010:824-827.

[89] Olby NJ, Vaden SL, Williams K, et al. Effect of cranberry extract on the frequency of bacteriuria in dogs with acute thoracolumbar disk herniation: A randomized controlled clinical trial. *J Vet Intern Med*. 2017;31(1):60-68. doi:10.1111/jvim.14613

[90] Chou H-I, Chen K-S, Wang H-C, Lee W-M. Effects of cranberry extract on prevention of urinary tract infection in dogs and on adhesion of *Escherichia coli* to Madin-Darby canine kidney cells. *Am J Vet Res*. 2016;77(4):421-427. doi:10.2460/ajvr.77.4.421

[91] National Center for Complementary and Integrative Health (NCCIH). Cranberry. NCCIH Publication No. D291. Available at: https://nccih.nih.gov/health/cranberry. Published 2016. Accessed December 29, 2018.

[92] Guay DRP. Cranberry and Urinary Tract Infections. *Drugs*. 2009;69(7):775-807. doi:10.2165/00003495-200969070-00002

[93] Al-Bedah AMN, Elsubai IS, Qureshi NA, et al. The medical perspective of cupping therapy: Effects and mechanisms of action. *J Tradit Complement Med*. April 2018. doi:10.1016/J.JTCME.2018.03.003

[94] Qureshi NA, Ali GI, Abushanab TS, et al. History of cupping (Hijama): a narrative review of literature. *J Integr Med*. 2017;15(3):172-181. doi:10.1016/S2095-4964(17)60339-X

[95] Wang Y-T, Qi Y, Tang F-Y, et al. The effect of cupping therapy for low back pain: A meta-analysis based on existing randomized controlled trials. *J Back Musculoskelet Rehabil*. 2017;30(6):1187-1195. doi:10.3233/BMR-169736

[96] Al Bedah AMN, Khalil MKM, Posadzki P, et al. Evaluation of wet cupping therapy: Systematic review of randomized clinical trials. *J Altern Complement Med*. 2016;22(10):768-777. doi:10.1089/acm.2016.0193

[97] Zhang Y-J, Cao H-J, Li X-L, et al. Cupping therapy versus acupuncture for pain-related conditions: A systematic review of randomized controlled trials and trial sequential analysis. *Chin Med*. 2017;12(1):21. doi:10.1186/s13020-017-0142-0

[98] Li J-Q, Guo W, Sun Z-G, et al. Cupping therapy for treating knee osteoarthritis: The evidence from systematic review and meta-analysis. *Complement Ther Clin Pract*. 2017;28:152-160. doi:10.1016/j.ctcp.2017.06.003

[99] Cao H, Zhu C, Liu J. Wet cupping therapy for treatment of herpes zoster: a systematic review of randomized controlled trials. *Altern Ther Health Med*. 16(6):48-54.

[100] Lee MS, Choi T-Y, Shin B-C, Han C, Ernst E. Cupping for stroke rehabilitation: A systematic review. *J Neurol Sci*. 2010;294(1-2):70-73. doi:10.1016/j.jns.2010.03.033

[101] Lu S, Du S, Fish A, Tang C, Lou Q, Zhang X. Wet cupping for hypertension: A systematic review and meta-analysis. *Clin Exp Hypertens*. September 2018:1-7. doi:10.1080/10641963.2018.1510939

[102] Kim S, Lee S-H, Kim M-R, et al. Is cupping therapy effective in patients with neck pain? A systematic review and meta-analysis. *BMJ Open*. 2018;8(11):e021070. doi:10.1136/bmjopen-2017-021070

[103] Ma S, Wang Y, Xu J, Zheng L. Cupping therapy for treating ankylosing spondylitis: The evidence from systematic review and meta-analysis. *Complement Ther Clin Pract*. 2018;32:187-194. doi:10.1016/j.ctcp.2018.07.001

[104] Kim J-I, Lee MS, Lee D-H, Boddy K, Ernst E. Cupping for treating pain: A systematic review. *Evidence-Based Complement Altern Med*. 2011;2011:1-7. doi:10.1093/ecam/nep035

[105] Bridgett R, Klose P, Duffield R, Mydock S, Lauche R. Effects of cupping therapy in amateur and professional athletes: Systematic review of randomized controlled trials. *J Altern Complement Med*. 2018;24(3):208-219. doi:10.1089/acm.2017.0191

[106] Cao H, Li X, Liu J. An updated review of the efficacy of cupping therapy. Malaga G, ed. *PLoS One*. 2012;7(2):e31793. doi:10.1371/journal.pone.0031793

[107] Lee J-H, Cho J-H, Jo D-J. Cervical epidural abscess after cupping and acupuncture. *Complement Ther Med*. 2012;20(4):228-231. doi:10.1016/j.ctim.2012.02.009

[108] Rehman A, Ul-Ain Baloch N, Awais M. Practice of cupping (Hijama) and the risk of bloodborne infections. *Am J Infect Control*. 2014;42(10):1139. doi:10.1016/j.ajic.2014.06.031

[109] Lee SY, Sin JI, Yoo HK, Kim TS, Sung KY. Cutaneous *Mycobacterium massiliense* infection associated with cupping therapy. *Clin Exp Dermatol*. 2014;39(8):904-907. doi:10.1111/ced.12431

[110] Iblher N, Stark B. Cupping treatment and associated burn risk: A plastic surgeon's perspective. *J Burn Care Res*. 2007;28(2):355-358. doi:10.1097/BCR.0B013E318031A267

[111] Kulahci Y, Sever C, Sahin C, Evinc R. Burn caused by cupping therapy. *J Burn Care Res*. 2011;32(2):e31. doi:10.1097/BCR.0b013e31820ab104

[112] Jing-Chun Z, Jia-Ao Y, Chun-Jing X, Kai S, Lai-Jin L. Burns induced by cupping therapy in a burn center in northeast china. *Wounds a Compend Clin Res Pract*. 2014;26(7):214-220.

[113] Seifman MA, Alexander KS, Lo CH, Cleland H. Cupping: the risk of burns. *Med J Aust*. 2017;206(11):500.

[114] Gerber M. Omega-3 fatty acids and cancers: A systematic update review of epidemiological studies. *Br J Nutr*. 2012;107(S2):S228-S239. doi:10.1017/S0007114512001614

[115] Wu S, Liang J, Zhang L, Zhu X, Liu X, Miao D. Fish consumption and the risk of gastric cancer: Systematic review and meta-analysis. *BMC Cancer*. 2011;11(1):26. doi:10.1186/1471-2407-11-26

[116] Burckhardt M, Herke M, Wustmann T, Watzke S, Langer G, Fink A. Omega-3 fatty acids for the treatment of dementia. *Cochrane Database Syst Rev*. 2016;4:CD009002. doi:10.1002/14651858.CD009002.pub3

[117] Molina-Leyva I, Molina-Leyva A, Bueno-Cavanillas A. Efficacy of nutritional supplementation with omega-3 and omega-6 fatty acids in dry eye syndrome: a systematic review of randomized clinical trials. *Acta Ophthalmol*. 2017;95(8):e677-e685. doi:10.1111/aos.13428

[118] Thien FC, De Luca S, Woods RK, Abramson MJ. Dietary marine fatty acids (fish oil) for asthma in adults and children. *Cochrane Database Syst Rev*. 2002;(2):CD001283. doi:10.1002/14651858.CD001283

[119] Eslick GD, Howe PRC, Smith C, Priest R, Bensoussan A. Benefits of fish oil supplementation in hyperlipidemia: a systematic review and meta-analysis. *Int J Cardiol*. 2009;136(1):4-16. doi:10.1016/j.ijcard.2008.03.092

[120] Gao H, Geng T, Huang T, Zhao Q. Fish oil supplementation and insulin sensitivity: A systematic review and meta-analysis. *Lipids Health Dis*. 2017;16(1):131. doi:10.1186/s12944-017-0528-0

[121] Siscovick DS, Barringer TA, Fretts AM, et al. Omega-3 polyunsaturated fatty acid (fish oil) supplementation and the prevention of clinical cardiovascular disease. *Circulation*. 2017;135(15). doi:10.1161/CIR.0000000000000482

[122] Lian W, Wang R, Xing B, Yao Y. Fish intake and the risk of brain tumor: A meta-analysis with systematic review. *Nutr J*. 2017;16(1):1. doi:10.1186/s12937-016-0223-4

[123] Zheng J-S, Hu X-J, Zhao Y-M, Yang J, Li D. Intake of fish and marine n-3 polyunsaturated fatty acids and risk of breast cancer: Meta-analysis of data from 21 independent prospective cohort studies. *BMJ*. 2013;346(jun27 5):f3706-f3706. doi:10.1136/bmj.f3706

[124] Ries A, Trottenberg P, Elsner F, et al. A systematic review on the role of fish oil for the treatment of cachexia in advanced cancer: An EPCRC cachexia guidelines project. *Palliat Med*. 2012;26(4):294-304. doi:10.1177/0269216311418709

[125] Lovegrove C, Ahmed K, Challacombe B, Khan MS, Popert R, Dasgupta P. Systematic review of prostate cancer risk and association with consumption of fish and fish-oils: Analysis of 495,321 participants. *Int J Clin Pract*. 2015;69(1):87-105. doi:10.1111/ijcp.12514

[126] Aucoin M, Cooley K, Knee C, et al. Fish-Derived Omega-3 Fatty Acids and Prostate Cancer: A Systematic Review. *Integr Cancer Ther*. 2017;16(1):32-62. doi:10.1177/1534735416656052

[127] Abdulrazaq M, Innes JK, Calder PC. Effect of ω-3 polyunsaturated fatty acids on arthritic pain: A systematic review. *Nutrition*. 2017;39-40:57-66. doi:10.1016/j.nut.2016.12.003

[128] Senftleber N, Nielsen S, Andersen J, et al. marine oil supplements for arthritis pain: A systematic review and meta-analysis of randomized trials. *Nutrients*. 2017;9(1):42. doi:10.3390/nu9010042

[129] Rizos EC, Ntzani EE, Bika E, Kostapanos MS, Elisaf MS. Association between omega-3 fatty acid supplementation and risk of major cardiovascular disease events. *JAMA*. 2012;308(10):1024. doi:10.1001/2012.jama.11374

[130] Bauer JE. Therapeutic use of fish oils in companion animals. *J Am Vet Med Assoc*. 2011;239(11):1441-1451. doi:10.2460/javma.239.11.1441

[131] Scott DW, Miller WH, Decker GA, Wellington JR. Comparison of the clinical efficacy of two commercial fatty acid supplements (EfaVet and DVM Derm Caps), evening primrose oil, and cold water marine fish oil in the management of allergic pruritus in dogs: a double-blinded study. *Cornell Vet*. 1992;82(3):319-329.

[132] Matthews H, Granger N, Wood J, Skelly B. Effects of essential fatty acid supplementation in dogs with idiopathic epilepsy: A clinical trial. *Vet J*. 2012;191(3):396-398. doi:10.1016/j.tvjl.2011.04.018

[133] Smith CE, Freeman LM, Rush JE, Cunningham SM, Biourge V. Omega-3 fatty acids in Boxer dogs with arrhythmogenic right ventricular cardiomyopathy. *J Vet Intern Med*. 21(2):265-273.

[134] Roush JK, Dodd CE, Fritsch DA, et al. Multicenter veterinary practice assessment of the effects of omega-3 fatty acids on osteoarthritis in dogs. *J Am Vet Med Assoc*. 2010;236(1):59-66. doi:10.2460/javma.236.1.59

[135] Moreau M, Troncy E, del Castillo JRE, Bédard C, Gauvin D, Lussier B. Effects of feeding a high omega-3 fatty acids diet in dogs with naturally occurring osteoarthritis. *J Anim Physiol Anim Nutr (Berl)*. 2012;97(5):no-no. doi:10.1111/j.1439-0396.2012.01325.x

[136] Fritsch DA, Allen TA, Dodd CE, et al. A multicenter study of the effect of dietary supplementation with fish oil omega-3 fatty acids on carprofen dosage in dogs with osteoarthritis. *J Am Vet Med Assoc.* 2010;236(5):535-539. doi:10.2460/javma.236.5.535

[137] Fritsch D, Allen TA, Dodd CE, et al. Dose-titration effects of fish oil in osteoarthritic dogs. *J Vet Intern Med.* 2010;24(5):1020-1026. doi:10.1111/j.1939-1676.2010.0572.x

[138] Roush JK, Cross AR, Renberg WC, et al. Evaluation of the effects of dietary supplementation with fish oil omega-3 fatty acids on weight bearing in dogs with osteoarthritis. *J Am Vet Med Assoc.* 2010;236(1):67-73. doi:10.2460/javma.236.1.67

[139] Hielm-Björkman A, Roine J, Elo K, Lappalainen A, Junnila J, Laitinen-Vapaavuori O. An un-commissioned randomized, placebo-controlled double-blind study to test the effect of deep sea fish oil as a pain reliever for dogs suffering from canine OA. *BMC Vet Res.* 2012;8(1):157. doi:10.1186/1746-6148-8-157

[140] Zicker SC, Jewell DE, Yamka RM, Milgram NW. Evaluation of cognitive learning, memory, psychomotor, immunologic, and retinal functions in healthy puppies fed foods fortified with docosahexaenoic acid–rich fish oil from 8 to 52 weeks of age. *J Am Vet Med Assoc.* 2012;241(5):583-594. doi:10.2460/javma.241.5.583

[141] Taha AY, Henderson ST, Burnham WM. Dietary enrichment with medium chain triglycerides (ac-1203) elevates polyunsaturated fatty acids in the parietal cortex of aged dogs: Implications for treating age-related cognitive decline. *Neurochem Res.* 2009;34(9):1619-1625. doi:10.1007/s11064-009-9952-5

[142] Freeman LM, Rush JE, Kehayias JJ, et al. Nutritional alterations and the effect of fish oil supplementation in dogs with heart failure. *J Vet Intern Med.* 12(6):440-448.

[143] Lourenço AL, Booij-Vrieling HE, Vossebeld CB, Neves A, Viegas C, Corbee RJ. The effect of dietary corn oil and fish oil supplementation in dogs with naturally occurring gingivitis. *J Anim Physiol Anim Nutr (Berl).* 2018;102(5):1382-1389. doi:10.1111/jpn.12932

[144] Corbee RJ, Barnier MMC, van de Lest CHA, Hazewinkel HAW. The effect of dietary long-chain omega-3 fatty acid supplementation on owner's perception of behaviour and locomotion in cats with naturally occurring osteoarthritis. *J Anim Physiol Anim Nutr (Berl).* 2012;97(5):no-no. doi:10.1111/j.1439-0396.2012.01329.x

[145] Corbee, R. J.; Booij-Vrieling, H. E.; Lest, C. H. A. van de; Penning, L. C.; Tryfonidou, M. A.; Riemers, F. M.; Hazewinkel HAW. Inflammation and wound healing in cats with chronic gingivitis/stomatitis after extraction of all premolars and molars were not affected by feeding of two diets with different omega-6/omega-3 polyunsaturated fatty acid ratios. *J Anim Physiol Anim Nutr (Berl).* 23532;96(4):679-688.

[146] Mueller RS, Fieseler K V, Fettman MJ, et al. Effect of omega-3 fatty acids on canine atopic dermatitis. *J Small Anim Pract.* 2004;45(6):293-297.

[147] Saevik BK, Bergvall K, Holm BR, et al. A randomized, controlled study to evaluate the steroid sparing effect of essential fatty acid supplementation in the treatment of canine atopic dermatitis. *Vet Dermatol.* 2004;15(3):137-145. doi:10.1111/j.1365-3164.2004.00378.x

[148] Bright JM, Sullivan PS, Melton SL, Schneider JF, McDonald TP. The effects of n-3 fatty acid supplementation on bleeding time, plasma fatty acid composition, and in vitro platelet aggregation in cats. *J Vet Intern Med.* 1994;8(4):247-252. doi:10.1111/j.1939-1676.1994.tb03227.x

[149] Westgarth S, Blois SL, D. Wood R, Verbrugghe A, Ma DW. Effects of omega-3 polyunsaturated fatty acids and aspirin, alone and combined, on canine platelet function. *J Small Anim Pract.* 2018;59(5):272-280. doi:10.1111/jsap.12776

[150] Calder PC. Omega-3 fatty acids and inflammatory processes: from molecules to man. *Biochem Soc Trans.* 2017;45(5):1105-1115. doi:10.1042/BST20160474

[151] de Godoy MRC, McLeod KR, Harmon DL. Influence of feeding a fish oil-containing diet to mature, overweight dogs: Effects on lipid metabolites, postprandial glycaemia and body weight. *J Anim Physiol Anim Nutr (Berl).* 2018;102(1):e155-e165. doi:10.1111/jpn.12723

[152] de Godoy MRC, Conway CE, Mcleod KR, Harmon DL. Influence of feeding a fish oil-containing diet to young, lean, adult dogs: effects on lipid metabolites, postprandial glycaemia and body weight. *Arch Anim Nutr.* 2015;69(6):499-514. doi:10.1080/1745039X.2015.1100866

[153] Tsuruta K, Backus RC, DeClue AE, Fritsche KL, Mann FA. Effects of parenteral fish oil on plasma nonesterified fatty acids and systemic inflammatory mediators in dogs following ovariohysterectomy. *J Vet Emerg Crit Care.* 2017;27(5):512-523. doi:10.1111/vec.12635

[154] Barrouin-Melo SM, Anturaniemi J, Sankari S, et al. Evaluating oxidative stress, serological- and haematological status of dogs suffering from osteoarthritis, after supplementing their diet with fish or corn oil. *Lipids Health Dis.* 2016;15(1):139. doi:10.1186/s12944-016-0304-6

[155] Boe C, Vangsness CT. Fish oil and osteoarthritis: Current evidence. *Am J Orthop (Belle Mead NJ).* 2015;44(7):302-305.

[156] Villani AM, Crotty M, Cleland LG, et al. Fish oil administration in older adults: is there potential for adverse events? A systematic review of the literature. *BMC Geriatr.* 2013;13(1):41. doi:10.1186/1471-2318-13-41

[157] Lenox CE, Bauer JE. Potential adverse effects of omega-3 fatty acids in dogs and cats. *J Vet Intern Med.* 2013;27(2):217-226. doi:10.1111/jvim.12033

[158] Smith CE, Freeman LM, Rush JE, Cunningham SM, Biourge V. Omega-3 fatty acids in Boxer dogs with arrhythmogenic right ventricular cardiomyopathy. J Vet Intern Med. 21(2):265-273.

[159] Begtrup KM, Krag AE, Hvas A-M. No impact of fish oil supplements on bleeding risk: A systematic review. Dan Med J. 2017;64(5).

[160] Lehrer J. The truth wears off: Is there something wrong with the scientific method. The New Yorker. 2010. pp. 52-7.

[161] Alahdab F. Farah W. Almasri J. et al. Treatment effect in earlier trials of patients with chronic medical conditions: A meta-epidemiologic study. Mayo Clin Proc. 2017. Epub before print. Available at: http://www.mayoclinicproceedings.org/article/S0025-6196(17)30836-4/pdf Accessed February 21, 2018.

[162] Tankersley Jr RW. Amino acid requirements of herpes simplex virus in human cells. J Bacteriol. 1964; 87:609–13.

[163] Griffith RS, Norins AL, Kagan C. A multicentered study of lysine therapy in Herpes simplex infection. Dermatologica. 1978;156(5):257–67.

[164] Griffith RS. Walsh DE. Myrmen KH. Et al. Success of L-lysine therapy in frequently recurrent herpes simplex infection. Treatment and prophylaxis. Dermatologica.1987;175(4):183-90.

[165] Collins BK. Nasisse MP. Moore CP. In vitro efficacy of L-lysine against feline herpesvirus type-1. Proc 26th Ann Meeting Amer Col Vet Opthalmologists. Newport, RI. 1995;141.

[166] Bol S. Bunnik EM. Lysine supplementation is not effective for the prevention or treatment of feline herpesvirus 1 infection in cats: a systematic review. BMC Vet Res. 2015:11:284.

[167] Chi CC. Wang SH. Delamere FM. et al. Interventions for prevention of herpes simplex labialis (cold sores on the lips). Cochrane Database of Systematic Reviews. 2015;8. Art. No.: CD010095.

[168] Mailoo VJ. Rampes. S. Lysine for herpes simplex prophylaxis. Integrative Medicine. 2017;16(3):42-46.

[169] WHO Guidelines for the Treatment of Genital Herpes Simplex Virus. Geneva: World Health Organization; 2016.

[170] Thomasy SM, Maggs DJ. A review of antiviral drugs and other compounds with activity against feline herpesvirus-1. Vet Opthalmology. 2016;19(Suppl 1):119-130.

[171] UC Davis Koret Shelter Medicine Program. Feline upper respiratory infection aka URI. 2015. Available at: https://www.sheltermedicine.com/library/resources/?utf8=%E2%9C%93&search%5Bslug%5D=feline-upper-respiratory-infection-aka-uri Accessed February 21, 2018.

[172] Slater M. Interpreting research (and making it work for you): Is lysine a good investment for shelters wanting to prevent URI in cats? Available at: https://www.aspcapro.org/blog/2017/05/03/interpreting-research-and-making-it-work-you-lysine-good-investment-shelters-wanting Access February 21, 2018.

[173] Niedziela K. Researchers question lysine use in FHV cases. Vet Pract News. 2016;28(1):36-7.

[174] Mira F, Costa A, Mendes E, Azevedo P, Carreira LM. A pilot study exploring the effects of musical genres on the depth of general anaesthesia assessed by haemodynamic responses. *J Feline Med Surg.* 2016;18(8):673-678. doi:10.1177/1098612X15588968

[175] Mira F, Costa A, Mendes E, Azevedo P, Carreira LM. Influence of music and its genres on respiratory rate and pupil diameter variations in cats under general anaesthesia: contribution to promoting patient safety. *J Feline Med Surg.* 2016;18(2):150-159. doi:10.1177/1098612X15575778

[176] Albright JD, Seddighi RM, Ng Z, Sun X, Rezac D. Effect of environmental noise and music on dexmedetomidine-induced sedation in dogs. *PeerJ.* 2017;5:e3659. doi:10.7717/peerj.3659

[177] Alworth LC, Buerkle SC. The effects of music on animal physiology, behavior and welfare. *Lab Anim (NY).* 2013;42(2):54-61. doi:10.1038/laban.162

[178] Kogan LR, Schoenfeld-Tacher R, Simon AA. Behavioral effects of auditory stimulation on kenneled dogs. *J Vet Behav.* 2012;7(5):268-275. doi:10.1016/J.JVEB.2011.11.002

[179] Snowdon CT, Teie D, Savage M. Cats prefer species-appropriate music. *Appl Anim Behav Sci.* 2015;166:106-111. doi:10.1016/J.APPLANIM.2015.02.012

[180] Engler WJ, Bain M. Effect of different types of classical music played at a veterinary hospital on dog behavior and owner satisfaction. *J Am Vet Med Assoc.* 2017;251(2):195-200. doi:10.2460/javma.251.2.195

[181] Bowman A, Scottish SPCA, Dowell FJ, Evans NP. 'Four Seasons' in an animal rescue centre; classical music reduces environmental stress in kennelled dogs. *Physiol Behav.* 2015;143:70-82. doi:10.1016/j.physbeh.2015.02.035

[182] Bowman A, Scottish SPCA FJ, Dowell FJ, Evans NP. The effect of different genres of music on the stress levels of kennelled dogs. *Physiol Behav.* 2017;171:207-215. doi:10.1016/j.physbeh.2017.01.024

[183] Conzemius MG, Evans RB. Caregiver placebo effect for dogs with lameness from osteoarthritis. *J Am Vet Med Assoc.* 2012;241(10):1314-1319. doi:10.2460/javma.241.10.1314

[184] Gruen ME, Dorman DC, Lascelles BDX. Caregiver placebo effect in analgesic clinical trials for cats with naturally occurring degenerative joint disease-associated pain. *Vet Rec.* 2017;180(19):473-473. doi:10.1136/vr.104168

[185] Beyerstein BL, Downie S. Naturopathy. In: *Science Meets Alternative Medicine: What the Evidence Says about Unconventional Treatments.* Amgerst, NY: Prometheus Books; 2000:141-163.

[186] American Council on Animal Naturopathy (ACAN). What is Animal Naturopathy? | Animal Naturopathy. Available at: https://www.animalnaturopathy.org/what-is-animal-naturopathy/. Published 2018. Accessed January 3, 2019.

[187] Atwood KC, IV. Naturopathy, pseudoscience, and medicine: myths and fallacies vs truth. *MedGenMed*. 2004;6(1):33.

[188] Atwood KC. Naturopathy: a critical appraisal. *MedGenMed*. 2003;5(4):39.

[189] American Association of Naturopathic Physicians (AANP). Definition of Naturopathic Medicine. Available at: https://www.naturopathic.org/content.asp?pl=16&sl=59&contentid=59. Published 2011. Accessed January 3, 2019.

[190] The Academy of Veterinary Homeopathy (AVH). Certification. Available at: https://theavh.org/certification/. Accessed January 3, 2019.

[191] American Association of Professional Psychics (AAPP). Certified Psychics | Psychic Readings. Available at: http://certifiedpsychics.com/. Accessed January 3, 2019.

[192] International Society for Astrological Research (ISAR). ISAR Certification Program. Available at: http://www.isarastrology.com/certification. Published 2018. Accessed January 3, 2019.

[193] Caulfield T, Rachul C. Supported by science?: What Canadian naturopaths advertise to the public. *Allergy Asthma Clin Immunol*. 2011;7(1):14. doi:10.1186/1710-1492-7-14

[194] Colquhoun D. Science degrees without the science. *Nature*. 2007;446(7134):373-374. doi:10.1038/446373a

[195] Calabrese C, Oberg E, Bradley R, Seely D, Cooley K, Goldenberg J. P04.62. Systematic review of clinical studies of whole practice naturopathic medicine. *BMC Complement Altern Med*. 2012;12(Suppl 1):P332. doi:10.1186/1472-6882-12-S1-P332

[196] Busse JW, Wilson K, Campbell JB. Attitudes towards vaccination among chiropractic and naturopathic students. *Vaccine*. 2008;26(49):6237-6243. doi:10.1016/j.vaccine.2008.07.020

[197] Wilson K, Busse JW, Gilchrist A, Vohra S, Boon H, Mills E. Characteristics of Pediatric and Adolescent Patients Attending a Naturopathic College Clinic in Canada. *Pediatrics*. 2005;115(3):e338-e343. doi:10.1542/peds.2004-1901

[198] Lee AC, Kemper KJ. Homeopathy and naturopathy: practice characteristics and pediatric care. *Arch Pediatr Adolesc Med*. 2000;154(1):75-80.

[199] Downey L, Tyree PT, Huebner CE, Lafferty WE. Pediatric Vaccination and Vaccine-Preventable Disease Acquisition: Associations with Care by Complementary and Alternative Medicine Providers. *Matern Child Health J*. 2010;14(6):922-930. doi:10.1007/s10995-009-0519-5

[200] Wilson K, Mills E, Boon H, Tomlinson G, Ritvo P. A survey of attitudes towards paediatric vaccinations amongst Canadian naturopathic students. *Vaccine*. 2004;22(3-4):329-334.

[201] Atwood K. Naturopathy vs. Science: Vaccination Edition. Science-Based Medicine Blog. Available at: https://sciencebasedmedicine.org/naturopathy-vs-science-vaccination-edition/. Published 2014. Accessed January 3, 2019.

[202] Zanowski GN. a fresh look at spay/neuter legislation. *J Public Heal Manag Pract.* 2012;18(3):E24-E33. doi:10.1097/PHH.0b013e318222a7f5

[203] Yen IF, Peng JenLung, Ryan W, Chyao ChungHuai, Tung KwongChung, Fei ChangYoung. Low sterilization of pets causes shelter overpopulation. *J Anim Vet Adv.* 2014;13(16):1022-1026. doi:10.3923/javaa.2014.1022.1026

[204] Mahlow JC. Estimation of the proportions of dogs and cats that are surgically sterilized. *J Am Vet Med Assoc.* 1999;215(5):640-643.

[205] Olson PN, Moulton C. Pet (dog and cat) overpopulation in the United States. *J Reprod Fertil Suppl.* 1993;47:433-438.

[206] Root Kustritz M. Effects of surgical sterilization on canine and feline health and on society. *Reprod Domest Anim.* 2012;47:214-222. doi:10.1111/j.1439-0531.2012.02078.x

[207] Root Kustritz M V. Pros, cons, and techniques of pediatric neutering. *Vet Clin North Am Small Anim Pract.* 2014;44(2):221-233. doi:10.1016/j.cvsm.2013.10.002

[208] Mckenzie B. Evaluating the benefits and risks of neutering dogs and cats. doi:10.1079/PAVSNNR20105045

[209] Hoffman JM, Creevy KE, Promislow DEL. Reproductive capability is associated with lifespan and cause of death in companion dogs. Helle S, ed. *PLoS One.* 2013;8(4):e61082. doi:10.1371/journal.pone.0061082

[210] Gibson A, Dean R, Yates D, Stavisky J. A retrospective study of pyometra at five RSPCA hospitals in the UK: 1728 cases from 2006 to 2011. *Vet Rec.* 2013;173(16):396-396. doi:10.1136/vr.101514

[211] Beauvais W, Cardwell JM, Brodbelt DC. The effect of neutering on the risk of mammary tumours in dogs--a systematic review. *J Small Anim Pract.* 2012;53(6):314-322. doi:10.1111/j.1748-5827.2011.01220.x

[212] Sorenmo KU, Shofer FS, Goldschmidt MH. Effect of spaying and timing of spaying on survival of dogs with mammary carcinoma. *J Vet Intern Med.* 14(3):266-270.

[213] Scarlett JM, Salman MD, New JG, Kass PH. The role of veterinary practitioners in reducing dog and cat relinquishments and euthanasias. *J Am Vet Med Assoc.* 2002;220(3):306-311.

[214] Patronek GJ, Glickman LT, Beck AM, McCabe GP, Ecker C. Risk factors for relinquishment of dogs to an animal shelter. *J Am Vet Med Assoc.* 1996;209(3):572-581.

[215] New JC, Salman MD, King M, Scarlett JM, Kass PH, Hutchison JM. Characteristics of shelter-relinquished animals and their owners compared with animals and their owners in U.S. pet-owning households. *J Appl Anim Welf Sci.* 2000;3(3):179-201. doi:10.1207/S15327604JAWS0303_1

[216] Knol BW, Egberink-Alink ST. Treatment of problem behaviour in dogs and cats by castration and progestagen administration: A review. *Vet Q.* 1989;11(2):102-107. doi:10.1080/01652176.1989.9694206

[217] Hart BL, Barrett RE. Effects of castration on fighting, roaming, and urine spraying in adult male cats. *J Am Vet Med Assoc*. 1973;163(3):290-292.

[218] Hart BL, Cooper L. Factors relating to urine spraying and fighting in prepubertally gonadectomized cats. *J Am Vet Med Assoc*. 1984;184(10):1255-1258.

[219] Patronek GJ, Sacks JJ, Delise KM, Cleary D V, Marder AR. Co-occurrence of potentially preventable factors in 256 dog bite-related fatalities in the United States (2000-2009). *J Am Vet Med Assoc*. 2013;243(12):1726-1736. doi:10.2460/javma.243.12.1726

[220] Gershman KA, Sacks JJ, Wright JC. Which dogs bite? A case-control study of risk factors. *Pediatrics*. 1994;93(6 Pt 1):913-917.

[221] Neilson JC, Eckstein RA, Hart BL. Effects of castration on problem behaviors in male dogs with reference to age and duration of behavior. *J Am Vet Med Assoc*. 1997;211(2):180-182.

[222] Maarschalkerweerd RJ, Endenburg N, Kirpensteijn J, Knol BW. Influence of orchiectomy on canine behaviour. *Vet Rec*. 1997;140(24):617-619. doi:10.1136/VR.140.24.617

[223] Hopkins SG, Schubert TA, Hart BL. Castration of adult male dogs: effects on roaming, aggression, urine marking, and mounting. *J Am Vet Med Assoc*. 1976;168(12):1108-1110.

[224] Wright JC, Nesselrote MS. Classification of behavior problems in dogs: Distributions of age, breed, sex and reproductive status. *Appl Anim Behav Sci*. 1987;19(1-2):169-178. doi:10.1016/0168-1591(87)90213-9

[225] Borchelt PL. Aggressive behavior of dogs kept as companion animals: Classification and influence of sex, reproductive status and breed. *Appl Anim Ethol*. 1983;10(1-2):45-61. doi:10.1016/0304-3762(83)90111-6

[226] Ni_ Za Nski W, Levy X, Ochota M, Pasikowska J. Pharmacological treatment for common prostatic conditions in dogs-benign prostatic hyperplasia and prostatitis: An update. 2014. doi:10.1111/rda.12297

[227] Berry SJ, Strandberg JD, Saunders WJ, Coffey DS. Development of canine benign prostatic hyperplasia with age. *Prostate*. 1986;9(4):363-373.

[228] Mukaratirwa S, Chitura T. Canine subclinical prostatic disease: histological prevalence and validity of digital rectal examination as a screening test. *J S Afr Vet Assoc*. 2007;78(2):66-68.

[229] Vet Audit Group RK. *Routine Neutering Complication Rate*. Available at: http://vetaudit.rcvsk.org/wp-content/uploads/sites/5/2018/09/POC-Results-Aug-2018.doc; 2018.

[230] Burrow R, Batchelor D, Cripps P. Complications observed during and after ovariohysterectomy of 142 bitches at a veterinary teaching hospital. *Vet Rec*. 157(26):829-833.

[231] Pollari FL, Bonnett BN. Evaluation of postoperative complications following elective surgeries of dogs and cats at private practices using computer records. *Can Vet J.* 1996;37(11):672-678.

[232] Howe LM. Short-term results and complications of prepubertal gonadectomy in cats and dogs. *J Am Vet Med Assoc.* 1997;211(1):57-62.

[233] Pollari FL, Bonnett BN, Bamsey SC, Meek AH, Allen DG. Postoperative complications of elective surgeries in dogs and cats determined by examining electronic and paper medical records. *J Am Vet Med Assoc.* 1996;208(11):1882-1886.

[234] Larsen JA. Risk of obesity in the neutered cat. *J Feline Med Surg.* 2017;19(8):779-783. doi:10.1177/1098612X16660605

[235] Hart BL, Hart LA, Thigpen AP, Willits NH. Long-term health effects of neutering dogs: comparison of Labrador Retrievers with Golden Retrievers. Coulombe RA, ed. *PLoS One.* 2014;9(7):e102241. doi:10.1371/journal.pone.0102241

[236] Villamil JA, Henry CJ, Hahn AW, Bryan JN, Tyler JW, Caldwell CW. Hormonal and sex impact on the epidemiology of canine lymphoma. *J Cancer Epidemiol.* 2009;2009:591753. doi:10.1155/2009/591753

[237] Hoffman JM, Creevy KE, Promislow DEL. Reproductive capability is associated with lifespan and cause of death in companion dogs. Helle S, ed. *PLoS One.* 2013;8(4):e61082. doi:10.1371/journal.pone.0061082

[238] Torres de la Riva G, Hart BL, Farver TB, et al. Neutering Dogs: Effects on Joint Disorders and Cancers in Golden Retrievers. Williams BO, ed. *PLoS One.* 2013;8(2):e55937. doi:10.1371/journal.pone.0055937

[239] Evans CD, Lacey JH. Toxicity of vitamins: complications of a health movement. *Br Med J (Clin Res Ed).* 1986;292(6519):509-510.

[240] Tilburt JC, Emanuel EJ, Kaptchuk TJ, Curlin FA, Miller FG. Prescribing placebo treatments: results of national survey of US internists and rheumatologists. *BMJ.* 2008;337:a1938. doi:10.1136/bmj.a1938

[241] Cabanillas F. Vitamin C and cancer: what can we conclude--1,609 patients and 33 years later? *P R Health Sci J.* 2010;29(3):215-217.

[242] Creagan ET, Moertel CG, O'Fallon JR, et al. Failure of high-dose vitamin c (ascorbic acid) therapy to benefit patients with advanced cancer. *N Engl J Med.* 1979;301(13):687-690. doi:10.1056/NEJM197909273011303

[243] Hemilä H, Chalker E, Douglas B, Treacy B. Vitamin C for preventing and treating the common cold. In: Hemilä H, ed. *Cochrane Database of Systematic Reviews.* Chichester, UK: John Wiley & Sons, Ltd; 2007:CD000980. doi:10.1002/14651858.CD000980.pub3

[244] Lipton MA, Ban TA, Kane F., Levine J, Mosher LR, WIttenborn R. Megavitamin and orthomolecular therapy in psychiatry. *Nutr Rev.* 1974;32(0):suppl 1:44-7.

[245] Nutrition Committee CPS. Megavitamin and megamineral therapy in childhood. *CMAJ.* 1990;143(10):1009-1013.

[246] Jarvis WT. Food Faddism, Cultism, and Quackery. *Annu Rev Nutr.* 1983;3(1):35-52. doi:10.1146/annurev.nu.03.070183.000343

[247] Sanders KM, Nicholson GC, Ebeling PR. Is high dose Vitamin D harmful? *Calcif Tissue Int.* 2013;92(2):191-206. doi:10.1007/s00223-012-9679-1

[248] Wilson MK, Baguley BC, Wall C, Jameson MB, Findlay MP. Review of high-dose intravenous Vitamin C as an anticancer agent. *Asia Pac J Clin Oncol.* 2014;10(1):22-37. doi:10.1111/ajco.12173

[249] Hansen KE. High-dose vitamin D: helpful or harmful? *Curr Rheumatol Rep.* 2011;13(3):257-264. doi:10.1007/s11926-011-0175-9

[250] Robinson AB, Hunsberger A, Westall FC. Suppression of Squamous Cell Carcinoma in Hairless Mice by Dietary Nutrient Variation. *Mech Ageing Dev.* 1994;76(2-3):201-14.

[251] Wu Q-J, Xiang Y-B, Yang G, et al. Vitamin E intake and the lung cancer risk among female nonsmokers: a report from the Shanghai Women's Health Study. *Int J cancer.* 2015;136(3):610-617. doi:10.1002/ijc.29016

[252] Mursu J, Robien K, Harnack LJ, Park K, Jacobs DR. Dietary Supplements and Mortality Rate in Older Women. *Arch Intern Med.* 2011;171(18):1625. doi:10.1001/archinternmed.2011.445

[253] Watkins ML, Erickson JD, Thun MJ, Mulinare J, Heath CW. multivitamin use and mortality in a large prospective study. *Am J Epidemiol.* 2000;152(2):149-162. doi:10.1093/aje/152.2.149

[254] Sesso HD, Buring JE, Christen WG, et al. Vitamins E and C in the prevention of cardiovascular disease in men. *JAMA.* 2008;300(18):2123. doi:10.1001/jama.2008.600

[255] Paulsen G, Cumming KT, Holden G, et al. Vitamin C and E supplementation hampers cellular adaptation to endurance training in humans: a double-blind, randomised, controlled trial. *J Physiol.* 2014;592(8):1887-1901. doi:10.1113/jphysiol.2013.267419

[256] Schürks M, Glynn RJ, Rist PM, Tzourio C, Kurth T. Effects of vitamin E on stroke subtypes: meta-analysis of randomised controlled trials. *BMJ.* 2010;341:c5702. doi:10.1136/BMJ.C5702

[257] Lippman SM, Klein EA, Goodman PJ, et al. Effect of Selenium and Vitamin E on risk of prostate cancer and other cancers. *JAMA.* 2009;301(1):39. doi:10.1001/jama.2008.864

[258] Klein EA, Thompson IM, Tangen CM, et al. Vitamin E and the risk of prostate cancer: the Selenium and Vitamin E Cancer Prevention Trial (SELECT). *JAMA.* 2011;306(14):1549-1556. doi:10.1001/jama.2011.1437

[259] Klein EA, Thompson IM, Tangen CM, et al. Vitamin E and the risk of prostate cancer. *JAMA.* 2011;306(14):1549. doi:10.1001/jama.2011.1437

[260] Martinez ME, Jacobs ET, Baron JA, Marshall JR, Byers T. dietary supplements and cancer prevention: Balancing potential benefits against proven harms. *JNCI J Natl Cancer Inst.* 2012;104(10):732-739. doi:10.1093/jnci/djs195

[261]Brasky TM1, White E1, Chen CL1. Long-Term, Supplemental, One-Carbon Metabolism-Related Vitamin B Use in Relation to Lung Cancer Risk in the Vitamins and Lifestyle (VITAL) Cohort. *J Clin Oncol*. 2017;35(30):3440-3448. doi: 10.1200/JCO.2017.72.7735

[262] Liberles SD. Mammalian Pheromones. *Ann Rev Physiol*. 2014;76:151-175.

[263] Yew JY. Chung H. Insect pheromones: An overview of function, form, and discovery. *Prog Lipid Res*. 2015;59:88-105.

[264] Wyatt TD. The search for human pheromones: the lost decades and the necessity of returning to first principles. *Proc Biol Sci*. 2015;282(1804):20142994.

[265] Pageat, P. Gaultier E. Current research in canine and feline pheromones. *Vet Clin No Amer Small Anim Pract*. 2003;33(2):187-211.

[266] CEVA Santé Animale. Available at: https://www.ceva.com/Products/Companion-animals/Behaviour. Accessed December 20, 2017.

[267] CEVA Animal Health. Available at: https://www.feliway.com/us/FELIWAY/The-Science-Behind-Feliway. Accessed December 27, 2017.

[268] Pageat P. (1995) U.S. Patent No. 5709863 A. U.S. Patent and Trademark Office. Available at: https://www.google.com/patents/US5709863. Accessed December 27, 2017.

[269] Beck A. CEVA Santé Animale. (2015) European Patent No. EP2954886 A1. Available at: https://www.google.com/patents/EP2954886A1?cl=en. Accessed December 27, 2017.

[270] Nouvel L. McGlone J. Sargeant's Pet Care Products, Inc. (2014). U.S. Patent No. 8741965 B2. U.S. Patent and Trademark Office. Available at: https://www.google.com/patents/US8741965. Accessed December 27, 2017.

[271] Pageat P. Institut de Recherche en Semiochimie et Ethologie Appliquee. (2014) Patent No. WO2014001836 A1. Availabe at: https://www.google.com/patents/WO2014001836A1?cl=en. Accessed December 28, 2017.

[272] Lundh A, Lexchin J, Mintzes B, Schroll JB, Bero L. Industry sponsorship and research outcome. *Cochrane Database of Systematic Reviews*. 2017, Issue 2. Art. No.: MR000033.

[273] Frank D. Beauchamp G. Palestrini C. Systematic review of the use of pheromones for treatment of undesirable behavior in cats and dogs. *J.Am.Vet.Med.Assoc*. 2010;36(12):1308-1316.

[274] Siracusa C, Manteca X, Cuenca R, del Mar Alcala M, Alba A, et al. Effect of a synthetic appeasing pheromone on behavioral, neuroendocrine, immune, and acute-phase perioperative stress response in dogs. *J Amer Vet Med Assoc* 2010;237(6):p. 673-81.

[275] Conti, LMC. Champion, T. Guberman, UC. et al. Evaluation of environment and a feline facial pheromone analogue on physiologic and behavioral measures in cats. J Fel Med Surg. 2015;19(2):165-70.

[276] Chadwin RM. Bain MJ. Kass PH. Effect of a synthetic feline facial pheromone product on stress scores and incidence of upper respiratory tract infection in shelter cats. *J Am Vet Med Assoc.* 2017 Aug 15;251(4):413-420.

[277] Landsberg GM. Beck A. Lopez A. et al. Dog-appeasing pheromone collars reduce sound-induced fear and anxiety in beagle dogs: a placebo-controlled study. *Vet Rec.* 2015 Sep 12;177(10):260.

[278] Contreras ET. Hodgkins E. Tynes V. et al. Effect of a pheromone on stress-associated reactivation of feline herpesvirus-1 in experimentally inoculated kittens. *J Vet Intern Med.* 2017 Dec 8.

[279] Jensen KT, Rabago DP, Best TM, Patterson JJ, Vanderby R. Early inflammatory response of knee ligaments to prolotherapy in a rat model. *J Orthop Res.* 2008;26(6):816-823. doi:10.1002/jor.20600

[280] Reeves KD, Sit RWS, Rabago DP. Dextrose Prolotherapy. *Phys Med Rehabil Clin N Am.* 2016;27(4):783-823. doi:10.1016/j.pmr.2016.06.001

[281] Rabago D, Slattengren A, Zgierska A. Prolotherapy in Primary Care Practice. *Prim Care Clin Off Pract.* 2010;37(1):65-80. doi:10.1016/j.pop.2009.09.013

[282] Rabago D, Nourani B. Prolotherapy for osteoarthritis and tendinopathy: A descriptive review. *Curr Rheumatol Rep.* 2017;19(6):34. doi:10.1007/s11926-017-0659-3

[283] Sit RW, Chung VC, Reeves KD, et al. Hypertonic dextrose injections (prolotherapy) in the treatment of symptomatic knee osteoarthritis: A systematic review and meta-analysis. *Sci Rep.* 2016;6(1):25247. doi:10.1038/srep25247

[284] Hassan F, Trebinjac S, Murrell WD, Maffulli N. The effectiveness of prolotherapy in treating knee osteoarthritis in adults: A systematic review. *Br Med Bull.* 2017;122(1):91-108. doi:10.1093/bmb/ldx006

[285] Hauser RA, Lackner JB, Steilen-Matias D, Harris DK. A systematic review of dextrose prolotherapy for chronic musculoskeletal pain. *Clin Med Insights Arthritis Musculoskelet Disord.* 2016;9:CMAMD.S39160. doi:10.4137/CMAMD.S39160

[286] Hung C-Y, Hsiao M-Y, Chang K-V, Han D-S, Wang T-G. Comparative effectiveness of dextrose prolotherapy versus control injections and exercise in the management of osteoarthritis pain: A systematic review and meta-analysis. *J Pain Res.* 2016;9:847-857. doi:10.2147/JPR.S118669

[287] Nagori SA, Jose A, Gopalakrishnan V, Roy ID, Chattopadhyay PK, Roychoudhury A. The efficacy of dextrose prolotherapy over placebo for temporomandibular joint hypermobility: A systematic review and meta-analysis. *J Oral Rehabil.* 2018;45(12):998-1006. doi:10.1111/joor.12698

[288] Morath O, Kubosch EJ, Taeymans J, et al. The effect of sclerotherapy and prolotherapy on chronic painful Achilles tendinopathy: A systematic review including meta-analysis. *Scand J Med Sci Sports.* 2018;28(1):4-15. doi:10.1111/sms.12898

[289] Krstičević M, Jerić M, Došenović S, Jeličić Kadić A, Puljak L. Proliferative injection therapy for osteoarthritis: A systematic review. *Int Orthop.* 2017;41(4):671-679. doi:10.1007/s00264-017-3422-5

[290] Sherwood JM, Roush JK, Armbrust LJ, Renberg WC. Prospective evaluation of intra-articular dextrose prolotherapy for treatment of osteoarthritis in dogs. *J Am Anim Hosp Assoc.* 2017;53(3):135-142. doi:10.5326/JAAHA-MS-6508

[291] Dehaan RL. My Experience With Prolotherapy In Animals An Alternative Answer to Anterior Cruciate Ligament and Hip Dysplasia Degeneration. *J Prolotherpy.* 2009;1(1):258.

[292] Vadalà M, Morales-Medina JC, Vallelunga A, Palmieri B, Laurino C, Iannitti T. Mechanisms and therapeutic effectiveness of pulsed electromagnetic field therapy in oncology. *Cancer Med.* 2016;5(11):3128-3139. doi:10.1002/cam4.861

[293] Hannemann PFW, Mommers EHH, Schots JPM, Brink PRG, Poeze M. The effects of low-intensity pulsed ultrasound and pulsed electromagnetic fields bone growth stimulation in acute fractures: a systematic review and meta-analysis of randomized controlled trials. *Arch Orthop Trauma Surg.* 2014;134(8):1093-1106. doi:10.1007/s00402-014-2014-8

[294] Yuan J, Xin F, Jiang W. Underlying Signaling Pathways and Therapeutic Applications of Pulsed Electromagnetic Fields in Bone Repair. *Cell Physiol Biochem.* 2018;46(4):1581-1594. doi:10.1159/000489206

[295] Gaynor JS, Hagberg S, Gurfein BT. Veterinary applications of pulsed electromagnetic field therapy. *Res Vet Sci.* 2018;119:1-8. doi:10.1016/j.rvsc.2018.05.005

[296] Griffin XL, Costa ML, Parsons N, Smith N. Electromagnetic field stimulation for treating delayed union or non-union of long bone fractures in adults. *Cochrane Database Syst Rev.* 2011;(4):CD008471. doi:10.1002/14651858.CD008471.pub2

[297] Galli C, Pedrazzi G, Mattioli-Belmonte M, Guizzardi S. The Use of Pulsed Electromagnetic Fields to Promote Bone Responses to Biomaterials *In Vitro* and *In Vivo*. *Int J Biomater.* 2018;2018:1-15. doi:10.1155/2018/8935750

[298] McCarthy CJ, Callaghan MJ, Oldham JA. Pulsed electromagnetic energy treatment offers no clinical benefit in reducing the pain of knee osteoarthritis: A systematic review. *BMC Musculoskelet Disord.* 2006;7(1):51. doi:10.1186/1471-2474-7-51

[299] Kroeling P, Gross A, Graham N, et al. Electrotherapy for neck pain. *Cochrane Database Syst Rev.* 2013;(8):CD004251. doi:10.1002/14651858.CD004251.pub5

[300] Gordon GA. Designed electromagnetic pulsed therapy: Clinical applications. *J Cell Physiol.* 2007;212(3):579-582. doi:10.1002/jcp.21025

[301] Negm A, Lorbergs A, MacIntyre NJ. Efficacy of low frequency pulsed subsensory threshold electrical stimulation vs placebo on pain and physical function in people with knee osteoarthritis: A systematic review with meta-analysis. *Osteoarthr Cartil.* 2013;21(9):1281-1289. doi:10.1016/j.joca.2013.06.015

[302] Hug K, Röösli M. Therapeutic effects of whole-body devices applying pulsed electromagnetic fields (PEMF): A systematic literature review. *Bioelectromagnetics.* 2012;33(2):95-105. doi:10.1002/bem.20703

[303] Gaynor JS, Hagberg S, Gurfein BT. Veterinary applications of pulsed electromagnetic field therapy. *Res Vet Sci.* 2018;119:1-8. doi:10.1016/j.rvsc.2018.05.005

[304] Buchner N, Rindler NM, Biermann S, Westermann HHF. The effect of pulsed electromagnetic field therapy on surface temperature of horses' backs. *Wien Tierarztl Monatsschr.* 2014;101(7):137-141.

[305] Scardino MS, Swaim SF, Sartin EA, et al. Evaluation of treatment with a pulsed electromagnetic field on wound healing, clinicopathologic variables, and central nervous system activity of dogs. *Am J Vet Res.* 1998;59(9):1177-1181.

[306] Shafford HL, Hellyer PW, Crump KT, Wagner AE, Mama KR, Gaynor JS. Use of a pulsed electromagnetic field for treatment of post–operative pain in dogs: A pilot study. *Vet Anaesth Analg.* 2002;29(1):43-48. doi:10.1046/j.1467-2987.2001.00072.x

[307] Pinna S, Landucci F, Tribuiani AM, Carli F, Venturini A. The effects of pulsed electromagnetic field in the treatment of osteoarthritis in dogs: Clinical study. *Pakistani Vet J.* 2013;33(1):96-100.

[308] Biermann NM, Rindler N, Buchner HHF. The effect of pulsed electromagnetic fields on back pain in polo ponies evaluated by pressure algometry and flexion testing - a randomized, double-blind, placebo-controlled trial. *J Equine Vet Sci.* 2014;34(4):500-507.

[309] Zidan N, Fenn J, Griffith E, et al. the effect of electromagnetic fields on post-operative pain and locomotor recovery in dogs with acute, severe thoracolumbar intervertebral disc extrusion: A randomized placebo-controlled, prospective clinical trial. *J Neurotrauma.* 2018;35(15):1726-1736. doi:10.1089/neu.2017.5485

[310] Singh S, Ernst E (Edzard). *Trick or Treatment? : Alternative Medicine on Trial.* London: Corgi; 2009..

[311] Carroll RT. *The Skeptic's Dictionary : A Collection of Strange Beliefs, Amusing Deceptions, and Dangerous Delusions.* Hoboken, NJ. Wiley; 2003.

[312] Rand WL. *Reiki Master Manual : Including Advanced Reiki Training.* Maharashtra, India. Vision Publications; 2003.

[313] Robinson J, Biley FC, Dolk H. Therapeutic touch for anxiety disorders. *Cochrane Database Syst Rev.* 2007;(3):CD006240. doi:10.1002/14651858.CD006240.pub2

[314] O'Mathúna DP. Therapeutic touch for healing acute wounds. *Cochrane Database of Systematic Reviews.* Chichester, UK: John Wiley & Sons, Ltd; 2016:CD002766. doi:10.1002/14651858.CD002766.pub5

[315] vanderVaart S, Gijsen VMGJ, de Wildt SN, Koren G. A systematic review of the therapeutic effects of reiki. *J Altern Complement Med.* 2009;15(11):1157-1169. doi:10.1089/acm.2009.0036

[316] Lee MS, Pittler MH, Ernst E. Effects of reiki in clinical practice: a systematic review of randomised clinical trials. *Int J Clin Pract.* 2008;62(6):947-954. doi:10.1111/j.1742-1241.2008.01729.x

[317] Ferraz GAR, Rodrigues MRK, Lima SAM, et al. Is reiki or prayer effective in relieving pain during hospitalization for cesarean? A systematic review and meta-analysis of randomized controlled trials. *Sao Paulo Med J.* 2017;135(2):123-132. doi:10.1590/1516-3180.2016.0267031116

[318] Joyce J, Herbison GP. Reiki for depression and anxiety. *Cochrane Database Syst Rev.* 2015;(4):CD006833. doi:10.1002/14651858.CD006833.pub2

[319] Rosa L, Rosa E, Sarner L, Barrett S. A close look at therapeutic touch. *JAMA.* 1998;279(13):1005. doi:10.1001/jama.279.13.1005

[320] Shahin M. The effects of positive human contact by tactile stimulation on dairy cows with different personalities. *Appl Anim Behav Sci.* 2018;204:23-28. doi:10.1016/J.APPLANIM.2018.04.004

[321] Beetz A, Uvnäs-Moberg K, Julius H, Kotrschal K. Psychosocial and psychophysiological effects of human-animal interactions: the possible role of oxytocin. *Front Psychol.* 2012;3:234. doi:10.3389/fpsyg.2012.00234

[322] Vormbrock JK, Grossberg JM. Cardiovascular effects of human-pet dog interactions. *J Behav Med.* 1988;11(5):509-517.

[323] Dudley ES, Schiml PA, Hennessy MB. Effects of repeated petting sessions on leukocyte counts, intestinal parasite prevalence, and plasma cortisol concentration of dogs housed in a county animal shelter. *J Am Vet Med Assoc.* 2015;247(11):1289-1298. doi:10.2460/javma.247.11.1289

[324] Mariti C, Carlone B, Protti M, Diverio S, Gazzano A. Effects of petting before a brief separation from the owner on dog behavior and physiology: A pilot study. *J Vet Behav.* 2018;27:41-46. doi:10.1016/j.jveb.2018.07.003

[325] Shiverdecker MD, Schiml PA, Hennessy MB. Human interaction moderates plasma cortisol and behavioral responses of dogs to shelter housing. *Physiol Behav.* 2013;109:75-79. doi:10.1016/j.physbeh.2012.12.002

[326] HAMA H, YOGO M, MATSUYAMA Y. Effects of stroking horses on both humans' and horses' heart rate responses. *Jpn Psychol Res.* 1996;38(2):66-73. doi:10.1111/j.1468-5884.1996.tb00009.x

[327] Lynch JJ, Fregin GF, Mackie JB, Monroe RR. Heart rate changes in the horse to human contact. *Psychophysiology.* 1974;11(4):472-478.

[328] Gruenstern J. Yunnan Baiyao-Miracle herb for your clinic. *Integr Vet Care J.* 2014;4(1):26-28.

[329] Xie H. Preast V. (2013). *Traditional Chinese Veterinary medicine: Fundamental Principles.* 2nd Ed. Reddick, FL: Chi Institute Press.

[330] Ogle CW, Dai S, Ma JC. The haemostatic effects of the Chinese herbal drug Yunnan Baiyao: A pilot study. *Am J Chin Med.* 1976;4:147–152.

[331] Ogle CW. Soter D. Cho CH. The haemostatic effects of orally administered Yunnan Baiyao in rats and rabbits. *Compar Med East and West.* 1977;5(2):155-160.

[332] Graham L. Farnsworth K. Cary J. The effect of Yunnan Baiyao on the template bleeding times and activated clotting times in healthy ponies under halothane anesthesia. *J Vet Emerg Crit Care.* 2002;12(4):279. (abstract only)

[333] Fan C. Song J. White CM. A comparison of the hemostatic effects of notoginseng and Yunnan Baiyao to placebo control. *J Herb Pharmacother* 2005;5:1–5.

[334] Epp TS. McDonough P. Padilla DJ. et al. The effect of herbal supplementation on the severity of exercise-induced pulmonary haemorrhage. *Equine Comp Exer Physiol.* 2005;2:17-25.

[335] Lee A. Boysen SR. Sanderson J. et al. Effects of Yunnan Baiyao on blood coagulation parameters in beagles measured using kaolin activated thromboelastography and more traditional methods. *Int J Vet Sci Med.*. 2017;5(1):53–56.

[336] Frederick J. Boysen S. Wagg C. Chalhoub S. The effects of oral administration of Yunnan Baiyao on blood coagulation in beagle dogs as measured by kaolin-activated thromboelastography and buccal mucosal bleeding times. *Can J Vet Res.* 2017;81(1):41-45.

[337] MacRae R. Carr A. The effect of Yunnan Baiyao on the kinetics of hemostasis in healthy dogs. ACVIM Forum, National Harbor, MD, 2017.

[338] Adelman L. Olin S. Egger CM. Stokes JE. Effect of oral Yunnan Baiyao on periprocedural hemorrhage and coagulation in dogs undergoing nasal biopsy. ACVIM Forum, National Harbor, MD, 2017.

[339] Ness SL. Frye AH. Divers TJ. et al. Randomized placebo-controlled study of the effects of Yunnan Baiyao on hemostasis in horses. *Am J Vet Res.* 2017;78(8):969-976.

[340] Huang WF, Wen KC, Hsiao ML. Adulteration by synthetic therapeutic substances of traditional Chinese medicines in Taiwan. *J Clin Pharmacol.* 1997;37(4):344-50

[341] Saper RB, Phillips RS, Sehgal A, Khouri N, Davis RB, Paquin J, Thuppil V, Kales SN. Lead, mercury, and arsenic in US- and Indian-manufactured Ayurvedic medicines sold via the Internet. *JAMA.* 2008;300(8):915-23.

[342] Debelle FD, Vanherweghem JL, Nortier JL (2008) Aristolochic acid nephropathy: a worldwide problem. *Kidney Int.* 74:158–169

[343] Calahan J. Howard D. Almalki AJ. et al. chemical adulterants in herbal medicinal products: A review. *Planta Med.* 2016 Apr;82(6):505-1

[344] Harris ESJ. Cao S. Littlefield BA. Craycroft JA. et al. Heavy metal and pesticide content in commonly prescribed individual raw Chinese herbal medicines. *Sci Total Environ* 2011;409:4297–4305.

[345] Coghlan ML. Deep sequencing of plant and animal DNA within traditional Chinese medicines reveals legality issues and health safety concerns. *PLOS Genetics.* 2012;8(4):e1002675.

[346] Shmalberg J. Hill RC. Scott KC. Nutrient and metal analyses of Chinese herbal products marketed for veterinary use. *J Anim Physiol Anim Nutr (Berl)*. 2013;97(2):305-14

347 How can Yunnan Baiyao capsules help with your sick dog? (March 2016) Available at: http://bit.ly/2ikEdWp Accessed August 21, 2017.

[348] Ernst, E. (2002), Adulteration of Chinese herbal medicines with synthetic drugs: a systematic review. *J Int Med*, 252: 107–113.

[349] Basko I. Behind the green door: "Tangled herbaceutical testing." *J Am Holistic Vet Med Assoc*. Apr-Jun 2003;22(1):31-35.

[350] Nahin RL, Barnes PM, Stussman BJ. Expenditures on complementary health approaches: United States, 2012. National Health Statistics Reports. Hyattsville, MD: National Center for Health Statistics. 2016.

[351] Bo Yang. Zhe-Qi Xu. Hao Zhang. et al. The efficacy of Yunnan Baiyao on haemostasis and antiulcer: a systematic review and meta-analysis of randomized controlled trials. *Int J Clin Exp Med*. 2014;7(3):461-482.

[352] Murphy LA, Panek CM, Bianco D, Nakamura RK. Use of Yunnan Baiyao and epsilon aminocaproic acid in dogs with right atrial masses and pericardial effusion. *J Vet Emerg Crit Care*. 2016 Sep 26. doi: 10.1111/vec.12529. [Epub ahead of print]

10 |
A Prescription for Science-Based Pet Care

*The first principle is that you must not fool yourself – and you are
the easiest person to fool.*

- Richard Feynman

What's It All About?

Throughout this book, I have tried to accomplish two basic tasks. First, I
wanted to provide you with useful, reliable information about some common
alternative therapies you might consider for your pets. I've tried to explain
the core ideas behind these practices, how they might work, what the scientific evidence says about them, and what risks they might pose. Some of this
information will likely stay relevant for a long time. At this point, it is pretty
unlikely that we will discover dramatic new evidence concerning homeopathy or chiropractic, which have been around and have been studied for decades.

Some of the specific information in this book, however, may be super-
seded by new evidence in the next five to ten years. The nature of science is
that our understanding evolves and improves over time. Particularly in areas
of active, ongoing research, such as probiotics and herbal medicine, we are
likely to see new discoveries and major shifts in our understanding in the

coming decade. I look forward eagerly to new evidence, and as someone convinced that the scientific process is our best hope for a reliable and useful understanding of the world, I see changing my mind over time not as a failure or admission that my viewpoint is wrong but as a validation of the methods of science and skepticism.

Fortunately, I've built some insurance against obsolescence into this book. Apart from informing you about specific CAM practices, my larger goal has been to give you strategies for evaluating such approaches on your own and making decisions about all the options for managing your pets' health. I have attempted to create not only a reference but a toolbox which you can draw from when confronted with claims and treatments I have not talked about.

To finish up, then, I would like to offer some general principles and strategies for evaluating therapies you may be considering using with your pets.

OUR CORE QUESTIONS

By now you're pretty familiar with the three questions we should ask about every treatment we consider for our pets. You also know a lot more about how to use these questions, the principles of the scientific method, and the warning signs of untrustworthy claims I have just discussed. Here is a quick summary of these core questions and how to use them when you encounter new treatment options for your animal friends.

What Is It?

The key to this question is to ask for clear, specific, plausible explanations for what a therapy involves and how it is supposed to work. You should ask about the specific ingredients in any remedy—what is in it and how much of each component. You should expect details, and these details should be consistent with a reasonable, science-based understanding of biology and health. If the answers to this question rely on vague language, mysteries, forces that can't be seen or explained, or other pseudoscientific principles, then the treatment should have one strike against it in your mind.

Does It Work?

The answer to this question should involve scientific evidence, not merely theory and anecdote. Remember that not all evidence is created equal. Here's a little visualization of the hierarchy to remind you.

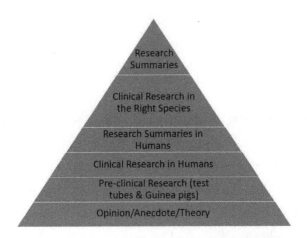

The closer to the top you get, the more confident you can be that the evidence reflects the true effects of a treatment. Even at the very top, with summaries of multiple studies looking at exactly the treatment you're considering in the right species with the same problem you are trying to solve, you still have to remember that not all studies are equally reliable. One nice thing about systematic reviews as a form of research summary is that they will usually consider the size of a study, the blinding of investigators and owners, the type of control treatment, and all the other details of how studies try to minimize bias and error. If this kind of research finds only low-quality studies, or finds that the better-quality trials don't see a benefit while the lower-quality ones do, this tells you our confidence in that treatment should not be set too high.

In keeping with our new appreciation of uncertainty, bear in mind that if someone qualifies their claims for a treatment or indicates that there is some uncertainty about it, this is a good sign. Weighing the risks and benefits of a therapy would be easiest if we had perfect and complete information, but this is almost never the case. Being aware of the degree of uncertainty about a treatment's effects makes you better able to make informed choices about using it.

Is It Safe?

The cardinal rule here is that any treatment that is having any effect at all is going to have some risk of side effects. If someone tells you a treatment is absolutely safe, they are either mistaken or dishonest, or the treatment does nothing. The evidence you need to decide if a medical therapy is safe comes from the same sources, and with the same caveats as the evidence for determining if it works. Anecdotes and lab animal studies are less reliable than good-quality clinical trials.

Placebos for Pets?

Nothing in medicine is perfect, and inevitably we always take some risk when we treat our pets' illnesses. However, with good, scientific information we can often determine that the risk is less than the likely benefit. Certainly, the risk we know about from research evidence is likely to be less than the unknown risk of untested treatments, whatever their advocates may claim. In the real world of veterinary medicine, where treatments typically become available in a storm of enthusiasm well before they have been through rigorous scientific testing, it is wise to be cautious about new treatment options and leery of jumping onto every bandwagon that rolls by.

GENERAL PRINCIPLES

Use Your Reason as Well as Your Heart

I have already alluded several times to the fact that our relationship with our pets is driven by love. We have powerful, personal connections to our animal companions, and this drives us to worry about them and to seek every possible means for protecting and preserving their health. Unfortunately, the intensity of this motivation can lead us to make desperate, ill-considered choices that may have the opposite of the effect we hope for. Even in the direst circumstances, when we are facing a life-threatening and incurable illness, we can make things worse if we don't think carefully and rationally about the treatments we choose.

A tragic example of this in human medicine involves something called the "Gonzalez Protocol." This is a "detoxification" regime recommended by some alternative practitioners for cancer patients, usually in humans but some elements of this therapy have also been recommended for pets by alternative medicine veterinarians. The protocol is a complex and burdensome mixture of extreme diet, supplements, coffee enemas, and manual therapies.

Despite the implausibility of this treatment, and the lack of any evidence other than anecdote to suggest it works, a clinical trial in people was actually conducted to evaluate the Gonzalez Protocol. And despite objections from experts in bioethics and from skeptics, the trial was approved by regulators for patients with advanced pancreatic cancer with the reasoning that this was a disease for which death in a short time was a virtual certainty, and conventional therapies have not been yet been found that do much to help these patients. This is the classic "nothing to lose" argument, and it is often made for alternative therapies that would otherwise be avoided for lack of any good reason to believe they work.

Unsurprisingly, the study found no benefit to patients form the Gonzalez Protocol.[1] What was surprising and disheartening, even to skeptics, was that patients who received this treatment died sooner than those getting conventional care, and they had significantly worse quality of life scores. This therapy managed to increase the suffering and shorten the lives of even the most desperately ill terminal cancer patients. There have been several other, less dramatic studies showing that the use of alternative therapies tends to be associated with worse outcomes in people with cancer. The "nothing to lose" argument is simply false.

The lesson for us, then, is that even when we are emotionally desperate and faced with the heartbreaking situation of a serious and untreatable disease in our pets, we should be cautious about grasping at straws. The urge to do something to relieve their suffering can easily lead us astray. And while

Placebos for Pets?

untested or unproven treatments may sometimes turn out to be helpful, you now know from the many examples we have looked at that they are more likely to do nothing much at all, and sometimes they can make things worse for the animals we love.

WATCH OUT FOR RED FLAGS

The Galileo Complex

I have talked a bit about plausibility, and the importance of considering how likely a claim is to be true given what we already know about the world. Unlikely and implausible claims about medical treatments sometimes turn out to be true, and these are celebrated as acts of inspiration and genius that make the story of science so exciting. We all know that Galileo suffered for his claims about the nature of the earth and the solar system, and we all know he was eventually vindicated as a genius. He was right, and most of the experts and authorities were wrong.

Most of us don't know the story of Dr. Sanden, who was famous in his time for his electric belt.

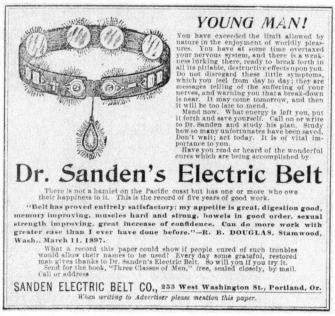

Image from Hood River Glacier, April 9, 1897, courtesy of History Museum of Hood River County

Dr. Sanden was one of the visionaries who harnessed the power of electricity to provide health benefits in the nineteenth century. Dr. Sanden's belt, and those of other electropathic practitioners, were sold in the tens of thousands, and testimonials proclaimed their benefits for many medical conditions, from kidney and liver problems to back pain to sexual dysfunction. Medical experts, electricians, and other conventional authorities of the time mocked Dr. Sanden and other proponents of electric belts, but they are certainly not mocked today.

In fact, they are not really thought of much at all today because, of course, their claims were nonsense and never supported by any reliable scientific evidence. This is the fate of most maverick geniuses who promote ideas that make little sense in terms of established scientific knowledge and that are rejected by most experts. Such claims are often dismissed not because of the closed-mindedness or lack of imagination of scientists but because they are far more likely to prove false than true, despite the exciting and inspiring exceptions.

Contrary to the claim often made by alternative medicine advocates that science does a poor job of fairly evaluating unconventional ideas, the scientific process can be surprisingly quick to overturn established beliefs when the evidence warrants it.

In the early 1980s, two Australian physicians started working on the idea that a stomach ulcer could be caused by a bacterial infection. Ulcers had long been blamed on stress and other factors, and it was thought at the time that the stomach was a sterile environment due to the highly acidic contents. Most physicians and experts would have found the idea that bacteria were a major cause of ulcers pretty unlikely. When Drs. Warren and Marshall proposed the idea, it was definitely met with skepticism. However, other scientists started checking their claims in new experiments, and research into the idea took off. Within about ten years, this unlikely hypothesis had become a widely accepted explanation for stomach ulcers. By 2005, only about twenty years from their initial publication, Drs. Warren and Marshall were awarded the Nobel Prize in medicine.[2]

This contrasts starkly with the situation for many alternative therapies, such as homeopathy or Chinese Medicine, in which ideas that are hundreds or thousands of years old and which have failed to prove themselves scientifically are not only still accepted but are central pillars of CAM practice.

Science is, in many ways, a more flexible and agile system than many of those whose proponents accuse it of being dogmatic and closed-minded.

The takeaway message, then, is that if an idea is implausible or requires us to reject well-established scientific knowledge, it is a safer bet that this idea is wrong than that it will instigate the next seismic paradigm shift in medicine. Iconoclastic figures who claim they have insights that most experts have not discovered or cannot understand are probably not a reliable source of advice for how to take care of your pet. For convenience sake, I like to call their attitude the Galileo Complex, and it is a clear warning sign that you may have encountered unreliable information.

The Dan Brown Gambit

A red flag related in some ways to the Galileo Complex is something I have named the Dan Brown Gambit, after the author of several novels that feature elaborate and secret conspiracies to hide explosive truths. This is the claim that a simple and brilliant idea that could lead to dramatic improvements in pet health is being actively suppressed by powerful and sinister forces threatened, economically or ideologically, by this idea.

These forces are often identified as Big Pharma, Big Pet Food, the Disease Industry or Medical/Industrial Complex, and many other such pejorative names. Basically, the claim requires us to believe that the reason a particular CAM therapy has failed to prove itself scientifically or has not been widely adopted is not because it simply doesn't work but because scientists, doctors, the government, and companies that make healthcare-related products are all banding together to suppress it.

This idea fails the basic test of plausibility, and purveyors of it never seem to come up with a "smoking gun" showing this is actually happening. It assumes the worst motives on the part of everyone who is not a believer in the therapy being defended, and it is unfair and insulting to honest veterinarians and scientists who are working to help make the lives of our pets better. I have no doubt individuals and companies have bias and self-interest and that sometimes these lead them to act in ways that aren't honest and in the best interest of veterinary patients. But the notion that complex and malign conspiracies explain the failure of many alternative therapies to achieve acceptance better than the lack of evidence to support these therapies is a pretty self-serving and unlikely idea.

The Dan Brown Gambit is closely related to the Shill Gambit, the accusation that anyone who criticizes an unconventional therapy must be paid in some way by some conventional medical industry to do so. I get accused of this all the time. Users of the Shill Gambit seem to believe that no one could possibly doubt their beliefs honestly and based on the evidence (or lack of it), so skeptics must be driven by greed or are simply ignorant and misinformed. This is not an especially fair-minded, or humble, point of view. Both the Shill Gambit and the Dan Brown Gambit are warning signs that you are dealing with claims not supported by solid, scientific evidence.

The One True Cause of Disease

This one I owe to Dr. Harriet Hall, the SkepDoc and a tireless advocate for science-based medicine. She has insightfully observed that proponents of CAM therapies often claim that scientific medicine only treats the symptoms of disease, not the "real" cause. This is pretty clearly untrue in many cases, from the use of antibiotics to eradicate the bacteria that causes stomach ulcers, to the use of vaccines to prevent infections and cancers caused by microorganisms, to discoveries and advice about exercise, nutrition, smoking, and many other preventative and therapeutic steps science-based medicine allows us to take to eliminate causes of disease.

But as you've now heard me say repeatedly, biology is complicated, and there is rarely a single cause for most health problems. Interactions between our genes, our environment, our activities, our age, and numerous other factors all shift our risk for specific health problems up or down on an ongoing basis throughout our lives, and the same is true for our pets. Anyone who offers a single, simple explanation for all disease, particularly if they then offer to sell you the cure, either does not understand biology or is not being honest.

The One True Cause of Disease, apart from being an intrinsically unlikely idea in itself, is also often identified as some mysterious "energy" or spiritual force than cannot be objectively observed or manipulated. This further weakens the plausibility of any treatment based on such a cause since, as I have discussed before, such mysterious and intangible ideas have to be accepted and acted upon on faith alone and can't be subjected to the study and manipulation of science. Since science has proven so much more successful at improving our health than systems based on intangible metaphysical theories, you will serve your pets' health better by steering away from treatments based on simplistic and mysterious explanations for illness.

"You Can't Prove It's Not True!"

People making unlikely or controversial claims should naturally be expected to provide evidence to support these. Surprisingly often, however, alternative medicine advocates try to shift this burden of proof to their critics. Rather than testing their treatments scientifically and accepting the results, positive or negative, or even providing compelling evidence that scientific testing isn't the best way to evaluative these treatments, CAM proponents often simply claim that it is unfair and closed-minded not to accept their claim if we can't provide conclusive proof they are false.

This doesn't really make much sense. If I claim that I am the president of the United States, or that you can fly if you hold my hand and we jump off the roof of a building, can I reasonably expect you to accept these claims unless you have clear and robust proof that I am lying or deluded? If not, then why is it any different if I claim I can cure your cat's cancer with a secret recipe of herbs or by laying my hands on him even if I have no scientific evidence for these claims? Because medicine is complex, and the outcomes of our actions are often delayed, indirect, and hard to assess, it seems easier to entertain implausible claims without evidence than it does when we are asked to jump off a roof, especially if these claims match what we believe or want to believe and sustain our hopes. But the burden of proof still rightly belongs with those making the claims, not with those asking for evidence for them.

CAM advocates are also frequently fans of the saying "absence of evidence is not evidence of absence." This aphorism basically means that if we haven't studied something, we can't definitively say whether it is true or false.

This is trivially correct and is a basic principle of skepticism. Since we proportion our confidence in a claim to the evidence for it, our confidence must be zero and our judgement neutral if there is zero evidence.

However, the use of this argument to defend unproven therapies has a few pretty serious flaws. For one thing, if there is no evidence, we can't judge a claim to be true any more than we can judge it to be false. The fact that we don't have studies of a treatment may mean we can't confidently say it doesn't work, but it certainly doesn't mean we have any good reason to think it does. Since claims in medicine often involve actively giving a treatment to your pet, an absence of evidence for safety or efficacy ought to encourage you to avoid the treatment, not to try it blindly.

The other major failure of this argument is that there is often an absence of evidence despite significant effort to find some. There have been, for example, hundreds of preclinical studies and clinical trials of homeopathy over several decades. The fact that we can't yet find convincing evidence for any useful activity is itself pretty good evidence that there is none to find. Sure, every single study might have been done wrong, or all of the scientific method might be so flawed that homeopathy could be curing nearly every disease it treats and we still aren't seeing this in clinical trials. But that notion is about as implausible and unlikely as you can get compared with the much more reasonable explanation that homeopathy simply doesn't work. Sometimes an absence of evidence for an effect can be evidence that there is probably no effect to find.

Learn to Accept Uncertainty

This is perhaps the most difficult, and possibly one of the most important principles I can give you. We all yearn for the world to be comprehensible and manageable. We all want to be able to understand why bad things happen to our pets so we can prevent or fix them. The reality of medicine is frustrating and uncomfortable; it is complex and full of nuance and uncertainty and our understanding is always incomplete and full of errors and grows painfully slowly. But decisions based on this imperfect reality will always be better than decisions based on a false belief that we fully understand nature and can reliably control it.

One of the great marketing advantages CAM has over science-based medicine is the appeal of simple explanatory narratives. Sometimes we get to take advantage of this in scientific medicine. Bacteria cause infections, antibiotics kill bacteria and the infections go away. This is a simple, satisfying story that can be told in a 25 or 30-minute office visit, and it gives pet owners a sense that they understand the problem and the solution. But sadly, real life, and real medicine, aren't usually that clear cut.

People want simple, clear explanations for what is wrong with their pets. They want to know what the chances are of the problem getting better. And they want to know what needs to be done. All of these things allow the pet owner to either feel more in control of the scary thing that is happening to their pet, or at least to adjust their expectations and emotions to the inevitable. What people do not want is to be told that the cause of their pet's illness is unknown, that the doctor cannot say with certainty what will happen, and that any treatment is an educated guess at best. Without a clear and comprehensible description of the problem, and without a straightforward treatment or prognosis, we begin to doubt the competence of veterinarians and other experts we turn to for help caring for our pets.

To be fair, I have seen some CAM practitioners admit to not knowing what is wrong or to not being sure if their treatments will work. But far more often, where the science-based medical approach calls for painful honesty about the uncertainty involved, the CAM approach allows for confident, simple explanations of the problem and confident treatment recommendations.

Not being tied to an objective, verifiable physical reality, vitalist approaches can give people what they want and need emotionally when their pets are sick, even if they can't actually offer anything of benefit to the patient. This is an advantage in terms of appealing to the public that scientific medicine cannot co-opt or undermine.

Of course, scientific medicine often has the advantage of being right about the real causes and the appropriate treatments, and this eventually trumps the lack of appealing simplicity in scientific explanations. Very few CAM therapies have established themselves as popular treatments for acute, life-threatening diseases because they simply cannot compete with scientific medicine in terms of results. But when it comes to the vague and the chronic complaints that science does not yet have clear answers to, and for which indeed there may not even be clear answers to be found, we shall have to accept the disadvantage of being honest about the complexity and uncertainty of these conditions. It is the price paid for holding out for real answers rather than simple, appealing, but ultimately unreliable stories.

Placebos for Pets?

I am not suggesting that the inevitable uncertainty found in science and medicine means we are without real, useful knowledge, nor that any unscientific explanations for the world should enjoy the same credibility as science has earned. The fact that science is incomplete and imperfect is undeniable. Unfortunately, some people take this fact as justification for throwing out the whole enterprise of trying to understand and acquire real facts and knowledge. If vaccines don't protect us completely, this means they are useless. If science doesn't know everything, then anything must be possible. These naïve arguments ignore the very clear fact that uncertainty and the impossibility of knowledge are not the same thing.

There are different kinds of uncertainty in science. One is the uncertainty of what we don't know. A big part of what makes science fun is that the universe is so vastly more complex than our little brains that we are never going to be in danger of running out of new things to learn and discover. I like to imagine my own ignorance as a vast abyss yawing before me. Every day I throw in a few grains of sand, but it shows no sign of being filled in. There is no denying that the surprising and unexpected is out there waiting for us.

But that is not the same thing as saying anything we can imagine is likely to be true. Most of our guesses about the nature of reality turn out to be wrong. Until science came along, this left us fighting over belief systems and led to a bewildering proliferation of different, interesting, and usually mutually incompatible mythologies to explain the world. Now, science is creating the kind of knowledge that works everywhere, in every culture, and that endures through time. Sure, such secure knowledge is only tidbits compared to the vastness of reality, and there is plenty that falls by the wayside.

But never before have we been able to have even this much enduring knowledge. Barring the complete collapse of human civilization, we are always going to know that the heart circulates blood, that emotions live in the brain not the heart, that smallpox *used* to be caused by a virus, and so on. What we don't know is an opportunity, not an invalidation of what we do know.

Another kind of uncertainty, though, is the uncertainty about what we know. Scientists like to say that all knowledge is provisional, tentative and subject to revision. This is true, but non-scientists tend to overread this and believe it means all knowledge is ultimately just opinion and is unreliable. Proponents of unlikely ideas like to make much of the fact that scientific explanations are "only theories," but this ignores the fact that those ideas that endure and are refined over time can reach a point where having confidence in their truth makes a lot more sense than doubting them.

A different flavor of uncertainty about the known is statistical or probabilistic uncertainty. I recently put my age, gender, total cholesterol level, and a few other factors into a nifty little calculator that told me I have a 3% chance of dying of a heart attack in the next 10 years. So does anyone know if I'm going to die of a heart attack or not? No, of course not. Much scientific research generates knowledge and conclusions that are statistical, that apply reliably to groups but don't give precise predictions for individuals. However, such knowledge is still useful in helping us decide what to do as individuals.

As I mentioned in Chapter 6, if you go to a casino in Vegas and play roulette, the odds are you're going to lose. Sure, you could win. Some people do. But most people don't. This is a truth, though it is only a statistical or probabilistic truth. Casinos make lots of money betting against you, and you're a lot more likely to be able to afford that Winnebago when you retire if you play the odds and don't play roulette. Even though statistical truths apply imperfectly to the individual, they are real and useful guides for our choices. The uncertainty of probabilities does not justify ignoring the odds and doing whatever we like, in Las Vegas or in medicine

Uncertainty is inevitable, in science as in all areas of human life. But this doesn't mean knowledge is an illusion and blind belief is as good as facts in deciding what to do or not to do. Human beings have changed our planet and our own lives, both for the better and for the worse, through the power of discovering and applying knowledge about the physical world. Such knowledge is limited, incomplete, tenuous, and also a lot better than just guessing or hoping. And science has generated more reliable, trustworthy knowledge in the past couple centuries than hunches, guesses, and trial and error managed in all the rest of human history. Accept uncertainty and place your bets, ladies and gentlemen. I'm placing mine on science.

It is in the admission of ignorance and the admission of uncertainty that there is a hope for the continuous motion of human beings in some direction that doesn't get confined, permanently blocked, as it has so many times before in various periods in the history of man.

- Richard P. Feynman

[1] Chabot JA, Tsai W-Y, Fine RL, et al. Pancreatic Proteolytic Enzyme Therapy Compared With Gemcitabine-Based Chemotherapy for the Treatment of Pancreatic Cancer. *J Clin Oncol*. 2010;28(12):2058-2063. doi:10.1200/JCO.2009.22.8429

[2] Marshall B. A Brief History of the Discovery of Helicobacter pylori. In: Suzuki H, Warren R, Marshall B, eds. *A Brief History of the Discovery of Helicobacter Pylori*. Tokyo: Springer; 2016.

FURTHER READING

CRITICAL THINKING AND PHILOSOPHY OF SCIENCE

- Burton, R. (2008) On Being Certain: Believing You're Right Even When You're Not. New York: St. Martin's Press
- Carroll, RT. (2000) Becoming a Critical Thinker - A Guide for the New Millennium. Boston: Pearson Custom Publishing.
- Gilovich, T. (1993) How We Know What Isn't' So: The Fallibility of Human Reason in Everyday Life. New York: The Free Press.
- Kahneman, D. (2011) Thinking, Fast and Slow. New York: Farrar, Straus and Giroux.
- Kida, T. (2006) Don't Believe Everything You Think: The 6 Basic Mistakes We Make in Thinking. New York: Prometheus Books.
- McKenzie, BA. Veterinary clinical decision-making: cognitive biases, external constraints, and strategies for improvement. J Amer Vet Med Assoc. 2014;244(3):271-276.
- Park, RL. (2001) Voodoo Science: The Road from Foolishness to Fraud. Boston: Oxford University Press.
- Sagan, C. (1995) The Demon-Haunted World: Science as a Candle in the Dark. New York: Random House.
- Shermer, M. (1997) Why People Believe Weird Things: Pseudoscience, Superstition, and Other Confusions of Our Time. New York: Holt, Holt & Company.

- Tavris C. Aronson, E. (2008) Mistakes Were Made (But Not by Me): Why we Justify Foolish Beliefs, Bad Decisions, and Hurtful Acts. Boston: Mariner Books.
- Burch, D. (2009) Taking the Medicine: A Short History of Medicine's Beautiful Idea and our Difficulty Swallowing It. London: Chatto & Windus.

EVIDENCE-BASED VETERINARY MEDICINE

- Cockroft, P. Holmes, M. (2003) Handbook of Evidence-Based Veterinary Medicine. Oxford: Blackwell.
- Ramey DW. (Ed.). Evidence-based veterinary medicine. Vet Clin North Amer: Equine Pract. 2007 Aug;23(2).
- Schmidt, PL. (Ed.). Evidence-Based Veterinary Medicine. Vet Clin North Amer: Small Anim Pract. 2007 May: 37(3).
- Smith RD. (2006) Veterinary Clinical Epidemiology. 3rd ed. Boca Raton, FL: CRC/Taylor & Francis.
- Case LP. (2014) Dog Food Logic: Making Smart Decisions for Your Dog in an Age of Too Many Choices. Wenatchee: Dogwise Publishing.

COMPLEMENTARY AND ALTERNATIVE MEDICINE

- Barker Bausell, R. (2007). Snake Oil Science: The Truth about Complementary and Alternative Medicine. Boston: Oxford University Press.
- Ernst, E. Singh, S. (2008). Trick or Treatment: The Undeniable Facts about Alternative Medicine. New York: W.W. Norton & Co.

- Ernst, E. Pittler, MH. Wider, B. (Eds.) (2006). The Desktop Guide to Complementary and Alternative Medicine: An Evidence-Based Approach. Philadelphia: Mosby Elsevier.

- McKenzie, BA. Is complementary and alternative medicine compatible with evidence-based medicine? J Amer Vet Med Assoc. 2012;241(4):421-6.

- Offit, P. (2013) Do You Believe in Magic?: The Sense and Nonsense of Alternative Medicine. New York: Harper Collins.

- Ramey, DW. Rollin, BE. (2004). Complementary and Alternative Veterinary Medicine Considered. Ames: Iowa State Press.

- Sampson, W. Vaughn, L. (Eds.) (2000). Science Meets Alternative Medicine: What the Evidence Says about Unconventional Treatments. New York: Prometheus Books.